D0395035

ONE COUPLE, FOUR REALITIES:
Multiple Perspectives on Couple Therapy

This book is the written product of a unique Harvard Medical School Conference on Couple Therapy. In the book, four demonstration sessions with the same couple are presented by those who conducted them; additional perspectives and approaches to the case are written by a number of other therapists. Three retrospective reports are provided by the couple and the editors. In an Appendix, the editors discuss ethical and therapeutic aspects of using video-taped demonstration interviews for clinical teaching.

ONE COUPLE, FOUR REALITIES:
Multiple Perspectives on Couple Therapy

Edited by

RICHARD CHASIN
HENRY GRUNEBAUM
MARGARET HERZIG

THE GUILFORD PRESS
New York   London

© 1990 The Guilford Press
A Division of Guilford Publications, Inc.
72 Spring Street, New York, NY 10012

Printed in the United States of America

This book is printed on acid-free paper.

Last digit is print number: 9 8 7 6 5 4 3

Library of Congress Cataloging-in-Publication Data

One couple, four realities : multiple perspectives on couple therapy /
   edited by Richard Chasin, Henry Grunebaum, Margaret Herzig.
      p. cm.
   Includes bibliographical references.
   ISBN 0-89862-437-1   ISBN 0-89862-029-5 (pbk.)
   1. Marital psychotherapy. I. Chasin, Richard. II. Grunebaum, Henry,
   1926- III. Herzig, Margaret.
   [DNLM: 1. Marital Therapy—methods. WM 55 058]
RC488.5.054 1990
616.89'156—dc20
DNLM/DLC
for Library of Congress
                                                          90-3037
                                                          CIP

Acknowledgments

Harvard Medical School's Division of Continuing Education sponsored the series of conferences on which this book is based. Throughout the past decade Harvard has entrusted the Cambridge Hospital and, specifically, Chasin and Grunebaum, to produce its annual major continuing education conference on couple and family therapy. We put that trust to a test in 1983 when we designed a most unusual conference. We had never seen or done anything like it. We thank Doug Jacobs, then head of the continuing education office at Cambridge Hospital's psychiatry department, who wholeheartedly supported the original conference which was co-sponsored by the Family Institute of Cambridge. The second showing in Boston as well as its later editions in San Francisco (with the Mental Research Institute, Palo Alto) and in New York (with the Ackerman Institute for Family Therapy) were co-directed skillfully by Judy Platt, current head of continuing education.

The cooperation of the psychiatry department at Cambridge Hospital was not totally surprising since it has always encouraged innovative couple and family therapy training and treatment under the leadership of John Mack, Lee Macht, and Myron Belfer. We are particularly grateful to Myron Belfer, chairman at the time of the conference, without whose encouragement this enterprise could never have materialized.

The conferences that we produced opened with presentations by four well-known teachers of therapy, each of whom had conducted a demonstration interview with the same couple. All of the invited therapists, Peggy Papp, Jim Framo, Norman Paul, and Carlos Sluzki, had many opportunites to show their work separately and under circumstances they fully controlled. When we proposed that they each interview one couple chosen by us, with cameras rolling, and allow this work to be shown and compared with that of their colleagues, they rose to our challenge. We are indebted to them (and to Jim Framo's co-therapist, Mary Framo) for the exposure they were willing to endure and for their cooperation in producing this book.

"Larry" and "Jennifer"—the couple interviewed—deserve our gratitude and the appreciation of all who have benefited and will benefit in the future from their willingness to share their lives so that others could learn. As we indicate in the Appendix to this volume, their respect for themselves as well as for the project helped us to learn more as teachers and conference conveners than we would have had we chosen a couple with less dedication to educational objectives and less concern for their own dignity and autonomy. We are also extremely grateful to the couple's families for their participation in the family of origin sessions.

The conference presentations would have been less engaging were it not for the moving and unforgettable videotapes of the interviews by Henry Felt. The conferences were enriched by the participation of experienced workshop leaders from three cities, some of whom have contributed to this volume. These contributors have shown extreme grace in enduring the long period from project conception to completion of this book.

Many individuals contributed thoughtful comments, editorial suggestions, and long hard hours at our increasingly compatible (perforce!) Macintosh and IBM word processors. We thank Joan Holt who has cheerfully helped to keep Henry's professional life organized, productive, and pleasant. We thank Ann Dailey, Katherine Baldwin, and Ellen Grabiner at Dick Chasin's office. Ann brought literary sophistication to her editorial assistance, Katherine was an "eagle eye" when proofreading, and Ellen contributed helpful comments and, in the redrawing of the couple's original genograms, her talent as an artist. Further gratitude goes to Dr. Adele Pressman whose help was critical at the outset of the venture and to Carole Samworth who added editorial polish near the very end.

Monica McGoldrick, Maggie Scarf, and Lyman Wynne read the book in its pre-publication stage and each gave us excellent advice. In addition, Monica McGoldrick and Randy Gerson helped design the formal genogram. David Chasin accomplished its final rendering; he and Manny Glossberg assisted in the cover design.

At Guilford Publications, Seymour Weingarten believed in this book from the start, although there were times when he may have wondered in what decade he would receive a completed manuscript. When the manuscript finally appeared, Scott Holmes, Denise Adler, Naomi Heep, and other staff went into brisk collaborative action.

Finally, we are grateful to our families, who bore the presence in our lives of this complicated and long-lived project and celebrated with us its gratifying completion.

Contributors

Walter Abrams, EdD, Middlesex Family Associates, Lexingon, MA.

Nicholson Browning, MD, Middlesex Family Associates, Lexington, MA.

Richard Chasin, MD, Family Institute of Cambridge, Watertown, MA; Harvard Medical School at Cambridge Hospital, Cambridge, MA.

Victoria M. Follette, PhD, Department of Psychology, University of Nevada–Reno, Reno Nevada.

James L. Framo, School of Human Behavior, United States International University, San Diego, CA.

Frances Givelber, LICSW, Department of Psychiatry, Harvard Medical School at Cambridge Hospital, Cambridge, MA.

Henry Grunebaum, MD, Department of Psychiatry, Harvard Medical School at Cambridge Hospital, Cambridge, MA.

Judith Grunebaum, MSSS, Department of Psychiatry, Harvard Medical School at Cambridge Hospital, Cambridge, MA.

Rachel T. Hare-Mustin, PhD, Department of Counseling and Human Relations, Villanova University, Villanova, PA.

Margaret Herzig, BA, Social Science Writer and Editor, Lexington, MA.

Neil S. Jacobson, PhD, Department of Psychology, University of Washington, Seattle, WA.

Sharon Lamb, PhD, Department of Human Development, Bryn Mawr College, Bryn Mawr, PA.

Natalie S. Low, PhD, Department of Psychiatry, Harvard Medical School at Cambridge Hospital, Cambridge, MA.

Peggy Papp, MSW, The Ackerman Institute, New York, NY.

Betty Byfield Paul, LISCW, Division of Continuing Education, Postgraduate Certificate Program in Marital and Family Therapy, Boston University School of Social Work, Boston, MA.

Norman L. Paul, MD, Department of Psychiatry, Harvard Medical School at Mt. Auburn Hospital, Cambridge, MA.

Sallyann Roth, MSW, Family Institute of Cambridge, Watertown, MA; Department of Psychiatry, Harvard Medical School at Cambridge Hospital, Cambridge, MA.

Carlos E. Sluzki, MD, Department of Psychiatry, Berkshire Medical Center, Pittsfield, MA.

Kathy Weingarten, PhD, Family Institute of Cambridge, Watertown, MA.; Department of Psychiatry, Children's Hospital and Judge Baker Children's Center, Harvard Medical School, Boston, MA.

Contents

PART IV.   Issues in Couple Therapy

PART V.   Retrospective Reports by the Couple
and the Editors

PART I

BACKGROUND

1

A Multitheoretical Approach to Couple Therapy:[1]

The Harvard Couple Therapy Conference and the Preparation of This Book

THE EDITORS

We are all curious about how other therapists would deal with the cases we see. Even if we are comfortable with our own theoretical orientation and style, we wonder what would be accomplished if different approaches were used with our clients. This curiosity finds little satisfaction in the clinical literature. There we find a plethora of case material, not about our own clients, but about cases carefully selected to illustrate the writer's espoused position. This book, however, will present the work of several different therapists with a *single case*, one that they did not select.

This book, and the conference on which it is based, reflect our belief that each of the many theoretical approaches taken by couple therapists reveals and conceals different aspects of a couple's relationship, highlighting certain realities while leaving others in obscurity. Common sense alone might lead us to conclude that a couple's relationship is too

---

[1]In this book the term "couple therapy" is used rather than "marital therapy" for several reasons. First, many couples seen in clinical practice are not married. For example, they may be heterosexual and living together without intending to get married or may be in a committed same sex relationship. Second, the term "marital therapy" may imply that a particular bond and a particular commitment between the couple can be assumed to be present when in fact the character of the bond and the commitment may be precisely what are in question. Finally, the couple whose case is discussed throughout this book were not married at the time of the interviews.

complex a human undertaking to be encompassed or comprehended by any single theory. Taken together, multiple perspectives may provide the most authentic and meaningful guide to understanding the forces that shape the couple's life together.

The Harvard Couple Therapy Conference of 1983 took this multitheoretical approach as its organizing theme. The idea for the conference was born of a brainstorming session between Richard Chasin and Henry Grunebaum, who for several years had designed annual continuing education conferences for Harvard Medical School at the Cambridge Hospital.[2] Their goal was to create a conference that would bring theory and "real" clinical life closer together. They were curious about how their colleagues would deal with a single case and had in mind as a prototype the Hillcrest Family Tapes.[3] They felt that another such exercise was well past due, since much had changed in family therapy since then.

Four therapists differing in style and approach—all well-known innovators in the field—were invited to conduct videotaped demonstration interviews with the same couple. Two of them, Peggy Papp and Carlos Sluzki, were regarded as both systemic and strategic. They tended to work with couples in the "here and now," concerning themselves principally with the nature of the current relationship. Papp frequently used role playing and often worked as part of a team, while Sluzki worked alone and used only verbal methods. The other two therapists, Jim Framo and Norman Paul, were both more psychodynamic in orientation. They typically focused on the past, and often worked directly with families of origin. Framo was known for his interest in object relations theory, while Paul was more concerned with ungrieved losses and their impact on relationships. All four of the therapists considered themselves to be "family systems therapists." Each was familiar with the work of the others and was intrigued, indeed challenged, by the opportunity that the conference presented.

The first part of the conference consisted of presentations by the four therapists of the videotaped interviews that each had recently conducted with the couple. As mentioned above, these interviewers did not select the case, rather, it was selected by the organizers of the conference. Thus, each therapist was confronted with a new case as we are regularly in our offices.

The second part of the conference involved workshops during which

---

[2]Margaret Herzig began work on this project in 1988, when she joined Chasin and Grunebaum in producing this book.

[3]The Hillcrest tapes of therapists Nathan Ackerman, Murray Bowen, Don Jackson, and Carl A. Whitaker were produced in 1968 by Birdwhistle and VanFlack at the Eastern Pennsylvania Psychiatric Institute in Philadelphia and are now available through Pennsylvania State University (Audio-Visual Services) at University Park, PA.

other experienced therapists discussed how *they* would have understood and worked with this same couple. In keeping with the theme of the conference, the workshop leaders used the same case to illustrate their ideas and to comment on the approaches taken in the four interviews. At the second, third, and fourth editions of this conference in Boston, San Francisco, and New York, a third component was added: a videotaped six-month follow-up interview of the couple by Chasin and Grunebaum (see Chapter 18). To distinguish the original four invited interviewers from the other therapists and interviewers, we will at times refer to them as "the presenters."

In early 1983, in preparation for the first conference, each of the four presenters conducted a videotaped demonstration interview. Each had been given a brief written clinical case report prepared by the couple's current therapist (see Chapter 2). In accordance with our efforts to approximate "real life," the case report did not provide a comprehensive history, but rather covered the sort of information that one therapist might give to another in a detailed referral call.

Each of the presenters used the interview formats to which they were accustomed. Papp and Sluzki met only with the couple, Papp for two hours and Sluzki for one hour. Paul and Framo, the two presenters known for their family of origin work, conducted two-generational meetings. Framo met with Jennifer and Larry for one hour, then, along with co-therapist Mary Framo, spent two hours with Jennifer, her parents, and her sister. Paul worked alone; he spent almost four hours with the couple and Larry's family of origin in various combinations. (Larry's brother would have liked to participate in the session, but was unable to attend.)

The order of the interviews was determined entirely by logistics. The interview with Peggy Papp took place in her New York office. Later that day Jim and Mary Framo saw the couple with Jennifer's family in Papp's office.[4] Later, Norman Paul saw the couple with Larry's family in his Boston office. Finally, Carlos Sluzki, then living in California, conducted his interview in Boston the day before the conference to spare him two trans-continental trips, one for the interview and one for the conference.

The four interviews were videotaped in their entirety. They took place at intervals over a six-week period during which the couple's ordinary therapy sessions were suspended in order to avoid "overload." At the conference each presenter was given an hour and a half to illustrate and

---

[4]Jim Framo was the only therapist to have any contact with the couple prior to the session. He met with them for lunch following their session with Peggy Papp. Jim and Mary Framo joined the couple, Peggy Papp, and Jennifer's family for lunch following Papp's interview with the couple. None of the other therapists had any contact with the couple prior to their session.

explain his or her work with the couple. Each used about 45 minutes of this time to show videotaped segments excerpted from the interview in which he or she participated. In asking the presenters to prepare material for this book, we suggested that they write about what they had presented at the conference. Thus their chapters consist largely of transcribed interview segments and their own commentary upon them.

It is important to state that the conference exercise was not designed to evaluate the relative efficacy of the four sessions. Such an experiment would surely have met with profoundly troubling methodological obstacles, such as how to unravel the effects of the order of the interviews. Rather, we attempted to design an educational experience for us (the conference organizers), for the therapists, for the conference participants, for the couple,[5] and now for the reader.

The case involves a young couple, Larry and Jennifer. Their backgrounds are not unlike those of many clients or, for that matter, many therapists. Both are middle-class and well-educated. One is Jewish, the other is part Jewish. They had been in couple therapy for four months when they agreed to participate in this exercise, seeing in four separate sessions well-known therapists representing different styles or schools of thought. We explained to them that the exercise was designed not to judge the effectiveness of the therapists, but rather to demonstrate the "real life" application of various approaches to a single clinical case. The couple agreed to participate for financial remuneration, to gain new perspectives on their relationship, and for the gratification of being part of an exciting learning adventure for themselves and for professionals. (See Appendix for descriptions of the process by which the couple was recruited and the contracts that they made with us.)

None of us involved in the conference suffered from the illusion that the interviewers and the couple behaved "naturally," exactly as they would in an ordinary clinical context. Having only a single session in which to illustrate their espoused theory and preferred methods, we expected that the interviewers would be inclined to pursue their strategies forcefully.[6] In the safety and solitude of their own offices, and given more than one session, we imagined that they would do other things as well. Would they become more like each other or more different?

Certainly the objective of obtaining a videotape for a conference is different from that of helping a couple.[7] In the videotaped interviews,

---

[5]The couple was invited to attend the conference and, in fact, did so.
[6]Argyris and Schon (1974) discuss the difference between one's espoused theory and one's theory in action.
[7]See Zinberg (1987) for a discussion of the ways in which an interview that is acknowledged to be for public consumption differs from a private interview.

much that was of interest was not asked or volunteered, for example, about the possibility of previously unacknowledged abuse, and about the couple's sexual relations. The interviews also differed from the usual first encounter in that comparatively little attention was paid to the therapeutic alliance. The interviewers did not need to be concerned about whether the couple would return and participate in a continuing therapeutic process. In more normal circumstances, they might have spent more time gradually getting to know the couple and establishing a mutually comfortable working relationship. Despite such differences, it will be evident that much relevant material was obtained.

Each time the conference was presented, it was very well-attended and well-received. We could have offered it in other regions of the country, but Larry and Jennifer had grown older and more established in their professional lives and they felt that repeated presentations of the videotapes would have infringed unduly upon their privacy. This book solves that problem by providing a broad-based dissemination of our findings without continued visual exposure of the couple.

The book is divided into five parts. Part I contains background material about the entire project. It includes a copy of the case report that was made available to the interviewers and two versions of the couple's genograms: One represents the "free-hand" genographic drawings that the couple themselves prepared for the interviewers; the other version presents their genograms in the standardized form to which readers of the clinical literature are accustomed (McGoldrick & Gerson, 1985). Part II consists of chapters by each of the presenters[8] who saw Larry and Jennifer, in the order in which the interviews were conducted. Parts III and IV present chapters written by a selected group of the therapists who served as workshop leaders at the conference. The chapters in Part III present alternative theoretical approaches to evaluation and treatment, and illustrate these approaches using the case of Larry and Jennifer. The chapters in Part IV use the case to illustrate general issues that therapists of any theoretical persuasion may need to consider in their work with couples.

Three retrospective reports are provided in Part V. The first was written by the couple one day after the last interview. The second presents a follow-up interview that Chasin and Grunebaum conducted with the couple six months later; and the third was written by the couple six years later. These reports reveal changes not only in the couple's relationship, but also in their thoughts and feelings about the four interviews as they were experienced over time. That we have available not only the thoughts of the interviewers and skilled commentators, but also those of the couple, is one of the unique features of the book.

---

[8]Norman Paul's chapter was written with Betty Byfield Paul.

We have also included an appendix which addresses some of the clinical and ethical issues that arise when clients become participants in videotaped demonstration interviews. Our extended relationship with the couple, and the moving personal impression they related to us in person and in the follow-up reports, drew our attention to the vital importance of these issues. Since a detailed discussion of these matters did not seem fitting as a chapter in the body of the book, we have chosen to present it as an appendix. We added this discussion primarily for teachers of therapy, but also for any reader who wishes to learn more about our specific arrangements with Larry and Jennifer and our general thoughts about the clinical and ethical dimensions of teaching exercises like the one described in this book.

The information in the case report, the genograms, the interview transcripts, and the retrospective reports has been slightly fictionalized to protect the privacy of the couple and their families.[9] Moreover, the transcript material in the four chapters by the interviewers has been slightly edited for readability. We judged that the reader would be content to be spared extremely awkward phrasing, repetitions, "ums," and "you knows," as well as many of the ellipses and brackets that conventionally flag every departure from strict transcription.

The conference was distinctive, in some ways predictable, in others surprising. The interviewers felt "on the spot," and at times anxious. It seemed evident that they were comparing themselves to one another, yet no competitive statements were ever made. The therapists in the audience became very involved with the case, for at least three possible reasons: (1) They could easily identify with Larry and Jennifer. It could have been them, or perhaps their children. (2) There was an element of suspense. No one knew how the case would turn out. (3) They could identify with the presenters struggling with a new case, just as they would have in their own offices. We believe that this same level of involvement is available to readers, whom we invite to think of themselves alternately as therapist and client, imagining what they might have thought, done, or experienced under the same circumstances. We will reserve further comments of our own for the retrospective section of the book and the Appendix, offering the reader at this point an opportunity to learn with a fresh and open perspective about the case and how the four presenters and the various discussants

---

[9]As we (the editors) worked with each chapter we made decisions about fictionalization, aiming to alter the details of the case while retaining authenticity regarding clinical issues. Then the couple reviewed all chapters to determine whether the level of fictionalization offered by the editors seemed adequate to protect their privacy. They made only one minor change. In their writing of the six-year retrospective report, they offered their own elements of fictionalization, all of which we accepted.

approached it. It is our intent to stimulate each reader to consider his or her own work in light of these approaches.

CHRONOLOGY

January–February, 1983
The four videotaped interviews were conducted.

February 10–11, 1983
The first conference was held, in Boston.

October 19, 1983
The six-month follow-up interview was conducted.

December 1–2, 1983
The second conference was held, in Boston.

February 3–4, 1984
The third conference was held, in San Francisco.

January 25–26, 1985
The fourth conference was held, in New York City.

January, 1988–December, 1989
The manuscript of the book was prepared for publication.

May, 1989
The couple prepared their six-year retrospective report.

REFERENCES

Argyris, C. & Schon, D. (1974). *Theory in practice*. San Francisco: Jossey-Bass.
McGoldrick, M., & Gerson, R. (1985). *Genograms in family assessment*. New York: W.W. Norton.
Zinberg, N. E. (1987). Elements of the private therapeutic interview. *American Journal of Psychiatry, 144, pp. 1527–1533.*

2

The Couple:
History and Genograms

THE HISTORY OF THE COUPLE[1]

Jennifer

Jennifer, 29, is the younger of two children of Dutch-born parents of mixed religious backgrounds. Her father is 79, her mother 61. She describes her father, one of 10 children, as the adventurous type, one who came to this country on his own. Her mother was the illegitimate daughter of a woman whose family history is dark with secrets and references to mysterious deaths. Jennifer was 16 before she knew her mother had any father. Her mother grew up in a "school for parentless girls" where her own mother occasionally visited her and condemned the hatefulness of men. Jennifer's mother came to the United States alone at age 17. She stayed with a "sorceress" aunt who held seances.

Jennifer's parents were introduced by her father's brother and sister-in-law. Jennifer, 8 years younger than her sister, describes her own conception as an accident. As a child, she felt unloved and unwanted. Her parents had expected a boy and Jennifer felt she disappointed them. She was supposed to be named after one of her father's brothers.

After Jennifer's birth, her mother and sister became "pals." They slept in her sister's room, while Jennifer shared a bed with her father until she was about six. As her mother impressed their father's frailty upon them (insisting he was older than most fathers and on the verge of death), Jennifer came to feel responsible for his survival. Jennifer recalls being

---

[1]A case report was prepared by the couple's therapist in 1982 for use by the therapists who conducted the demonstration interviews. That report is reprinted here with minor editing and with alteration of specific details as deemed appropriate by the editors and the couple to protect the couple's privacy.

unable to sleep for fear that her father might stop breathing if she didn't watch the rise and fall of his chest. She feared something terrible might happen if she fell asleep.

Jennifer tells of a long childhood history of medical problems, multiple allergies of unknown etiology, and numerous digestive disorders, including chronic constipation. Her mother administered regular enemas, which Jennifer despised and later viewed as yet another one of her mother's many ways of "controlling me and invading every aspect of my life."

Jennifer never felt accepted. She has distinct memories of her mother trying to suffocate her. Her sister says she observed the mother hitting Jennifer's head against her crib. Jennifer feared her mother wanted to kill her. "Everything had to be perfect. I was terrified of my mother's rage." She vividly remembers that when she was 5, her father, using plaster of Paris, cautioned her not to put any of it in her mouth because it was poison. She scooped a handful into her mouth and ran off. She recalls that she was testing her parents to see if they would save her or, as she suspected, stand by and watch her perish. Her father rushed after her and made her vomit.

"Preoccupied with death," in her early years she drew pictures of graveyards and dead animals. She listened to requiem masses. She loved to draw and "escaped" into music and art.

Jennifer remembers her father "running after her sister and beating her with his belt," while she took refuge behind the couch. Jennifer says, "I was the target of my mother's wrath; my sister bore the brunt of my father's anger." She wondered why her father didn't protect her from her mother; she also felt that the sisters couldn't protect each other because they had to watch out for themselves. When she was 6 years old, Jennifer moved into her sister's room and her mother moved back with her father. Shortly thereafter, Jennifer's sister, at 16, said she was pregnant (she wasn't) and left home to marry her boyfriend and escape the family. Jennifer experienced terror and abandonment. Jennifer's sister divorced her first husband, by whom she had two daughters. She remarried and has a 4-year-old son from this second marriage.

Jennifer's father worked as a foreman at a shoe factory. Her mother began working in a bakery when Jennifer was about 15. She remembers home as a place always kept dark, where feelings were not allowed. Jennifer's mother derided and scorned men. She described sex as something horrible which women occasionally granted men in order to keep their interest. She also prohibited talking at the table. There was a lock on the telephone and when Jennifer did receive a call, her parents listened in. Jennifer recalls "night inspections" when her mother entered her room and searched under her bed for books. Jennifer often read library books about suicidal children. She felt "powerless and controlled."

Around the time Jennifer turned 13, in the seventh grade, she started to "hang out with hoods." She'd go off to school in her schoolgirl clothes carrying her flute case. Her schoolwork put her at the top of her class. After school she'd change in the girls' room, don black clothes and a stolen black leather jacket, tease her hair, and put on makeup. The switchblade in her pocketbook was part of the uniform. She'd arrive home in this costume, alarming her parents. They insisted she was "two people, a schizophrenic," and sent her to a psychiatrist. Jennifer resented the fact that they wouldn't talk to her themselves but sent her "to be fixed up." She liked being two different people. It was acting, something she felt very good at. She felt safe. Unlike the other members of the tough crowd, Jennifer wasn't sexually active and worried that her pals would kick her out. Her "hood" era ended after seventh grade.

In high school Jennifer withdrew from boys. She remembers having many superficial friends but no real ones. An outstanding student, a real perfectionist, she looked to her teachers for acceptance and recognition.

When time came for college, Jennifer's main goal was to get away. She wanted to go to UCLA, but her parents drew a circle with a 500-mile radius. She flew to the farthest allowable point: a university in Pennsylvania. Once at college, Jennifer felt "independent" and found the freedom exciting. She avoided communicating with her parents other than on a superficial basis. As a freshman she became engaged to a businessman six years her senior, whom she didn't know very well. Often away on business, he eventually disappeared without a word. Jennifer went to great lengths to trace him only to discover he had married another woman. She then "entertained suicidal thoughts and came close to committing suicide."

Larry and Jennifer met in 1972 and began a long relationship with many distinct phases. She saw Larry as "the rescue squad." Nonetheless, she liked the feelings of "power and being needed" that came with always having a lot of different men calling on her.

Larry

Both sets of Larry's Jewish grandparents moved from western Russia to New York City. His father, now 59, was the youngest of nine siblings. The paternal grandfather died when Larry's father was 4 years old. The grandmother remarried a man whom the father remembers as severe and harsh, and who forbade the children to study in the house. Larry's father was obliged to sit on the fire escape and read by the light of a street lamp. His sisters quarreled and several did not speak to each other for years. Larry's father received his business degree after 9 years of night school.

According to Larry's mother, her family of origin was "closer." There were three sisters and a brother. Larry knew his maternal grandmother well. His grandmother died when Larry was 5; his grandfather, when Larry was 15. This grandfather owned a large house in the Bronx; the first 10 years of Larry's life were spent in this house, which was shared by the maternal grandparents, Larry's family, and the family of a maternal aunt. Larry was close in age to two of his cousins, whom he describes as more like brothers than his own brother, who was five years older. He remembers that all the cousins were pushed together by their parents in spite of their individual differences.

Larry, 29, describes himself as gregarious, unlike one of his shyer cousins whom his mother insisted he include in his friendships and activities. When Larry was 9, his family moved to Westchester. He quickly made new friendships, many of which endure to this day. He recalls participation in a special progress class and skipping the eighth grade. His mother cautioned him not to express his delight in his promotion since his cousin, who was with them, had not been similarly advanced.

In high school, Larry loved sports and spent hours playing with his friends. "I was smart but didn't study. I was an underachiever." Teachers reassured his parents that he would apply himself as soon as something caught his interest. Larry had no particular "love" in high school, but had a girlfriend whenever the other members of his group of friends had girlfriends. During Larry's last year in high school, his brother got married. Until that time, Larry felt he hardly knew his brother. "I was introduced to my brother at his wedding." Larry and his brother are in related professional fields.

At his brother's wedding Larry met his sister-in-law's cousin who became his "first love." Larry spent his first two college years at school in Connecticut. He was a desultory scholar until he realized that he wanted to transfer to a school closer to his girlfriend, then at the University of Pennsylvania. Larry's grades rapidly improved, but he was not accepted at the University of Pennsylvania. The romance cooled. Nonetheless, he did transfer to another university in Pennsylvania (where he met Jennifer).

Larry describes his family as warm and loving. Family gatherings include many relatives with everyone talking at once, arguing, and teasing. During his childhood, Larry's extended family lived nearby. The doors of their houses, and of their refrigerators, were always open and the children felt at home everywhere. Larry describes his father as a quiet man, who acquiesces to his mother's wishes and instructions and his mother as more boisterous and intrusive. Larry's escape from people pressure was effected by closeting himself in his room with a television set. The voice of the TV was an environmental constant in the household. Larry indicated that when his mother shouted, people sided with his quiet father. His mother now comes to visit Larry and Jennifer dragging a suitcase full of chickens to stock their refrigerator. She busies herself in the kitchen. Larry relates that if, on the phone, she hears he has a cold, "she won't hang up until I swear I'm all right at least eight times."

It took Jennifer a long time to get used to the large family and active gatherings. Nevertheless, she feels safer with Larry's mother and father than with her own and has come to confide in them.

The Couple

Jennifer, at 29, is a postdoctoral fellow in genetic engineering at MIT. Larry, also 29, is doing research at Massachusetts General Hospital. They met 10 years ago as undergraduates at a university in Pennsylvania. Jennifer was beginning her sophomore year and Larry had just transferred in his junior year when they met at a dance. They began a relationship that continues into the present. For the last five years, they have lived together. At three different times they have decided to marry, but these engagements ended when Jennifer changed her mind. In September 1982, they began couple therapy with a psychiatry resident at a local teaching hospital.

Their first five years together (1972–1977) were turbulent. They lived together the first summer after they met and for various short periods through the following five years. Jennifer became involved with a number of other men while continuing her relationship with Larry. She saw him as someone she relied on. Larry thought of Jennifer as mixed up and in need of care. He recalls times when she went out with someone else and he waited in his car outside her house until she returned. At one point, she lived with another man whom, unknown to Larry, she promised to marry. Larry feels that the pattern for the ensuing years was set during this rough beginning. Jennifer was identified as the one who could not make a commitment to their relationship.

Larry graduated in 1974 and attended graduate school at Harvard University in physics, earning his PhD. Jennifer received a master's degree in biology after two years at Yale University before moving to the Boston area to continue graduate work for her PhD. The relationship continued through these years, often maintained by long-distance visits and calls.

When Jennifer moved to Boston in 1977, she moved in with Larry.

One month later, investigation of a persistent pain in Larry's foot revealed a rare type of bone cancer. An amputation of his left foot was performed immediately. Until that time, Larry, who loved sports, had spent much of his free time playing basketball. Although his life and the life of the couple were profoundly affected by his diagnosis and surgery, they rarely discussed it. Larry withdrew from everyone. During that time, Jennifer interceded and fielded phone calls from concerned friends and relatives. Larry embarked on a painful course of chemotherapy. After several months of the projected year of chemotherapy, he refused further treatment. Since the surgery he had become addicted to Percodan. Larry and Jennifer set out on a car trip to Canada during which time he withdrew himself from the narcotic.

Thereafter, Larry decided he had enough troubles of his own and would no longer tolerate the vagaries of the couple's established pattern. Now he would be more "self-centered." He wondered if the experience of their earlier years together had not caused him to lose trust.

Larry grew up a perpetual television viewer. With the loss of his foot, television sports substituted for his own participation and the television never fell silent. This became a source of one of Jennifer's main complaints: that she only wins Larry's attention during commercials. She feels excluded from Larry's thoughts and from his daily activities. Both acknowledge that Larry is more talkative with his friends. He also enjoys talking on the telephone whereas Jennifer often will not even answer the phone. They do not consider their sexual relationship "a major problem." Nevertheless, sex, initially terrific, is now felt to be tepid and mechanical.

They spend their days primarily at work. Jennifer works late hours at the lab. Larry watches TV and works at his computer. They tend to eat quick dinners away from home, doing little cooking. Jennifer performs most of the household chores and is known as the one more interested in keeping the house neat. Larry, the driver and auto mechanic, can be called on to rescue Jennifer if she has car trouble. He goes out at night to pick Jennifer up at her lab in Cambridge. He has always been her "protector," performing tasks from which she shrinks, such as returning her overdue library books. He now feels she must learn to do these things for herself, no longer supporting her conviction that she cannot. "Jennifer's a half-empty person, I'm a half-full person," Larry maintains.

The Therapy

Having spent ten years together, Jennifer and Larry were not sure where their life together was headed. Jennifer was in her second year of individual psychotherapy and Larry had never considered entering therapy. Jennifer initiated the idea of going into couple therapy and Larry agreed to try it. He says that he agreed to go primarily to please Jennifer, but also for them as a couple. Weekly sessions began in September 1982. At that time, they expressed their desire to improve communication with each other and to identify and resolve their problems. Jennifer and Larry intend to stay together and expect they will some day marry, but they feel entrenched in repeated, unsatisfying patterns.

Early in therapy, they enumerated their problems: Jennifer bemoaned Larry's incessant television watching which she saw as an evasion of communication with her. She contrasted his reluctance to talk to her with the general amiability and good humor he exhibits with friends. Larry felt that their problems were problems with Jennifer. Jennifer needs too much attention; she doesn't like festivities, parties, or his friends. Moreover, she is "poor at doing nothing" and always has to busy herself with work. Larry points out that despite Jennifer's expressed wish that he tell her of his daily doings, she is not interested in what he did or what he wants to talk about. He feels she is too self-absorbed to pay attention to his disclosures. On occasion, Jennifer asks Larry to explain something to her and then is angered by what she feels is his condescension or use of overly technical terms. Larry says that Jennifer is too competitive.

It soon became apparent that the plea for communication, in fact, contained rules. When Larry brought up that Jennifer had been "unfaithful," Jennifer wanted to change the subject. Larry also claimed that Jennifer believes that explaining actions ("I must have been angry at you") justifies them.

In therapy sessions several themes have emerged. Distance is very important to both Jennifer and Larry. Initially, Jennifer maintained distance by her involvement with other men. After Larry lost his foot, he withdrew and became the keeper of distance. Larry began by taking care of Jennifer; when he needed care, roles changed. This occurred not only with major events, but also in daily exchange.

Jennifer admires Larry's independence, rebelliousness, self-sufficiency, and intelligence. Larry likes Jennifer's intelligence, industry, and large capacity to feel emotion. Her need to be taken care of, however, is stated as the problem.

Helplessness is difficult for them to tolerate. For Jennifer to be helpless in the face of Larry's troubles is for her to feel guilty, responsible, and a failure. Especially in times of Larry's need, Jennifer needs "absolution" and attention. Larry isolates himself when he feels helpless. He "ignores" problems he cannot resolve. He feels helpless and falls silent when he fears intrusion or believes that he won't be heard.

When Larry fulfills one of Jennifer's needs, she may find herself furious, feeling empty and scared as though she's lost something. She prefers the position of giver: givers are empowered, getters vulnerable.

In carrying out an assignment to spend four hours together without TV or work, Jennifer worked at home while Larry studied. The assignment was repeated with emphasis on no work. Both read. They were surprised to realize they didn't use that time to talk. Distance was maintained. As Jennifer said to Larry, "I miss you most when we are together."

GENOGRAMS

Editors' note: The couple's genograms are presented here in two forms: first in Figures 2.1 and 2.2, as they prepared them, and second, in Figures 2.3 and 2.4, in a more standardized form. (See reference to McGoldrick and Gerson, chapter 1, this volume.) We include Larry's and Jennifer's own productions as indicators of their dramatic differences in style. Of course both sets of genograms have been altered to conceal the couple's true identities.

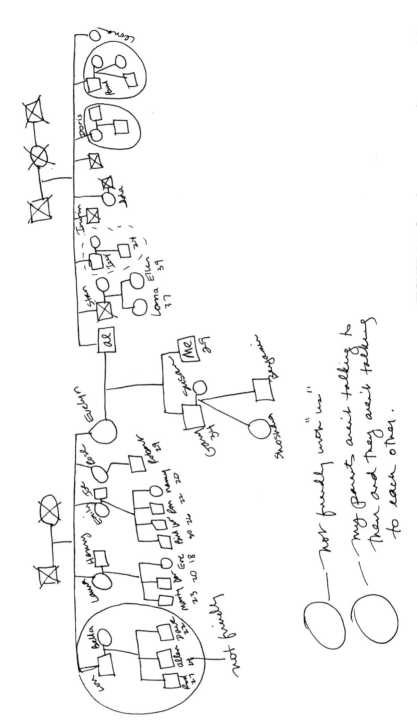

FIGURE 2.1. Larry's genogram, as he prepared it.

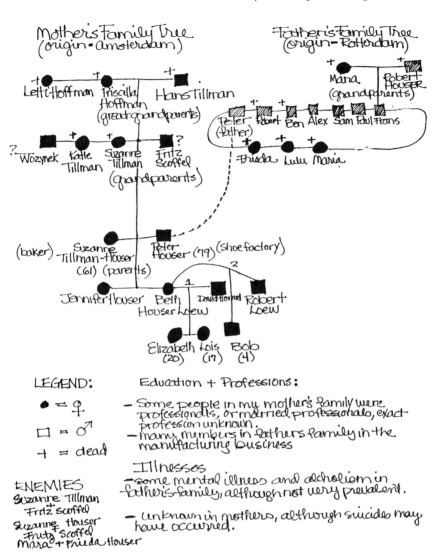

FIGURE 2.2. Jennifer's genogram, as she prepared it.

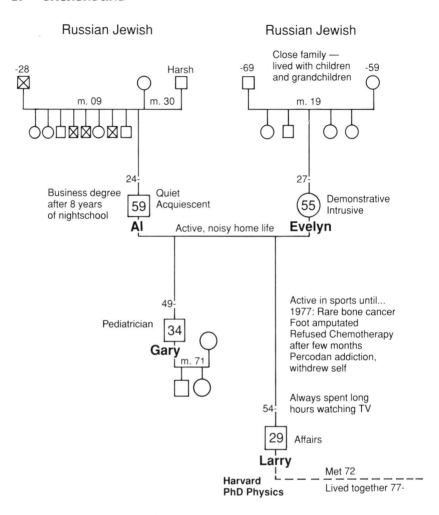

FIGURE 2.3. Larry's genogram, prepared by Monica McGoldrick and Randy Gerson.

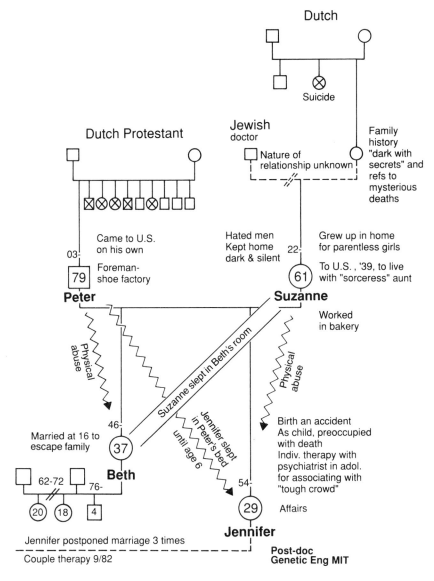

FIGURE 2.4. Jennifer's genogram, prepared by Monica McGoldrick and Randy Gerson.

PART II

THE FOUR DEMONSTRATION INTERVIEWS

3

The Use of Structured Fantasy in Couple Therapy

PEGGY PAPP

THEORETICAL APPROACH

The approach to couple therapy that I describe in this chapter involves identifying and exploring with the couple a central theme around which their presenting problem is organized, and the position of each partner in relation to this central theme. By "central theme," I mean a highly charged emotional issue around which conflict recurs. Generally, each partner takes a reciprocal position in relation to this theme and then polarizes his or her position. This results is an escalating cycle of interaction which neither partner is capable of controlling or stopping. The couple usually comes for therapy when this cycle has escalated beyond the point of endurance for one partner.

Reciprocal arrangements in marital relationships have been observed and written about extensively by therapists of different persuasions for many years. Some of the more common reciprocal patterns include the following: A wife who craves affection pursues an emotionally detached husband who distances; a strong, competent mate who constantly rescues a helpless weaker one; or an overly responsible spouse who tries to reform an irresponsible spouse. Such reciprocal arrangements have been variously described as "interlocking collusion" (Winch, Ktones, & Ktones, 1954), "bilateral reciprocity" (Dicks, 1967), "need complementarity" (Mittlemann, 1944, 1948), "hidden contracts" (Sager, 1976), "patterns of reciprocal overadequacy" (Bowen, 1978), and "unconscious deals" (Framo, 1982). The genesis of such arrangements is attributed to different sources depending upon the theoretical orientation of the therapist.

Reciprocity is not always problematic; indeed, it is necessary.

(Imagine two pursuers together, or two distancers. The pursuers would consume each other; the distancers would never meet.) Reciprocity becomes problematic only when it is thrown off balance in some way. The triggers for upsetting balance can come from either inside or outside the marital system. Developmental life events such as a career change, children leaving home, or the death of a parent can alter the reciprocity. A husband can lose his job due to an economic depression, putting him in a dependent position in relation to a wife who heretofore had depended on him. Or the trigger can come from within the relationship as one or the other spouse becomes dissatisfied with the way the reciprocity is being negotiated. For example, the original arrangement of "I will rescue you if you will remain dependent on me" may be upset if the spouse who is being rescued begins to feel controlled and withdraws from the rescuer. The rescuer then responds to the withdrawal by increasing the rescue attempts, the rescuee responds to the increased rescue attempts by withdrawing further, and so on.

When working with couples, I do not concern myself with the origins of this reciprocity but with the way the partners negotiate to maintain it. Most of these negotiations take place, not on the apparent or verbal level, but on what I call the "ulterior level." This level has been given different names by different therapists: Selvini-Palazzoli, Boscolo, Cecchin, and Prata (1978) refer to it as the "analogical level"; Watzlawick (1978), as the "right-brain hemisphere"; and Whitaker, in his usual picturesque language in conversation, as the "underbelly of the relationship." This is the level where covert contests, secret agendas, and hidden power struggles take place (see also Paul, Chapter 5, Framo, Chapter 4, and Givelber, Chapter 9, this volume).

Information regarding this level cannot be obtained directly, as it is beyond the couple's awareness. The partners are only aware of the increased tension, growing distance, or inexplicable outbursts. They define the problem either in vague, general terms such as "We are always fighting," or in isolated individual terms such as "She is always nagging," or "He constantly withdraws."

Over the years, in my search to comprehend this level, I have experimented with defining the marital relationship metaphorically rather than literally. Metaphors provide a complete gestalt in which disconnected patterns can be seen in relation to one another. Behavior, interaction, and perception can be linked simultaneously. Explanatory language tends to isolate and fragment, to describe one event as followed by another in a linear fashion. Figurative language, in contrast, tends to synthesize and combine, creating a holistic picture.

The metaphors are created through the use of guided fantasies. The clients are asked to close their eyes and have a fantasy about their problem. They are to imagine themselves in symbolic forms attempting to solve it. They are then asked to act the fantasy out with one another using as few words as possible. This is done through pantomime, physical positioning, and gesture. This technique is called "structured fantasy" and is a derivative of "family sculpting" (Duhl, Kantor, & Duhl, 1973). Over the years, I have experimented with many variations on sculpting (Papp, 1976a, 1976b, 1980; Papp, Silverstein, & Carter, 1973). At this point I use it primarily as a diagnostic tool. The fantasies allow the couple to communicate in images rather than words, and therefore provide a different kind of information. The images are then used as metaphors for what happens in their daily lives; they provide a way of speaking to the couple in their own language. As the session unfolds, and later, when I review the videotapes I have made of the fantasies, I try to ascertain (1) what the central theme is around which the current problem is organized, (2) what the reciprocal positions are that each partner takes in relation to this theme, and (3) what consequences would ensue if the couple changed these positions.

In thinking systemically, one must take into account the consequences of change. If one partner changes his or her position, it upsets the reciprocal arrangement. For example, if the husband's position is that of a "cop" who tries to reform his wife, and the wife's position is that of a "criminal" who indulges in delinquent behavior, if the "criminal" reforms, the "cop" is left, at least temporarily, without a familiar position. The goal of therapy is to rebalance positions to restore a workable reciprocity.

The Case of Larry and Jennifer

I knew from the written history of Larry and Jennifer that Larry had had his foot amputated because of cancer five years earlier, and that this event had triggered a shift in the relationship: Larry, formerly the pursuer, became more occupied with his own struggles and less preoccupied with Jennifer. During the first 45 minutes of my session with them, we discussed the effect of the amputation on their relationship, the changes that had occurred as a result of it, and many other aspects of their lives. For the purpose of this chapter, I will focus on the later part of the session, during which I employed the technique of structured fantasy to explore the central theme of the relationship.

Since I can appreciate that it is no easy task to come in off the street, sit in front of a stranger, and have fantasies, I always take some time in the beginning to make the couple comfortable. If they are to let their imaginations go, it is important for them to relax both their minds and bodies.

PAPP: What we're going to do now is an exercise that, hopefully, will help us understand, in a different way, what the basic problem is, and maybe point to some directions for change. I'd like you to get just as comfortable as possible. Just forget the words, if you can, and get into a position that is very, very comfortable. Now if you'll just close your eyes, and breathe deeply. Take a few deep breaths. Just let it all out and relax all the tension. Now, this is going to be an exercise in play. Actually it's like a game that children play. From time to time you may think it's silly because adults often think that children's games are silly. But if you remember, as a child, you had a very vivid imagination. You had fantasies and dreams that were uncensored. In those fantasies and dreams the images that would come to you would be very vivid and colorful. You may remember that as a child when you saw people in these fantasies and dreams they often took different forms. They took symbolic forms, they did not appear as people, but they may have appeared as objects, animals, somebody in history, caricatures. For example, if your father was authoritarian one day you may have seen him in a dream or fantasy as a policeman who came to take you to jail. If your mother was cross with you, you may have seen her as a witch— another day you may have seen her as an angel.

With this preparation, the couple begins the task of creating fantasies that symbolize their relationship. In this case, Larry began.

LARRY: She [Jennifer] can be a little girl.

PAPP: How little?

LARRY: Oh, about 12, and I'm about 12.

PAPP: OK. And where are you?

LARRY: With my friends.

PAPP: All right.

LARRY: And we're playing basketball.

PAPP: And what is Jennifer doing?

LARRY: She's on the side, with her girlfriends.

PAPP: OK. Would you sit over there, Jennifer? Let's say you're on the side.

JENNIFER: OK. (*Jennifer sits.*)

PAPP: We're going to make a play of this.

LARRY: OK. I'm trying to play with my friends and stay in the game.

PAPP: Yes.

LARRY: And the girls are bothering us. They're not letting us play, they're running on the court. I'm with my friends and I'm dribbling. (*He dribbles an imaginary ball. Jennifer interferes.*)

PAPP: OK. And how does she bother you?

LARRY: They try and kick the ball, and they run out in front of us so we can't play. (*He begins to play. Jennifer tries to get his attention. He pushes her away.*)

LARRY: Then I take the ball and I tell my friends, "Look, we can't play with these girls over here." So we just take the ball and we go over and sit down because we're not going to hit girls — so all of us go and sit down and start complaining about how they're not going to let us play.

PAPP: OK. And what does she do then? What does Jennifer do?

LARRY: They just run around until we . . . we're ignoring them. Finally, we can't ignore them anymore and we start playing with them. So we end up playing with them, and we don't play basketball that day. We walk off the court and I'm upset that we didn't get to play that day, but I'm also interested in the girls.

PAPP: Well, let's see what her game is. Let's see you play her game. What is it?

LARRY: Well, we have a ball and we throw it back and forth and they try and get it from us.

PAPP: Oh, I see.

LARRY: Because we're trying to show how much better at sports we are than them. So I get the ball and throw it back, and I get it back, and she's trying to get it from me. That's the fun. I hold it. (*Jennifer tries to get the ball but he pushes her away.*) I push her away, so you get some physical contact with the girls that way.

PAPP: Uh huh. And you keep throwing the ball back [and forth].

LARRY: Yes, we just keep throwing the ball back, and then we run away, and then she gets the ball, and I run after her and tackle her and put her on the ground and get the ball back.

PAPP: So, in the game that you play with her, it's her trying to get the ball away from you. It's her still trying to interfere with your game with the boys.

LARRY: Right. Although we are intentionally throwing the ball back to each other so they will try to get it from us.

PAPP: OK. Let's do that.

LARRY: OK. So I throw the ball back. (*He catches it and throws it back and forth.*)

PAPP: Are you enjoying this game?

LARRY: Yeah.

PAPP: Because you're showing them how much better you are than she is?

LARRY: But what it does is . . . there's this problem between us now. Some of us get more attention from the girls running after us than the other guys that are sort of just standing over there. The girls are really more interested in a few of us who . . . there are selected boys who the girls run after more and want to be run after by.

PAPP: And you're one of those boys?

LARRY: Yeah.

PAPP: So your other friends are angry and jealous of you?

LARRY: They're not jealous, but they're sort of standing there hoping the girls will run after them.

PAPP: Uh huh. Well, how come they run after you? Why are you the one that is selected?

LARRY: Um. I'm not the one . . . me and three others are selected and about five others are standing there, not . . .

PAPP: Not playing. Uh huh.

LARRY: And we throw the ball, I throw the ball to them because I see they feel bad and hopefully the girls will run after them. But they stay by either me or my other friend, waiting for us to get the ball back.

PAPP: Uh huh. OK. Now, what is the problem with this for you? What's your predicament?

LARRY: Um . . . well, the predicament is that we're not playing the game that we intended to play, and they've sort of come in between the male friendships that we have.

PAPP: OK, now . . .

LARRY: But the good part is that we get to interact with girls.

There are many different ways to analyze this fantasy. A few elements stood out for me. One was the context of adolescence, an awkward stage in male–female relationships. In that context, communication is mainly through teasing, showing off, and physical games. Larry is better at the game than Jennifer is and likes to show off. When he plays with her, he throws the ball over her head so that she can't catch it. He doesn't throw it to her so they can play together as equals. He keeps her on the periphery as an admiring observer. But she is also an interrupting observer, and he is ambivalent about her interruptions. On one hand, it interferes with his finishing his game with the boys, and on the other, he knows it is his only way of making contact with the girls.

Then I asked a question which I always ask when conducting the choreography: What would happen if this didn't change?

PAPP: Show me your worst fantasy about what will happen if you never finish the game with the boys.

LARRY: Um. Well, I go home and we haven't played that day.

PAPP: So you feel a sense of frustration?

LARRY: Yeah. I feel that we were prevented from . . . I've been planning this game for the last two days at school, and we've been arguing with each other about who would win, and we didn't get to play that day. We have to do it another day.

PAPP: How would that end? Say that you get into a battle with the other guys, there's a lot of friction, you're feeling frustrated because you didn't get to play your game, so then how would that end?

LARRY: Well, either we'd all get on our bikes and ride away as fast as we could and find another place to play, or we'd end up just sitting around with the girls after a while, just trying to interact with them and not really . . .

PAPP: Let's say that you get on your bikes and you ride away and you find another place to play. Will you act that out?

LARRY: So, we're all riding along, saying, "Weren't those girls stupid? I hope we got away from them." And some of the guys say, "Yeah, good thing we got away from them," while we're looking back to see if they're following.

PAPP: Oh, you're kind of hoping that they are following?

LARRY: Depends on the day. You know, if I really wanted to play that day . . .

PAPP: Let's say it's a day you really wanted to play.

LARRY: I hope they don't . . . so I tell my friend Jack, "Hurry up!" because he's always the slowest on the bicycle, "Hurry up before they see where we are going."

PAPP: So let's say you find a place to play, and the girls aren't there. Then what would happen?

LARRY: Well, I'm totally into the game, and um, and there's competition. And it enhances, I think, our friendship, that those of us on the same team are really working together toward a common goal, against those on the other team. It doesn't matter who's on our team, we switch a lot of times, but at that instant we're all working together, and if I make a really good play my friends say "Good shot," or some one of my friends makes a great play or I make a good pass. It's rewarding.

PAPP: So this is an experience that brings you closer to your friends, because you feel it's competitive and it's very gratifying.

LARRY: And it's testing myself. I was always interested in competition, either games, Monopoly, or sports. And it's the test. And I was always fairly proud of my physical abilities, and . . .

PAPP: Now let's say that Jennifer follows you. (*Jennifer follows him.*) Then what would happen? She's there and you can't find a place without her.

LARRY: Guys, forget it, I mean, we're stuck with them.

PAPP: What are you going to do with . . .

LARRY: Well, this was when I was 12. So we'd all maybe go to her basement and sit down. So I'll sit down and we start talking about nothing important, and, uh . . .

PAPP: Is your mind still back there where you wanted to be with the boys?

LARRY: No.

PAPP: No?

LARRY: No. And, we're interacting with everybody in the room there, about 25 of us, all sitting around, and fooling around and kicking each other, running and talking. And they're complaining about other girls at school.

PAPP: Let's see you play with each other, like you're saying.

LARRY: Well, you have to sit here. (*Jennifer sits next to him. They shove each other alternately, laughing.*) Yeah, we'd be sitting, and I'd say, "Why did you ruin our game?" (*Larry shoves her.*)

JENNIFER: Because it was fun. (*She shoves back.*)

LARRY: Sometimes they would punch real hard . . .

PAPP: M'hm.

LARRY: . . . and I would hit 'em back.

PAPP: Let's leave that there for now.

Larry's worst fantasy is that if he didn't get to finish the game he would not be able to test himself with his friends. Competition rewards and challenges Larry. He says he was always interested in games—"it's testing myself." But on the other hand, when Jennifer interrupts his game, he gets to have contact with her, even though the contact is adolescent (pushing, hitting, teasing, etc.)

Before turning to Jennifer's fantasy, I would like to define the kind of information I seek. I want to know how each person perceives the solution to the problem, what their specific dilemma is in trying to solve it, and what would happen if they solved it, or if they *never* solved it. I'm looking for the consequences of change, because therein lies the resistance. As George Bernard Shaw says, there are two tragedies in life: One is not to get your heart's desire, and the other is to get it. I'm trying to figure out what would happen either way. Jennifer's fantasy follows:

JENNIFER: OK. Again, we're both children, I'd say anywhere from 10 to 13 years old. I guess it's safer that way. I'm living on a farm somewhere, out in . . . I don't know where exactly it is, maybe in New England. I'm very lonely as a child, and I have lots of animals and horses and cows and sheep on the farm. I always fantasize about having a real playmate. I always wanted a real playmate. I've dreamt about it and wanted to have one, and one day, it's a summer day, I wake up in the morning with this really good feeling that something exciting is going to happen today. The chickens are making all sorts of noises because they want to be fed, and the roosters are making their normal sounds and crowing, and the birds are out, and I'm going out to feed the animals on the farm. I guess it's sometime probably in the spring or the summer. The weather's very warm and there are flowers out. I see this little boy. He's hiding behind the thicket. (*Larry hides beside a bookcase.*) He's just standing there, and he's not doing anything. He's just totally immobile, he seems to be paralyzed with fear. I walk over to him and try to establish some kind of contact. (*She walks over to him and motions to him.*) I sort of motion to him to want to play with me, and try to bring him out of the thicket . . .

PAPP: What does he do?

JENNIFER: . . . and he withdraws. He turns away, and he looks scared. (*Larry moves closer to the bookcase.*) He looks like he's frightened of me. I approach him, a little bit closer this time, and he's still very frightened. So I think, well, maybe he's just scared to play with me. My fantasy is that he was dropped off by his family, he was orphaned, they didn't want him, and I want to play with him and initially, maybe, I think he can't talk because he doesn't say anything. I'm talking to him, and motioning to him to play with me, to ride the horses with me. But he doesn't say anything.

PAPP: Let's do that.

JENNIFER: He still . . .

PAPP: Keep motioning to him.

JENNIFER: OK . . .come on, let's . . . (*Jennifer motions to him repeatedly and he shakes his head.*)

PAPP: And then?

JENNIFER: And then, well, I try the other approach. I try taking him by the hand to come with me. (*Jennifer takes his hand.*)

PAPP: What does he do?

JENNIFER: He still stays there. (*He pulls his hand away.*) He's scared. He doesn't seem to want to come with me. (*He shakes his head.*)

PAPP: What do you think he's afraid of?

JENNIFER: I think he's been hurt, so he's afraid of people. He seems to be afraid of people. He's very, very shy, very afraid and . . .

PAPP: What else do you do to try to get to him?

JENNIFER: Well, what I try to do is make him less afraid. I go and get the horse because I think this would be a good lure. I bring the horse out with me. (*She shows the horse and gets on.*) I get on and ride around a little bit. (*Jennifer moves in a circle.*) I'm sort of prancing around on the horse. I figure this will be a nice attraction for him. It looks like a lot of fun, maybe he will be interested in doing it with me.

PAPP: What does he do?

JENNIFER: He starts coming towards me, but very, very gradually . . . and I still try to get him interested in playing with me. Initially it's really not very successful, I mean he's still withdrawing, and he's still . . .

PAPP: Well, keep on . . . (*Larry approaches a little.*)

JENNIFER: . . . reluctant to come and play with me, so I try to grab him again. I'm smiling at him and talking to him and I'm showing him that there's butterflies flying around now, and flowers all over. I'm picking the flowers and trying to catch the butterflies. I'm trying to get him to join in with me in my activities, and he still seems a little bit reluctant.

PAPP: Keep on. (*Larry approaches a little.*)

JENNIFER: So I'm catching the butterflies. I'm having a good time. (*Jennifer moves around.*) I'm smiling and laughing and trying to get him to come with me.

PAPP: Then what happens?

JENNIFER: The resolution is that finally he comes out of this withdrawal.

He smiles at first, and he follows me around. He doesn't . . . it's not very obvious that he wants to interact with me at first, but then he starts following me around.

PAPP: And then?

JENNIFER: It looks like so much fun. I'm catching butterflies. (*Jennifer moves again and stoops to pick flowers.*) And I'm picking flowers and throwing them up in the air. Then you start following me and doing the same thing. You start smiling and laughing, and then we become good pals.

PAPP: So, there's not a problem in this?

JENNIFER: Well, there was when he was hiding. But the solution was that he started reacting.

PAPP: Uh huh. You were able to get him to do that?

JENNIFER: Yeah, and the horses and the flowers . . .

PAPP: OK. Let's take it back to before the solution. Let's say that he never comes out. Let's say that he's just there, and he never comes out, no matter what you do. Try a lot of things to get him involved. (*Larry returns to his corner. When Jennifer beckons, he signals to her to leave him alone.*)

JENNIFER: Come on. He's still not coming. So the thing . . . the bad part of the fantasy . . . the worst thing that could happen in this fantasy is that his family finds him and they pick him up and I never see him again. Or he runs away and I can't find him anymore. He disappears. He might run off into the thicket and I can't find . . .

PAPP: Let's have you just pretend to disappear. (*Larry turns his back.*) He goes off into the thicket and disappears. Then what would happen to you?

JENNIFER: I'd be devastated because it was like . . . he was very hopeful that I could bring him out, I mean it was my feeling that perhaps if I tried hard enough I could bring him out, and make him interact.

PAPP: Would you go looking for him again?

JENNIFER: I would look for him. I would look for him again and I'd be there the next day, and the day after, to see if I could find him.

PAPP: You'd keep trying to find him? You wouldn't give up on him?

JENNIFER: No.

PAPP: OK. Let's sit down and talk about this for a few minutes.

Notice the difference in the contexts of their fantasies. Jennifer's is extremely poetic and lyrical, in comparison to Larry's very earthy fantasy of sports, competition, and challenge. In both fantasies they are children, even younger children in Jennifer's fantasy than in Larry's. She sees herself as the rescuer and Larry as a scared, lost little boy. She is very intent on drawing him out and repairing the hurt caused by others. This is her challenge. Her greatest fear is that he will disappear and she will not have accomplished her task of healing him.

In Jennifer's fantasy I am struck by a contradiction. From reading the history, and from the discussion at the beginning of the session, I knew that Jennifer had had a problem with commitment. In the beginning of their relationship, Larry was pursuing her and she was always running away from him. Whenever they were about to settle down together, she would feel trapped or would leave. I wondered when I read the history, what she was running from, assuming, in my systemic way, that there was something Larry did that drove her away. In the fantasy she presented, the positions have been reversed. One obvious explanation of this reversal would be that Larry's vulnerability to cancer and the amputation of his foot brought out Jennifer's commitment to him and her desire to care for him. I wanted to discuss this issue with the couple.

JENNIFER: I guess my fantasy would be to want to draw him out and make him feel that it's safe to express these feelings.

PAPP: You would like to make him feel it's safe in the courtyard, and in the barnyard, and that none of the animals are going to hurt him, that . . .

JENNIFER: Right, and I'm not going to hurt him.

PAPP: How could she make you feel it was safe?

LARRY: Um . . .

PAPP: And that she's not going to hurt you?

LARRY: Well, as you can imagine with our rocky beginning with trust, it's not easy to come by . . . so I really don't know what it is she has to do to, to help that along.

PAPP: Do you have any ideas about that, about how you could draw the little boy out so that he wouldn't be afraid of you, or afraid to trust you?

JENNIFER: Maybe by making it known to him that I'm more committed than I . . .

PAPP: How would you go about doing that?

JENNIFER: Possibly by getting married, although we've discussed this before and it's just sort of a symbol of commitment. I mean, the real commitment has to come from within, and you have to feel it, so a marriage certificate is really not the answer.

LARRY: . . . I think it's fairly obvious that the best way to be trusted is to become trustworthy, and that's the best way . . .

PAPP: But then you're afraid that being trustworthy will lead to being trapped, is that right? (*To Jennifer*)

JENNIFER: Right.

PAPP: Suffocated and . . . all right, let's stand up once more and let's say that you're in the barnyard again and you win him over. (*Larry retreats to the bookcase.*)

JENNIFER: OK. He's coming out now. (*Larry comes out, willingly.*) Look, now we're playing together, right?

PAPP: M'hm.

JENNIFER: Oh, we're riding the horses, and picking flowers, and now we're going to go over to the garden.

LARRY: I'll be picking flowers?

JENNIFER: M'hm.

PAPP: Let's see you do that, let's act it out.

JENNIFER: OK. (*Larry and Jennifer pick flowers.*)

PAPP: You're picking flowers together . . .

JENNIFER: . . . and catching butterflies. Put the flowers here, catching butterflies, riding the horses, and let's see, what else are we doing? We're just running around in the field. There are a lot of rolling hills, and we're just running around and chasing each other, sort of playing games, chasing each other back and forth.

PAPP: At what point would you begin to feel suffocated or trapped?

JENNIFER: I guess when he would start controlling all the game playing. (*Larry pulls Jennifer to one side and indicates what flowers to pick. She resists. They struggle, briefly.*)

PAPP: Let's see you control the game playing. Start doing things again.

JENNIFER: OK. We're picking flowers. (*They begin picking flowers.*)

PAPP: At what point in your daily life does he begin to control the game playing?

JENNIFER: When I feel like he's telling me what to do, and how to conduct certain things, and I guess how I should feel is the thing that really gets me upset. He tells me how I should feel. That is even beyond controlling the games, that's controlling the feelings. I'll be very upset one day coming home from work, something happened, an experiment was a complete disaster, a fiasco, whatever, and I'll be really distressed. And I'll come home and he'll say, "Oh, that's not a big deal, you shouldn't feel upset. You know, you do this all the time, and it's nothing." He's not allowing me to feel upset or feel angry or feel sad and that's when he starts to control my emotions.

PAPP: And then how does he also control your behavior, do you feel?

JENNIFER: Well, then I start feeling, well, maybe he's right. I shouldn't be upset and I shouldn't feel angry, and I shouldn't feel . . . and I'm taking these things too seriously, and I start doubting how I should feel about a certain situation and it gets me very confused.

PAPP: And at that point you begin to feel trapped, suffocated, as though he's imposing something on you?

JENNIFER: Yeah. That's very true. I think at those times I don't know whose feelings they are. If they're mine, or if they've been imposed on me. Somebody told me how to feel and therefore I feel this way, and I don't know who's really feeling these feelings.

LARRY: There's a slight dichotomy there. I mean, she comes to me for advice and I tell her it's not such a big deal, don't get so upset, it's silly to get so upset about everything that comes along in life; you'll be upset all your life, all the time. And the next day, usually she says, "You know, it was ridiculous for me to be upset about that, it ruined my whole night and it doesn't matter that much today."

JENNIFER: But at the time you made me feel silly, for having those feelings.

LARRY: I didn't make you feel silly, I told you if it were me I'd . . .

PAPP: Within this fantasy, what would be the answer to that problem? Let's say that he begins to try and control the game. Let's see. What, what would be the answer, Jennifer, to that problem? Would you start again playing the game? (*They pick flowers. They begin to mime an argument about which flower to pick.*)

JENNIFER: I guess the compromise would be for me to control one game, for him to control another game, or allow me to finish the game I started, and then, if he wants to do another game, then he can be the leader in that game.

PAPP: Do you think you could get him to do that?

JENNIFER: I'll try. (*Larry and Jennifer argue again. He relents for a moment, picks one of her flowers, and then drags her toward his patch.*)

PAPP: So you got him to do that. You got him to do it for a few minutes, anyway. Do you think in reality it would be hard to have that happen, or not?

JENNIFER: Yeah, well, it doesn't in reality. I mean in reality what happens is there's a slight compromise, but I don't feel satisfied with it. I mean, for example, I might want him to go somewhere with me, something that he doesn't necessarily want to do. I'm just trying to think of a specific example. Going, say, to one of my laboratory parties. You know, he's not too thrilled about the idea, but he says, "Oh, OK, we'll go, we'll go," and what he'll do is he'll come with me but he'll say, "Let's go now." He'll leave early or something like that so it's not a full compromise, it's sort of a partial compromise.

PAPP: You feel the compromises are not full?

JENNIFER: Right, now if he would . . .

LARRY: I think it's more: "I'll do it but I'm not overtly happy doing it."

JENNIFER: Right, that's the other thing too, he's doing it reluctantly.

LARRY: I don't pretend all evening that I'm happy, she senses it.

JENNIFER: I sense that he's not happy. He's just doing it because he thinks or feels like he has to, or I would make him feel guilty if he didn't do it.

Jennifer's dilemma is now clear. If she draws the little boy out, and he stays and really participates with her, she is afraid he will control her game. In daily life when she tells him her problems, instead of just listening and sympathizing with her feelings, he tries to solve her problems. He tells her what to do and how to feel. She then mistrusts her own thoughts and feelings. This is probably the point at which she feels suffocated and wants to escape. Even when Larry compromises, he does so reluctantly. Jennifer still feels he's controlling the game. Of course, she contributes to this by acting confused and doubting herself.

If we look at the fantasies together, we see two people controlling or interrupting each other's games. Each does this in a different way. According to Larry, in their daily life Jennifer always chooses the most inappropriate moment to try to get him involved with her. He comes home from work very tired and drained. He feels he has nothing left over to give Jennifer, and all he wants to do is watch television—usually sports. Just as someone is about to make a basket, Jennifer says something like, "Oh, Larry, have you noticed the dog's depressed?" (Speaking of displacement!) Then he says, "Yes, why don't you take the dog to a dog psychiatrist?" Or she will snuggle up in bed and "make nice" to him, just as someone is about to score in the game.

In the interview, I returned to Larry's fantasy and asked him what he would have to do to stop Jennifer from interrupting his game. Sometimes a different solution arises within the context of fantasy.

PAPP: OK. Now let's go back to when you feel Jennifer is interrupting your game. You're on the basketball court again.

LARRY: Right.

PAPP: You'll get your Actor's Equity card after this, OK? Will you play basketball again?

LARRY: Yeah, I'll be playing basketball. And I'll come out and say, "Look, I'll tell you what, just let us finish five more points, finish the game, and then we'll play with you, OK? In fact, we like to play with you, but let us finish the game first." They would say, "OK," and then they'd wait two points and then they would bother us again.

PAPP: In other words, you don't feel that she would comply, if you tried to draw some kind of a . . .

LARRY: It probably wouldn't work, I'd want five points, and she'd interrupt me in two.

PAPP: Uh huh. Listen, act that out. Try it and let's see what would happen. (*He starts to play the game. She doesn't interrupt but he keeps looking over his shoulder at her.*) You keep looking at her. Would your mind be on her if you were playing?

LARRY: Yeah, I'd play lousy. The girls would destroy my game even if they were standing there. I'd be showing off.

PAPP: You're showing off for her?

LARRY: Yeah, I'd really try to do things that I couldn't, to show off.

PAPP: I see. When you're watching television do you show off for her by showing her your expertise about the game?

LARRY: Mmm . . . no.

PAPP: You don't talk to her and say, "Look at that guy, you know what he just did," and give her a kind of running commentary like that?

LARRY: No, she's not interested.

PAPP: You're not interested?

JENNIFER: Yeah.

LARRY: She wants to know if Joe Namath was a good center fielder.

PAPP: I see. But keep on trying. Let's see how you'd go about doing this. You've still got your mind on her. (*Larry begins shooting baskets again.*)

LARRY: I missed a shot because of them and then they interrupt after two points.

PAPP: You would play a lousy game even if she didn't interrupt for five minutes because you'd be so preoccupied with what she was doing.

LARRY: That's right. I know that she's annoyed so I don't enjoy it as much.

PAPP: M'hm.

JENNIFER: That puts a damper on it.

PAPP: So that's not a solution. Find a solution.

LARRY: Well . . .

PAPP: Change the picture so there's a solution.

LARRY: Um. I don't know a solution, because I never like to play with girls in, um, that way.

PAPP: Just within this setting, and within this moment, try something different, maybe that you've never tried before, but find a solution.

LARRY: OK. (*Larry pulls Jennifer aside for a talk and gestures "five points" to her. She holds up five fingers, he nods and pats her shoulder.*)

PAPP: In other words, you would really sit down with her and explain to her how long it's going to be. You'd really convince her to stay out of it. Then you would be able to carry on?

LARRY: Yes.

Larry has come up with at least one solution that is different from simply ignoring her. He will sit down and talk with her and they will agree on a certain amount of time for him to complete his game.

Next I asked them to have another fantasy, this time hoping that they would see themselves in still more symbolic forms. In their first fantasies, they were simply younger versions of themselves. In their second fantasies I wanted them to move to a more symbolic level. Larry began:

LARRY: I'm Thomas Jefferson. And I really have a lot of important things to do.

PAPP: Yes, you would, as Thomas Jefferson.

LARRY: [I have to] meet with the Continental Congress. But my wife is very frail . . .

PAPP: She's your wife?

LARRY: Yeah. And I'm there, and I know that the country needs me. It's in a mess and I have to write the Declaration of Independence. But I really don't want to do it because she's back in Virginia, sick.

PAPP: (*To Jennifer*) Would you come over and lie on the couch and be sick?

JENNIFER: OK. (*She lies on the sofa.*)

LARRY: But I'm in Philadelphia. I'm sitting, writing, and doing a decent job. When I get to work I do a very good job on things. But there's always this thing in the back of my mind. I'm wondering how she is, and there are no phones, letters are very slow and they get lost, and I just want to leave and get back, but I can't . . .

PAPP: But you're always preoccupied with her. What is your fantasy about what is happening to her?

LARRY: Well, that she's in bed and sick and not doing very well.

PAPP: And what would your nightmare be . . . your worst nightmare?

LARRY: Well, obviously that she would be dead, and I wouldn't know it until I got back . . .

PAPP: M'hm.

LARRY: . . . and I wouldn't be there.

PAPP: And then you would reprimand yourself for not having been there?

LARRY: Yeah.

PAPP: OK, let's say that you go back home to take care of her. You leave your job and go back home. You stop writing the Declaration of Independence.

LARRY: Yeah. Franklin can do that. (*Larry goes over to Jennifer and leans over her.*) I say, "How are you doing?" and then I sort of sit there. I get her up and I sort of carry her outside. We're sitting on the porch.

PAPP: You got her well, but now you feel you didn't write the Declaration of Independence.

LARRY: Now I'm here, and I say, "Franklin can't write English. He's smart, but it's got to be something that can stand throughout history."

PAPP: I see.

LARRY: Little kids are going to read it in third grade, and . . .

PAPP: So, she's taken you away from work that you feel is extremely important?

LARRY: Right.

PAPP: Mmm.

LARRY: So, I have the solution, you know. I take her and put her in the carriage and we both go back to Philadelphia.

PAPP: Let's see that. You put her in the carriage. (*Larry helps Jennifer up, gently guiding her to the carriage.*)

LARRY: I take her, put her in the carriage, and we drive to Philadelphia, and then I sit down and I start writing. Now she's sick but she's here.

PAPP: That would be OK if you took her with you?

LARRY: Yeah.

PAPP: If you involved her in your problems?

LARRY: She wouldn't be involved, she would be doing her own stuff.

PAPP: Uh huh. But you would be able to keep your eye on her and know that she was safe. And you'd feel you had fulfilled your obligation to her?

LARRY: Yeah.

PAPP: When you were Jefferson before, and she was lying on the bed, would you go back to that, please? (*Jennifer lies down on the sofa again.*) What was it that prevented you from this solution? What prevented you from going back?

LARRY: Um, what prevented me?

PAPP: Uh huh.

LARRY: Wanting to be in history books. I don't know . . . that slowed me because it's a very long trip up and back and it was critical that it get done fairly quickly, because Washington was getting beaten . . . and he needed money.

PAPP: In reality how do you feel your preoccupation or worry or concern about Jennifer prevents you from doing what you really want to do, what you feel is important?

LARRY: Well . . .

PAPP: Does she interfere with your work in some way or your concentration, or . . .

LARRY: Um, I guess. You know, but that's true with any couple, you can't always do something without regard for the other.

PAPP: It's true. I was just wondering at what point in your life you feel this takes away from something that's very important to you.

LARRY: In the beginning years, she was always of primary importance. My career and school were always secondary. I'd cut classes to go visit her.

PAPP: I see, so now you're feeling the conflict because your own things are becoming more important?

LARRY: Right. And she might take it that I care less about her, but I don't think it's true. I've just grown as an individual, and I just feel that in order to interact, to be happy with her, you have to be happy with yourself first. And although my career is still secondary, it is not as far away. I wouldn't neglect it totally.

PAPP: I see, it has become more important . . . OK.

This second of Larry's fantasies carries out the theme of his first fantasy: Jennifer interrupts his game. But in this second fantasy a new theme appears, the theme of rescue. Rescuing was a very prevalent aspect of Larry and Jennifer's relationship in its early years. Larry bailed Jennifer out of every kind of difficulty, on the assumption that she had emotional problems that she could conquer if he just hung in there long enough. Notice that in both of Larry's fantasies Jennifer is the one in the "down" position. In the first he is a basketball hero while she is an admiring fan on the sidelines. In the second, he is a famous statesman while she is sick and needy. He is competent and able to stand on his own. She is helpless without him.

The second fantasy also reveals an important change that has taken place in the relationship. Jennifer no longer takes precedence over everything else in Larry's life. He is no longer willing to sacrifice himself for her as he did in the past. He thinks more about his own needs and goals now. Jennifer's second fantasy follows:

JENNIFER: I would like to be somebody like a famous composer, for instance . . . Mozart.

PAPP: You're Mozart?

JENNIFER: Right, I'm Mozart and I'm sitting at the piano. (*Jennifer sits.*) And I'm feverishly composing a requiem mass, OK?

PAPP: Uh huh.

JENNIFER: And you know, I have this premonition that this is it for me. Anyway, that there aren't many days left in my life. And my wife, Larry, is yelling at me for not spending enough time with her. And she's ridiculing me for writing this composition.

PAPP: OK, will you act that out?

JENNIFER: OK. (*Jennifer plays the piano and Larry interrupts pointing to the time, gesturing to her to stop. She continues to play. He persists.*)

PAPP: So, now you're in the position of the one who doesn't want to be involved, to give more of yourself, your time?

JENNIFER: M'hm.

PAPP: When, in reality, does this happen?

JENNIFER: When I feel like I'm under a lot of pressure to get something done, that it is very important. When I have a deadline and I feel like Larry might be needing me for something else, you know, like he might need to plan a party for his office, or to work out some kind of household problem, you know, that I haven't gotten around to doing, and I feel this tremendous conflict. I feel like I'm neglecting him, or the house, or whatever, because I'm concentrating on my work, because I have something to do.

PAPP: Figure out a solution to that within this fantasy. Do something different.

JENNIFER: OK.

PAPP: Begin the fantasy again.

JENNIFER: OK. (*Jennifer begins playing the piano. Larry interrupts. Jennifer gestures with five fingers.*) Just five minutes . . .

LARRY: Five points, five minutes. (*They all laugh.*)

PAPP: Five points, five minutes . . . yes.

Isn't it interesting that they both saw themselves as immortal men? Jefferson, the intellectual giant, and Mozart, the artistic giant. Wow! What a marriage that would be!

There is a striking difference between Jennifer's first and second fantasies. In her second fantasy, she totally reverses her position. Rather than Jennifer pursuing Larry for more emotional involvement, he is now pursuing her. She places Larry in the one-down position of a wife begging for time and attention from a creative genius who doesn't have time to give. I suppose the reason she cast herself as a male genius rather than a female genius is because there are few (if any) models of women geniuses with meek "wife-like" spouses to care for them.

Be that as it may, in this fantasy Larry is interfering with Jennifer's game—or her life work. In daily life, it seems she is torn between being a good partner to Larry and developing her own potential. In her fantasy, she settles the question the same way Larry did, by asking for five more minutes—which is hardly time to write a research grant, let alone a requiem mass!

There are innumerable ways one can interpret and use this kind of material. It provides a rich source of areas to explore and questions to ask in future sessions. But how does one select a central theme from the many different themes revealed in these fantasies? There is the theme of control, for example, with each trying to control the other person's game. There is the theme of emotional closeness and distance, with each shifting positions in an effort to regulate intimacy. There is the theme of competitiveness, as evidenced in the last fantasies. Jefferson and Mozart are a formidable couple. Who deserves the spotlight? Which one should give in to the other? All of these themes are potentially of crucial importance, but I must choose a starting point. Generally I begin with the theme that, at the moment, seems the most relevant to the presenting problem. I keep the others in mind as reference points throughout therapy.

In this case I chose the theme of control around which to design an initial task, because both Larry and Jennifer complained of the other person interrupting or controlling his or her game. The task was designed in the form of a game, reflecting the theme of games used in their fantasies. I call such tasks "pre-change tests." I tell the couple that these tasks are not for the purpose of producing any major change; rather, they indicate if the system is ready to change, and if so, in what direction. Who should change, in what way, and how fast?

I always keep the pre-change test simple. In this case, I suggested that they monitor each other very carefully for one week. When Larry sensed Jennifer needed emotional contact, he was to find a way to give it without making her feel that he was controlling her game (her thoughts or feelings). This was presented as a challenge to him since he had indicated that he liked to test himself. In doing the task Larry would, I hoped, find a variety of ways of responding to Jennifer without her feeling trapped or controlled.

Jennifer was to monitor Larry very carefully to discover the moment that he was most receptive to involvement, and at that moment, she was to communicate to him very clearly what she needed from him. This was presented as a challenge to her. The competitiveness between Larry and Jennifer was brought into service in the design of the tasks. They were both to "keep score" by writing down when the other person either succeeded or failed in carrying out the instructions I had given them.

One problem in attempting to illustrate my approach to Larry and Jennifer in this chapter is that I was not able to give them the tasks directly. I generally give such tasks in the second session. The first session is devoted primarily to using the fantasies to gather information and form a hypothesis. It is impossible for me to detach myself enough to study and compare the fantasies while I'm in the middle of guiding them. My comparative analysis is best accomplished when viewing the videotapes after the session. Since it was impossible for me to have a second interview with the couple, I gave the suggestion for the task to their therapist who was free to use it or not use it, at her discretion.

Regrettably, I have no follow-up for the suggestion; thus this report of an opening intervention is, in a sense, incomplete. However, fuller expositions of my approach as it has been applied in other cases are available elsewhere (Papp, 1976a, 1976b, 1980, 1982; Papp, Silverstein, & Carter, 1973).

Conclusion

The process of structuring fantasies can be an enjoyable and freeing experience for both the therapist and the couple. The couple is allowed to caricature their relationship and express through caricatures thoughts and feelings they may be unable or unwilling to express in a purely verbal exchange. The fantasies provide the therapist with rich personal metaphors through which to explore the couple's relationship on several different levels. When the partners respond to interactional questions such as, "Where do you go when she does that? Does she follow you? How do you stop her? Show me how she reacts to that," the therapist is able to see patterns of interaction in the form of actual movement. The couple's thinking about their relationship is reached through questions such as, "What is the difficult predicament in this for you? What do you believe would happen to him if you don't save him? What is your nightmare about this, supposing it never changes?" Answers to such questions reveal the couple's perceptions of themselves and one another, their expectations, assumptions, attitudes, and fears. An understanding of both the interactional patterns of the relationship and the inner perceptions and thoughts of each partner about it provides the therapist with a holistic picture on which to base a variety of interventions.

Structured fantasies can be useful not only in the first session as a diagnostic tool, but throughout therapy as a barometer of change. When the fantasies are seen sequentially and compared, they reveal more precisely than words can the ways in which positions and perceptions have shifted. Fantasies can also serve as a guide for the therapist in constructing interventions and can spur self-initiated experimental change in the couple.

REFERENCES

Bowen, M. (1978). *Family therapy in clinical practice*. New York: Jason Aronson.

Dicks, H. W. (1967). *Marital tensions*. New York: Basic Books.

Duhl, F., Kantor, D., & Duhl, B. (1973). Learning, space, and action in family therapy: A primer of sculpture. In D. Bloch (Ed.), *Techniques of family psychotherapy: A primer*. New York: Grune & Stratton.

Framo, J. (1982). *Explorations in marital and family therapy*. New York: Springer Publishing Company.

Mittlelmann, B. (1944). Complementary neurotic reactions in intimate relationships. *Psychoanalytic Quarterly, 13*, 479–491.

Mittelmann, B. (1948). The concurrent analysis of married couples. *Psychoanalytic Quarterly, 17*, 182–197.

Papp, P. (1976a). Brief therapy with couples groups. In P. Guerin (Ed.), *Family therapy: Theory and practice*. New York: Gardner Press.

Papp, P. (1976b). Family choreography. In P. Guerin (Ed.), *Family therapy: Theory and practice*. New York: Gardner Press.

Papp, P. (1980). The use of fantasy in a couples group. In M. Andolfi & I. Zwerling (Eds.), *Dimensions of family therapy*. New York: Guilford Press.

Papp, P. (1982). Staging reciprocal metaphors in a couples group. *Family Process, 21*(4), 453–467.

Papp, P., Silverstein, O., & Carter, E. (1973). Family sculpting in preventive work with well families. *Family Process, 12*(2), 197–212.

Sager, C. (1976). Marriage contracts and couple therapy. New York: Brunner/Mazel.

Selvini-Palazzoli, M., Boscolo, L., Cecchin, G., & Prata, G. (1978). *Paradox and counterparadox*. New York: Jason Aronson.

Watzlawick, P. (1978). *The language of change*. New York: Basic Books.

Winch, R. F., Ktones, T., & Ktones, V. (1954). The theory of complementary needs in mate selection. *American Sociological Review, 19*, 241–249.

4

Integrating Families of Origin into Couple Therapy

JAMES L. FRAMO

My approach to psychotherapy is based on my belief that family of origin issues are fundamental to people's intimate or relationship problems. Although many therapists subscribe to this belief, I have taken the uncommon step of bringing in the families of origin of clients for face-to-face family meetings. Family of origin sessions evolve out of several contexts in which I do treatment: family therapy, marital therapy, couples' group therapy, and family-oriented individual therapy. Sometimes single individuals who are not regular clients and who wish to work on issues with parents and siblings request family of origin sessions. The involvement of the family of origin usually has powerful effects on the original problems for which clients entered treatment (Framo, 1982; Framo, 1990; Framo, Weber, & Levine, in press).

My work with families of origin is the logical outcome of the idea that hidden transgenerational forces exercise a critical influence on present intimate relationships (see Paul, Chapter 5, and J. Grunebaum, Chapter 10, this volume). Current marital and parental difficulties are largely reparative efforts to correct, master, defend against, live through, or cancel old conflicts from the original family. These conflicts and transference distortions from the past are lived anachronistically through the spouse and children. Most people do not "see" their intimate partners as they really are: Old ghosts stand in the way. People try to handle their old anxieties *through* a current relationship; they attempt to make an interpersonal resolution of intrapsychic conflict. Jennifer and Larry are not unique in this respect.

The theoretical basis of my work with families of origin, more fully explicated elsewhere (Framo, 1970, 1976), is as follows:

1. The human need for a satisfactory object relationship constitutes a fundamental motive of life (Fairbairn, 1954). This object relationship

approach is contrasted with Freud's theory in which instinctual gratification is fundamental (see Givelber, Chapter 9, this volume).

2. Unable to give up their parents or change them in outer reality, infants incorporate (introject) the frustrating aspects of their relational world. They retain these introjects as enduring psychological representatives of their caretakers.

3. Intrapsychic conflicts arise from experiences in the original family. In an effort to resolve these conflicts, the individual shapes his or her current relationships into patterns similar to those of the original family.

4. One's mate or children are perceived largely in terms of one's own needs; for example, they may be seen as carrying one's denied, split-off traits. Mates select each other to recover lost aspects of their primary object relations, aspects that they re-experience in the other by projective identification (Dicks, 1967). A main source of marital disharmony is that spouses project disowned aspects of themselves onto their mates and then fight them in the mates (see Low, this volume).

5. By having sessions with his or her family of origin, the adult takes the problems back to their original sources, thereby making available a direct route to etiological factors. These sessions serve diagnostic as well as therapeutic purposes in that both the old and new families can be cross-referenced for similar patterns.

6. Dealing with the real, external figures loosens the grip of the internalized representatives of these figures and exposes them to current realities. The parents and siblings of today are not the parents and siblings of the past; indeed, they never were as they were perceived to be. The original transference figures can also be objects of transference today; few adults ever get to see their parents as real people.

7. Having gone backward in time, the individual can then move forward, treating the spouse as a person in his or her own right.

8. Not only do family of origin sessions help to resolve problems in the current family, but coming to terms with parents and siblings before they die can also be a profoundly liberating experience for the individual and other family members. There are usually positive changes in the individual and marital systems levels, as well as in the family of origin relationships.

When clients are prepared to deal face to face with critical and heretofore avoided issues with parents and siblings, they can clear away some of the filters and cobwebs that exist between them and their intimate others. Furthermore, past bitterness toward parents and siblings can be dissipated, allowing clients to achieve that ultimate stage: forgiveness of their parents (and siblings). Clients are then freed from spending their lives expiating guilt or enduring self-hatred. Self-esteem can be raised. In my view, family of origin therapy is the ultimate form of brief therapy. One session with one's parents and siblings, conducted with skill, determination, and care can bring about more changes than an entire course of individual or couple therapy. As typified by this case, however, most people are terrified of meeting with parents and siblings and telling the truth. Jennifer's resistance was apparent, palpable, and normal. Since I usually conduct family of origin sessions with a female cotherapist, I asked Mary Framo to join me for that part of the interview.[1]

Before we met with Jennifer and her family of origin in New York in January of 1983, Henry Grunebaum had sent us the background information presented in this book, so we knew something about the couple and their families. I was arbitrarily assigned to Jennifer's family of origin. Norman Paul saw Larry's.

The night before we left for New York to do the interview I got a phone call from Jennifer's sister, Beth, who told me that she was a mental health professional, that her mother was very defensive, and that if her mother were confronted in any way she (the mother) would "go berserk or leave the room."[2] She said that she had a lot of anger toward her mother and that her mother had "abused" Jennifer. Then Beth said, "I want you to know that when I come to that session I will not deal with my parents about anything important; I will not deal with any issues. I will stick strictly to superficialities." I told Beth that in the session she would be free to deal with whatever she wanted. Following that reassurance, she agreed to attend.

The next day, I saw the couple alone, and then Mary Framo joined me in the session with Jennifer and her family. I told the couple in the beginning that I would be dealing only briefly with their relationship and that the bulk of the time would be spent in preparing Jennifer for her family session. Larry understood that Norman Paul would be seeing him with his family at a later date.

Most of this chapter will focus on the interview with Jennifer's family of origin and my attempts to prepare Jennifer for it, but I will briefly summarize here my initial impressions of the couple and some of the issues that emerged in my interview with them alone.

I found Jennifer and Larry to be delightful, likeable, and cooperative. Furthermore, despite the difficulties they had, I saw a strong bond and much caring between them. They seemed to be in a committed relationship.

---

[1] I would like to express my appreciation to Mary Framo for her invaluable participation in the family of origin session.

[2] *Editors' note:* After reading the manuscript of this chapter, Beth told us that she recalls telling Jim Framo that it was her father, not her mother, who might "go berserk or leave the room."

It was immediately apparent that Jennifer was the pursuer in the relationship and Larry the distancer (see Fogarty, 1979).[3] Jennifer spoke of Larry not sharing his feelings with her and withdrawing from emotional closeness; she was hungry for love and closeness. She said, "I might as well be a piece of furniture as far as he is concerned." She indicated that Larry's distance forced her to withdraw, and then she felt lonely and isolated. Incidentally, Jennifer said that one of the reasons she was attracted to Larry was because of his family—that they were open and close with each other, so unlike her own family (Napier, 1978). Jennifer's sense of inner emptiness could only be filled by others; she felt that if she could only get to Larry she would be complete, but she couldn't reach him. She intended him to be her rescuer.

One of the difficulties with pursuers is that when they do get close to someone they often feel suffocated, tied down, and trapped, and then have to break away for freedom. But then they feel forsaken and lonely, and have to push for fusion and closeness again. This is what Fairbairn calls the "in-and-out program" whereby one either fears losing one's personality by absorption, or feels depressed and cut off (Guntrip, 1952). Separateness means being rejected, being unloved, being a nothing.

Larry said of Jennifer, "She is no good at doing nothing and always has to be busy at work." Jennifer is a workaholic like her sister; both were reared by Dutch parents with a strict work ethic. Larry also said that Jennifer is very competitive, and one can see that in her relationship with her sister.

I spent some time dealing with the impact of Larry's cancer and the loss of his foot. Jennifer's need to be taken care of (and Larry's need to be protective of her) was thrown out of kilter when Larry was seriously ill and she was forced to take care of him (reviving the feeling that she had when she was expected by her mother to take care of her father).

Some new information came out in the couple's interview. Jennifer described how Larry once hit her and tried to strangle her; Larry did not remember this, but said that if it did happen it was when she saw other men years ago. Larry also revealed that he had been involved with other women. This news shocked and hurt Jennifer.

In the following excerpt from the couple interview, I not only addressed Jennifer's deep inner sense of unworthiness and her feeling of being in the way, but I also began to deal with her reluctance to address significant issues with her family. Ordinarily, I have many weeks in which to help my clients overcome their initial resistance to a session with their original families, to get a detailed family history, to prepare

---

[3]Although Larry was allegedly the distancer, in truth they both alternated in these roles. As Fogarty says, inside every distancer is a pursuer and inside every pursuer is a distancer.

the client, and to develop an agenda of issues. In this special case, I had only a few minutes to prepare Jennifer. Her sister had already warned me not to deal with anything meaningful, and Jennifer felt just about the same way. Her fear was evident in statements such as, "I did not think we were going to have family therapy," or "I didn't think we were going to deal with anything personal."

JIM FRAMO: Jennifer, I get the impression that you're the kind of person who goes through life saying, "Pardon me for living."

JENNIFER: Sort of. Yeah, I guess I do. I always feel like I'm not worthy or that I don't deserve things, or that I need to prove myself all the time, prove my worthiness.

JIM FRAMO: Prove your existence? Do you have a right to a life?

JENNIFER: (*shrugs her shoulders*) Yeah, I guess it comes out sometimes . . . I just remember feeling the helplessness . . . (*long pause*)

JIM FRAMO: What are you experiencing right now, at this moment?

JENNIFER: I guess what you said . . . I feel like I don't have the right to exist or something and that's an old theme that comes back.

JIM FRAMO: OK, let's hear about that old theme.

JENNIFER: Well . . . these things come from my childhood. I always felt that I shouldn't have been around, and that people would have been happier if I weren't there, and . . .

JIM FRAMO: You mean you never felt *valued*?

JENNIFER: Valued, needed, useful, appreciated, or wanted . . . I guess I just felt like it was an accident that I appeared on the scene, and that it was my fault if unpleasant things happened after I was born.

JIM FRAMO: How much of this have you shared with your family, what you're telling me now?

JENNIFER: Not much, not much at all.

JIM FRAMO: You've never told your parents that you felt this way?

JENNIFER: Maybe indirectly, but never directly.

JIM FRAMO: Never directly. Can you?

JENNIFER: No, I don't think so. It would be very hard for me to do it. Maybe someday I'd like to be able to do it.

JIM FRAMO: But we have an unparalleled opportunity here. I'm going to be interviewing you with your family. Here's your chance.

JENNIFER: I just think under these circumstances, that it's being taped and everything, that I would feel much too uncomfortable, and put on the spot.

JIM FRAMO: Yeah, I see.

JENNIFER: I couldn't do it. I know that an audience will be viewing this.

JIM FRAMO: Yes. Let me give you a point of view about that. You see, ordinarily when I work with a couple I work with them for a number of months. I usually have a long period of time to prepare people for the session that you're about to have. So, in a sense, it's kind of artificial to have just a short period of time to prepare you for something that ordinarily I take months to do.

JENNIFER: Uh huh.

JIM FRAMO: But we'll try. This is my specialty, seeing people with their family of origin. I get calls from people around the country who say, "I want to bring in my family." Sometimes at great expense they bring them from all over the country.

JENNIFER: Sure.

JIM FRAMO: What they are saying to me, in essence, is, "I want to come to terms with my parents before they die."

JENNIFER: Uh huh.

JIM FRAMO: Otherwise, after they're gone, like, you have to suffer unending guilt, you know.

JENNIFER: But I'd like to do that on my terms. I think when I'm ready.

JIM FRAMO: I hear you.

JENNIFER: I'm not sure today is the right time.

JIM FRAMO: I hear what you are saying.

JENNIFER: You see?

JIM FRAMO: The only problem with that is, first of all, most people *don't* do it. They say they're going to, but they never get around to it because it's frightening!

JENNIFER: Uh huh, it sure is.

JIM FRAMO: Secondly, it's somewhat easier when there is a third party present who's objective and not emotionally involved. Someone to help facilitate it.

JENNIFER: But this wasn't . . . the purpose of this whole thing wasn't family therapy. It's couples therapy.

JIM FRAMO: Well, but they're involved with each other. . . . I see your anxiety.

JENNIFER: You know what I mean?

JIM FRAMO: I see your anxiety.

JENNIFER: OK.

JIM FRAMO: Let me put it this way. I want you to imagine for a moment that you're standing by the grave of your mother and father. What would you wish you had said to them before they died?

JENNIFER: I don't know. I guess I can't even think about it.

JIM FRAMO: Try.

JENNIFER: I guess I don't want to right now.

JIM FRAMO: Do you have a sense that it's all been said, that there would be nothing left unsaid?

JENNIFER: No, I don't think anything's been said, really. But I just don't think that I will allow myself to do it right now. I just . . . I feel too inhibited.

JIM FRAMO: I hear you.

JENNIFER: And I have incredible control mechanisms (*she laughs*).

JIM FRAMO: I hear what you're saying.

JENNIFER: So I don't think I can do it. I just feel uncomfortable about it. It might be too overwhelming for me to do it.

JIM FRAMO: Uh huh.

JENNIFER: I guess I feel that my desire to protect myself is so strong that I probably won't allow myself to do it.

JIM FRAMO: See, what I'm talking about is not telling your parents off or getting angry at them. I'm talking about getting to know them as people. Very few of us ever get to know our parents as real people.

JENNIFER: But it has to be reciprocated. I mean, I don't want to be the one who's going to make myself vulnerable, and then not have it reciprocated.

JIM FRAMO: So you wouldn't anticipate that you'd get anything back?

JENNIFER: (*Pause*) It's a fear.

JIM FRAMO: Uh huh. May I ask you, what did you plan to talk about with your mother and father and sister when they came? What were your thoughts? What were you going to do at that time?

JENNIFER: I had a lot of anxiety about it and I was hoping that we would just talk about things that weren't that personal. You know, you might have some sort of drama in mind for us that we would act out. Perhaps a scene where somebody forgot the car keys, and who would get angry at whom, and what would be going on, or something like that.

JIM FRAMO: I see. So you . . .

JENNIFER: I didn't think it was going to be family therapy, like you're asking, "OK, what are the problems here?"

JIM FRAMO: No, what I'm talking about isn't family therapy. I'm not here to treat your family.

JENNIFER: Yeah.

JIM FRAMO: What I'm here to do, basically—my cotherapist and I are going to do it together—is to help facilitate communication among all your family members. We're not treating you all. It's to help you all to deal with each other. We're creating the setting in which to do that. But your fantasy about what it was going to be like was that we were just going to act out a scene of some sort?

JENNIFER: Yeah.

JIM FRAMO: And we wouldn't get into anything personal?

JENNIFER: No, because I figured you only had about an hour's time so that, you know, you wouldn't get into anything personal. And I know how my mother reacts to things, she sloughs things off.

JIM FRAMO: Yes, your sister called me and told me that.

JENNIFER: Right. And she wouldn't want to get into anything very deep, she'd be evasive, and . . .

JIM FRAMO: Well, your sister went a little farther. She said that your mother would go berserk . . .

JENNIFER: Uh huh.

JIM FRAMO: . . and she might walk out of the room . . .

JENNIFER: Well, that's very possible.

JIM FRAMO: . . . .if she were confronted. So your sister had the same plan that you did. Namely, she said, "I really only want to talk about superficialities."

LARRY: I think that her mother, and you'll see, is more reasonable than they say, in my opinion. But I only know her as an outsider.

JIM FRAMO: She's more reasonable, you say?

LARRY: Yeah, I think.

JIM FRAMO: Than what? Than they are portraying?

LARRY: She certainly evades big issues, there's no question about it, but I think that there's some element of . . .

JIM FRAMO: The impression that I got is that she's very fragile and can't tolerate the truth, or ever being confronted.

JENNIFER: Right. Either she'll deny it or she'll walk out of the room. If it feels like she's sitting in the hot seat and her denial is not going to work, she'll walk out of the room.

JIM FRAMO: First of all, we have no intention of attacking your parents. I mean, we're very protective towards parents. Let me get a little bit of history from you, OK?

JENNIFER: OK, sure.

Jennifer's father was 79 years of age and her mother 61 at this time. She told me she felt a little closer to her father, but not close, really, to either. She said that her father beat her sister and mother beat her when she was a child. She was terrified of her mother's rages. The mother and sister were in alliance, and the mother told Jennifer it was her job to take care of the father because he was old and fragile; Jennifer felt responsible for her father's survival. She said there was never any emotion expressed in the family, there was little affection, and the house was always dark. Her parents were "polarized" in their marriage. Mother told Jennifer that men were no good and were only interested in one thing. Jennifer said that she and Beth were competitive and hated each other as kids, although Beth mothered her. She and her sister could not protect each other from the beatings; they had to watch out for themselves. She felt "powerless and controlled." As a child she was preoccupied with death, drew pictures of graveyards, and listened to requiem masses.

I was cautioned by Jennifer not to get into her mother's background, because the mother was illegitimate and had been raised in an institution. Her mother, she said, would not talk about that. Jennifer was not willing to confront her parents with any of her true feelings, and it was difficult to find anything important that we could talk about. In view of the fact that Jennifer usually had no difficulty talking about her feelings, this was surprising. I knew, however, that we would get beyond her fear and anxiety once she and the family got caught up in the process. I also knew that most people, still under the influence of the intense affect associated with the early images of their parents, see them as more crazy, threatening, and monster-like than they really are. This is borne out by Larry's statement that Jennifer's mother is more reasonable than one would conclude from Jennifer's portrayal of her.

Later in this first session, Jennifer agreed that there were two safe areas she was willing to discuss: her father's background and her relationship with her sister. At the end of this discussion, when Jennifer felt she would be in control of how much she was willing to risk, she was less apprehensive about the session.

JIM FRAMO: Growing up. What was it like as a kid?

JENNIFER: Oh, growing up. We [Jennifer and her sister] hated each other. We couldn't stand each other. We were continually competing and fighting, although she took care of me quite a bit in the beginning. My mother didn't want to mother me, so my sister got that responsibility.

JIM FRAMO: She resented it?

JENNIFER: Yeah.

JIM FRAMO: Your sister had to take care of you?

JENNIFER: Oh yeah, she did. She was like my mother, really. So when she left to get married, I felt very abandoned by her.

JIM FRAMO: But you fought a lot?

JENNIFER: We fought a lot. When I got older we started fighting more. I mean we used to have fights and some of them were knock-down battles. Other times it was very indirect. She would do something and then I'd get angry and then two weeks later I'd do something to get back at her.

JIM FRAMO: Did you ever feel love toward her as a kid?

JENNIFER: (*Looks down, with a thoughtful and perplexed expression*) I don't really remember. It's funny, it's very vague in my mind.

JIM FRAMO: What's your relationship like with your sister these days, as adults?

JENNIFER: Superficial. We see each other during holidays, usually, and there's very little exchange of words. It's just sort of, "Hi, how're you doing?"

JIM FRAMO: You never talk about the family, and your parents, and things like that?

JENNIFER: Sometimes. It's very rare. I think what happens is that we get to the point where we build up our relationship into a deeper one. Like we'll communicate on a deeper level. We'll talk a little bit about what happened in the past, comparing notes, so to speak. You know, "What was Dad doing to you and why wasn't he doing that to me, and what was Mom doing to you?" Things like that. We'll compare notes quite a bit, but then we build up to a certain point where we get close, and then something gets in the way. There are these barriers that all of a sudden present themselves.

JIM FRAMO: Have you sisters ever hugged each other?

JENNIFER: During holidays (*laughs*).

JIM FRAMO: Holidays only?

JENNIFER: Holidays only. It's permitted then.

JIM FRAMO: What's your relationship like with your mom these days?

JENNIFER: (*Looks down, sighs*) Strained again. Very strained. I don't confide in her about anything personal. I usually don't tell her what's going on in my private life. It's all very superficial.

JIM FRAMO: How does she feel about Larry?

JENNIFER: I think she feels threatened by him. I think she feels that, in many ways, he took her daughter away. (*Smiles*)

JIM FRAMO: How about you and Dad now?

JENNIFER: It's funny, it's hard to talk to him. It's just very hard to talk to him about anything. He sort of goes off on tangents and . . .

JIM FRAMO: I get the impression, though, that it's impossible to talk with Mom, but it's just difficult to talk with Dad. Is that correct?

JENNIFER: Hmm. These are difficult questions. They require thought. It's difficult to talk to Dad. I think it's almost impossible to talk to him, too. Because I'll tell him things and then, 10 minutes later, he'll start talking about something else . . .

JIM FRAMO: I see.

JENNIFER: . . . and then I feel like, "Well, I didn't get anywhere, so what's the use?"

JIM FRAMO: You never told him that?

JENNIFER: No.

JIM FRAMO: As a matter of fact, you never told your parents anything that was really in your heart. (*Pause. Jennifer shakes her head in agreement.*) You know, it's interesting how people go through life about this. They'll tell their spouse, they'll tell their friends, they'll tell their siblings, they'll tell their therapist, they'll tell Dear Abby, and they won't tell the people that need to be told.

JENNIFER: Uh huh.

JIM FRAMO: Everybody but the people that need to be told.

JENNIFER: Well, obviously, it feels unsafe to do it.

JIM FRAMO: Yeah, I know.

JENNIFER: Otherwise, we'd do it.

JIM FRAMO: I know, you really have to feel you're in a protected place to do it. When I prepare people for these sessions, I try to get them to come up with an agenda of things that they want to deal with.

JENNIFER: Uh huh.

JIM FRAMO: And I haven't heard one thing that you feel prepared to deal with, with your family.

JENNIFER: Because I didn't think we would be doing family therapy . . .

JIM FRAMO: I see.

JENNIFER: . . . or a family type of thing. The focus was supposed to be couples. I thought that what you might want to do with the family is get background information. Like what was it like eating dinner at my house or what was it like going out to the movies, which we never did. That kind of thing.

JIM FRAMO: So, those are the safe things that you'd want to talk about.

JENNIFER: Right.

JIM FRAMO: Daily events that weren't loaded, or emotional in any way.

JENNIFER: Right. Absolutely.

JIM FRAMO: That's what you'd prefer?

JENNIFER: Yeah . . . it would make it a lot . . .

JIM FRAMO: OK, but I wonder if we could at least set a minimal agenda. Would you be interested at all in bettering your relationship at least with your sister?

JENNIFER: Yeah, I feel safer with that.

JIM FRAMO: You feel safer with that. Larry, do you have an overall picture of the whole family?

LARRY: Yeah. I think they all have things below the surface that they don't let out. They're not very warm people, although they're extremely friendly. They've always been very nice to me. In the beginning years, everything was a secret. Her mother would take her aside and they'd talk about nothing, really, say clothes. But in order to do that, she had to take her and close the door to the bedroom. Everything . . . The house is dark.

JENNIFER: Don't forget that you are a man. We have secrets from men.

LARRY: Oh, yeah.

JIM FRAMO: From men?

JENNIFER: Sure.

JIM FRAMO: What do you mean, "The house is dark"? The shades are pulled down?

LARRY: The shades are pulled, the lights are out except in the kitchen.

JIM FRAMO: Why?

JENNIFER: They like it dark. I don't know. They're just very sheltered people. That's why I'm amazed that they are coming here.

JIM FRAMO: Gee, what are they going to do with these bright lights [for the videotaping]?

JENNIFER: Probably freak out (*laughs*).

JIM FRAMO: Oh, my.

LARRY: I mean, they're very intelligent people.

JIM FRAMO: Well, they must be, they've got two Ph.D. daughters.

LARRY: Her father was kicked out of the house at 13. He was one of 10 children. He was never shown any love, in Holland, in the old country, and he was on his own after age 13. His mother said, "Don't come back." And she stuck him in an apprenticeship.

JIM FRAMO: Is that right?

LARRY: Yeah.

JIM FRAMO: Wow. (*To Jennifer*) Would your father be interested in talking about his background?

JENNIFER: Oh, yeah.

LARRY: Yes.

JENNIFER: He loves talking about his background.

LARRY: He loves talking about that.

JIM FRAMO: Great. That's something we can talk about. OK, go on.

JENNIFER: My mother would not want to.

JIM FRAMO: Why?

JENNIFER: She had a horrible background. At least that is how it was presented.

JIM FRAMO: What do you mean?

JENNIFER: Well, she was illegitimate and abandoned. She was put in an orphanage type of situation.

JIM FRAMO: She didn't know her father?

JENNIFER: No. She doesn't want to know, but I want to find out. I'm curious about that.

JIM FRAMO: Didn't she ever even speculate about who her father was?

JENNIFER: She doesn't want to. As far as she knows, he's dead. That's what she keeps telling me.

JIM FRAMO: Did she ever know who he was?

JENNIFER: She knows his name. That's it.

LARRY: She said he came to the house with . . .

JENNIFER: That was somebody else, that was a Jewish doctor who came to the house.

LARRY: But she suspects that's . . .

JENNIFER: . . . that he might have been my grandfather.

JIM FRAMO: He's a Jewish doctor?

JENNIFER: Yeah.

JIM FRAMO: Well, was she brought up when the Nazis were there?

JENNIFER: No, no.

LARRY: Yes, they were actually.

JENNIFER: No, but she came over when she was 17.

LARRY: They left in 1939, on the last ship over, so I wondered that myself.

JENNIFER: Yeah.

JIM FRAMO: Oh, I see. How about her mother? Is her mother still alive?

JENNIFER: Oh, no.

JIM FRAMO: Did she keep in contact with her mother?

JENNIFER: Very, very minimally.

JIM FRAMO: Did she have any other relatives, aunts, uncles, anybody?

JENNIFER: Not a close family at all, a small family, not close.

LARRY: Her aunt, grandmother's sister . . .

JENNIFER: Katie, you mean? Yeah, but she was already dead.

LARRY: Yeah. She committed suicide.

JIM FRAMO: Who? Your mother's aunt?

JENNIFER: Yeah.

JIM FRAMO: Has your mother ever talked about her family at all?

JENNIFER: Hardly at all. She doesn't like to talk about them.

JIM FRAMO: Is that a closed subject that we have to stay away from?

JENNIFER: It's a delicate, very, very delicate area.

JIM FRAMO: So, in other words, only if she wants to volunteer.

JENNIFER: Right. I wouldn't push her to talk about anything because . . .

JIM FRAMO: You wouldn't push her to talk about anything?

JENNIFER: Right, she'll automatically get defensive and she'll start denying things.

JIM FRAMO: What are the safe subjects with Mom?

JENNIFER: (*Laughs*) There aren't too many.

LARRY: That's the problem with her family. All the discussion is superficial, usually boring.

JENNIFER: You could talk about my father's background. He loves that. With my mother you could talk about . . . uh . . .

JIM FRAMO: Holland? Would she have any memories of her homeland?

JENNIFER: No. (*Looks to Larry for suggestions*)

JIM FRAMO: I can't even tell her I was in Amsterdam once?

JENNIFER: You could tell her that.

JIM FRAMO: That I was in Leiden?

JENNIFER: That they would love.

LARRY: You could talk, I think, about what happened when they were growing up.

JIM FRAMO: What happened when who was growing up?

LARRY: Jennifer.

JENNIFER: (*Looking shocked and frightened*) With my mother? *No,* don't ever mention that!

LARRY: Like who was working, and how you did in school.

JIM FRAMO: Well, I understand that there was some question that you might have been somewhat abused as a small child. I take it that that's a subject that you would never want to bring up.

JENNIFER: Well, not on camera and tape. I just feel too uncomfortable about it. I mean, I feel like I don't have control over the situation and I don't like that.

JIM FRAMO: Suppose we were not on camera, and we were having a session without it being taped?

JENNIFER: It'd probably be easier, but still difficult.

JIM FRAMO: Would you be able to do it at all, ever? Under any circumstances?

JENNIFER: I hope so! That's why I'm in therapy right now. I'm working towards that. I mean that's one of the issues I want to resolve.

JIM FRAMO: I personally believe that at some point you have to work out some stuff with your parents. Because sometimes, you know, we have childhood perceptions that are distorted. Sometimes they're based on childhood memories, and when you can get the facts, you might get a different picture. Some things might have been going on in your mother's life that you didn't know about.

JENNIFER: I'm sure.

JIM FRAMO: And people usually end up, when they do this, with a much more sympathetic view of their parents.

JENNIFER: I do have that, too.

JIM FRAMO: Sure.

JENNIFER: There's another side of me that is extremely sympathetic and I feel sorry for both my mother and my father, especially my mother. There's a lot of anger, but there's also a lot of empathy and sympathy.

JIM FRAMO: Right. I hear you, but what I'm getting at, Jennifer, is that the piece of gold in this for you is that maybe if you work some stuff out with them directly, face to face, you won't have to go through life feeling that you have no right to existence. Instead you might feel that you're a person and you have a right to live and enjoy life.

JENNIFER: But is that contingent on working things out with my family or is that contingent on working things out with myself?

JIM FRAMO: With your therapist? (*Smiles*)

JENNIFER: Yeah.

JIM FRAMO: Well, my bias is to work it out with your family.

JENNIFER: Uh huh.

JIM FRAMO: It's painful, and it's difficult, but everybody I've known who's done it ends up saying, "You know what, it wasn't nearly as bad as I thought it was going to be." Anyway, during the session you can decide how much you want to risk.

JENNIFER: OK, as long as I'm given that control.

JIM FRAMO: Yes, you're in control. I won't push you beyond where you want to go.

JENNIFER: Uh huh.

JIM FRAMO: I'm just going to allow the opportunity for things to come out.

JENNIFER: OK, that's great. That's reasonable.

JIM FRAMO: We're going to see your family for the first hour and then we're going to take a break. Then we're going to have one more hour. Sometimes during the break things can happen. People often decide they might want to go a little step further.

JENNIFER: Or retreat.

JIM FRAMO: Yes.

LARRY: We have realized for a long time that this interaction with her family is necessary.

JENNIFER: Um hm.

LARRY: I think she would . . . although it's very frightening.

JENNIFER: It's terrifying.

JIM FRAMO: I was scared to death to do it with my family. I've done it with my own family. I would never ask anybody to do what I wouldn't do. But it's scary as hell to tell the truth to your parents.

LARRY: But I think it's worthwhile.

JIM FRAMO: You're going to do it too, Larry.

JENNIFER: He doesn't have as many ghosts in the closet as I do.

JIM FRAMO: Well, he's got some things. Don't forget that mother who was always hovering over him. (*They all laugh.*) Anyway, thank you very much. Larry, I really appreciate your contribution to this and I hope at some point you'll get a chance to watch the videotape of her family, as she will get a chance to watch a videotape of your family.

LARRY: I'd love to.

We cotherapists saw Jennifer and her mother, father, and sister for two hours, with a break between the two hours. As usual, the first hour was used to get acquainted. As expected, the family members all dealt with superficial external events, and avoided anything personal or revealing. In response to my question, "What was it like to grow up in this family?" Beth said her father was more structured and her mother more flexible. The mother (Suzanne) said her husband was strict and did not want the children to talk during meals. Father (Peter) indeed did speak freely of his background, saying that his own father spoke to his children twice a year. The mother thought she and Jennifer were more alike, and Beth said that she and Father were similar emotionally, but that she and her mother were close. (During the session Beth was very protective of her mother, not at all expressive of the hostility she had mentioned in her phone conversation with me the night before; See footnote 1.) The father repeatedly said to Jennifer, "We don't know what your problem is. You don't tell your mother and father what you think. I know something is on your mind."

Just at the point when Jennifer was about to tell her parents what she really thought, an electrical transformer in the room blew out and the room filled with smoke. It couldn't have been timed better. Larry, waiting outside, got the battery from his car to run the television apparatus. We took a break while the equipment was being repaired, then we saw the family for another hour, and they finally got down to work. And the truth, avoided for so long, began to be told.

Early in the second portion of the family session, the mother said she did not realize that Jennifer did not feel close to her, and she went on to talk about what a difficult child Jennifer had been. As a baby, she had been sick a lot and cried and screamed a great deal. Mary and I resonated with her statement about how difficult it is to raise children, and I said that a screaming baby can make you so upset and frustrated at times that you might feel like strangling the kid. What I was doing here was giving the mother permission to talk about any physical abuse she might have inflicted on Jennifer. Actually, the mother did say she spanked Jennifer a lot, so I asked Jennifer if she remembered being spanked as a child. Jennifer said she did, and added that she had been afraid of her mother. "I felt she did not want me around." The mother looked shocked. We speculated that the mother must have had a difficult life, which prompted the mother, against everyone's prediction, to talk about how she was raised in an institution in Amsterdam, where they were very strict. We encouraged her to talk about her deprivation.

I hypothesized that the hatred Jennifer felt toward her mother was related to her own self-derogation. I believed that when Jennifer could see her mother as a real human being and understand what her mother had had to struggle with, she could mitigate her ambivalence about her. As a function of a new and different, honest interchange between this mother and daughter, the tenacity of Jennifer's attachment to her negative introject of her mother might be loosened. The mother's listening and not collapsing or counterattacking could create a profound experience for the family. Then, when Jennifer could forgive her mother, she could forgive herself.

I have heard many adult children say in family of origin sessions that we should take their side, and almost invariably, they say later that they are grateful that we tried to explain the parents' behavior and that we did not join them in attacking or belittling the parents. Jennifer was not atypical in this regard. Later in the session there was an exchange in which it was clear that Jennifer felt that we were trying to justify her mother's cruelty to her and that we were siding with her mother. Nonetheless, at this point I took a chance and assumed that if we continued to refrain from criticizing the mother, inwardly Jennifer would be relieved. The worst mistake a therapist can make in family of origin sessions is to demean or denigrate parents. Nonetheless, had there been more time we would have given more recognition to Jennifer's painful memories of those early years.

When Jennifer began to open up with her hurt and anger, both parents tried to explain these feelings in terms of her jealousy of Beth. Her father kept saying, "I know there is something on your mind that is bothering you," and then rambled on so much that Jennifer attempted to stop him by protesting, "You ask me, but you don't give me a chance to talk." The father kept asking, "Are you jealous of Beth?" Here is a short interchange from the transcript:

JENNIFER: No, it's not jealousy of Beth, it's anger at Mom, for always going with her.

MOTHER: Like when Beth and I used to go shopping? Well, you were seven then.

JENNIFER: Uh huh, I was a little kid.

MOTHER: Beth was more advanced with everything, so we used to go shopping and do different things.

JIM FRAMO: I once asked Jennifer, "Do you have any pleasant memories of you and Mom?" And she said, "After Beth left, my mother and I would go shopping together."

MOTHER: Isn't that something! (*Smiles*)

JIM FRAMO: She remembers that very pleasantly.

JENNIFER: Because I don't remember us doing anything together before that. It was as if as soon as I appeared on the scene, Beth became my mother and you became pals with Beth, and you walked off with her. And I took care of Dad. (*Laughs*)

SISTER: And I felt displaced. I had been close to my father prior to Jennifer's birth, and my earliest recollections involve memories of my father that were affectionate and warm. I remember a lot of very young, very early interactions, more with my father than with my mother. Jennifer was born and was a difficult baby and suddenly I felt a sense of wanting to parent her and be stroked by my mother for being very responsible and very much the first-born child. But at the same time I felt alienated from my father. I felt suddenly that my father had become very close to Jennifer. He and I had a fractured relationship at that point. And that's when my mother and I got very close. (*Framo notices an anguished expression on Jennifer's face.*)

JIM FRAMO: Beth, excuse me. I get a sense that you're . . . Jennifer, you're really struggling with something right now. What is it?

JENNIFER: No. I'm just feeling all these things over again.

JIM FRAMO: Yeah.

JENNIFER: You know, what my sister is saying is very true. It's just the feelings I'm getting from it.

JIM FRAMO: What are those feelings?

JENNIFER: I'm feeling sort of, you know, abandoned by my mother and sort of saddled with my father, in some kind of weird relationship. It was clearly undefined to me what our relationship was supposed to be because I slept with my father.

JIM FRAMO: Um hm.

JENNIFER: So I didn't know what my role was going to be or what I was supposed to do.

JIM FRAMO: But age six is pretty young.

JENNIFER: Yeah, but still, I mean I was a confused child . . . I guess. I didn't know . . .

JIM FRAMO: You thought your mom turned you over to your father?

JENNIFER: Yeah. It was almost like, OK, she turned me over to my father and she went with my sister. I mean, she went shopping with her and did things with her.

MOTHER: Jennifer, I . . .

JENNIFER: Well, you two did everything together.

MOTHER: But there was nothing together. Beth was in school all of the time, she had so many friends. I mean, I hardly had anything. . . . You were in first, second grade when we moved, and I was not with Beth at all. It was always you and I, always. See, I can't even . . . uh . . . isn't that funny?

FATHER: Bring it out now, Jennifer, because we are all together.

MARY FRAMO: Can I make a suggestion? Let these gal's work it out, it's their problem.

At one point, we began dealing with the relationship between Jennifer and her sister, not only because it felt safer to Jennifer, but also because I was using Beth as a transitional route to the mother. Here is an excerpt from the transcript of the interchange between the sisters.

JIM FRAMO: One of the things I noticed, Jennifer, is that when you were dealing with your parents a few moments ago it was very difficult for you and you kept looking to Beth for support.

JENNIFER: Uh huh.

JIM FRAMO: Like it's safer.

JENNIFER: It probably is.

JIM FRAMO: The barriers that exist between you and Beth . . . how could they be broken down?

FATHER: I was always trying to get them closer together, to understand each other a little more because it hurts us.

JIM FRAMO: See, I'm wondering what gets in the way. Is it the past? Is it that she had Mom at one point and you felt you didn't?

JENNIFER: I'm sure that there are multiple factors. I mean not just one thing. I think we were both very competitive, won't you agree, Beth?

SISTER: Yeah.

JENNIFER: In terms of wanting to be on top, wanting to be the most noticed, wanting to be, you know . . .

SISTER: (*To Jennifer*) I'll probably oversimplify it, but if I could sum it up in terms of our adolescence—our respective adolescences, because we were light-years apart—I would say that I was the bad girl and you were the good girl. I was more overtly rebellious and defiant, and I was going to do it my way no matter what. I think you tried very hard to be perfect, very hard to please.

JENNIFER: Uh huh.

SISTER: I remember thinking at some point in my life that I could never be perfect enough so I would give up on being perfect and just do it my way. If anybody liked it that was OK, and if they didn't like it that was OK too. I was just going to do it my way, because I could never be as quote, unquote "good" as you. You were very good.

JENNIFER: Uh huh.

JIM FRAMO: So you were the good kid.

JENNIFER: (*Laughs*) At least on the surface.

JIM FRAMO: Well, maybe you figured, "I'd better be good."

JENNIFER: Uh huh, I think so.

FATHER: In kindergarten, already she had beautiful handwriting. Beautiful pictures she'd draw for us.

JIM FRAMO: Are you two competing these days?

JENNIFER: Subconsciously, maybe.

SISTER: I don't feel any sense of competitiveness towards you.

JIM FRAMO: How *do* you feel towards her these days? Now?

SISTER: I feel we have closeness when we get into periods of communication, that the communication is very rich and very meaningful, and I feel like I really know Jennifer. But I feel a sense of frustration because we have these moments when we're very close, and then suddenly there's a big block of time when we don't communicate with each other.

JIM FRAMO: During that period are you angry at each other? The period in which you don't communicate?

SISTER: I don't feel a sense of anger, I feel a sense of . . .

JIM FRAMO: Distance?

SISTER: Distance, because . . .

JIM FRAMO: Do you (To Jennifer) feel anger?

JENNIFER: (To Beth) Sometimes I feel like you're mad at me for something, rather than I'm mad at you.

JIM FRAMO: Do you ever check it out and ask her, "I get the sense that you're angry with me, am I right or not?"

JENNIFER: Well, it could be that I'm really angry and it's safer to have somebody angry at me. (Laughter)

SISTER: What do you think you might be angry at me about? Because I'm not angry at you.

JENNIFER: I don't know . . . I'm not really sure what it is.

Following this interchange the two sisters spoke of their being workaholics. Beth works seven days a week and Jennifer starts at 6:00 in the morning and works until 10:00 at night. They said that their relationship is superficial, that they are both so busy, and that Beth hates to talk on the phone; finally, Beth said that she is so busy she finds it hard to "block in" time for Jennifer. All of this suggests that the distancing between the sisters is related to the remoteness between the parents and children, or perhaps between the parents themselves in this disengaged family. (There is probably a connection between these family of origin dynamics and the closeness–distance conflict Jennifer has with Larry.)

In the next part of the interview we got the sisters to truly meet and touch. One could see the accumulated anguish and dramatic relief in both sisters as they hugged, cried, and comforted each other. Their embrace induced the parents to cry. It took thirty years for the emotions and unhappiness in this family to be expressed; they required the right conditions for release. I asked Mother to hug Jennifer and she did so, awkwardly, partly because she was restricted by a microphone wire. We tried to build on this breakthrough for the future, but Father kept trying to make a patient out of Jennifer. Mother and Jennifer tried to work out their different perceptions, and Jennifer hung on a bit to her resentment, feeling that we did not pay enough attention to the depth of her pain and maltreatment. At the end, however, she recognized that the session was a beginning.

JIM FRAMO: Jennifer, does your sister ever come through for you at a time when you need her? And Beth, does she ever come through for you when you need her?

SISTER: I haven't expressed an "I need" feeling for quite a while.

JIM FRAMO: When there is a crisis in your life, you wouldn't call on Jennifer?

SISTER: No.

JIM FRAMO: And vice versa?

JENNIFER: Well, what happened when Larry's foot was amputated? How did you find out about his foot, through Mom?

SISTER: Yes.

JENNIFER: I mean, that was a time when I was angry at you, and it was my fault, in a sense, because I didn't tell you I needed you. But I remember you didn't call or anything and everybody else was calling and sending flowers and phoning.

JIM FRAMO: Why couldn't you get on the phone to Beth and say, "I need you"?

JENNIFER: Fear of being let down, maybe. I don't know.

JIM FRAMO: *(To Beth)* Would you turn her down?

SISTER: No, absolutely not.

JIM FRAMO: Well, tell her that. I think she needs to hear it.

SISTER: Jennifer, any time you need me I'm available for you.

JENNIFER: Same here. You came through for me this time [by coming to the session]. . . . *(Jennifer's voice breaks)*

SISTER: *(Smiling)* Well, as I said, I know you'd do it for me. I just know you love me like I love you. If you say, "I need this from you," there's absolutely no debate about that. It's "Yes. How, when, and where." *(Beth looks to Framo)*

JIM FRAMO: *(To Beth)* Go over and hug her. *(Beth rises and walks directly to Jennifer and embraces her. Both stand up. Jennifer sobs deeply as she clings to Beth for several minutes. The following verbal exchanges occur during the embrace. They are barely audible.)*

SISTER: I'm here for you.

JENNIFER: Same here, Beth.

SISTER: How are you feeling?

JENNIFER: *(Tentatively)* OK.

SISTER: Sad?

JENNIFER: Well, yeah. *(pause)* How are you feeling?

SISTER: Close.

JENNIFER: That's good. (*The sisters look at each other's faces but keep holding each other.*) You're not crying, so I feel silly.

SISTER: Silly's a judgment. You're just feeling very intense feelings. It's been a long day today. (*She brushes Jennifer's hair away from her teary face. The two end the embrace. Jennifer and both her parents are crying.*)

JIM FRAMO: I have only one handkerchief.

JENNIFER: Rip it in half.

JIM FRAMO: I noticed your dad was crying.

MARY FRAMO: Mom too.

JIM FRAMO: . . . and [your] Mom. Mom, could you do the same thing? (*Jennifer and Mother embrace, both struggling with tears.*) I wish I had more handkerchiefs. (*The crying continues for a while.*) I think that this has been long overdue in this family. How much harder it is to state positive feelings than negative ones. They're always so much more embarrassing. (*To Mother*) Suzanne, before this meeting I was told that you would be very difficult to deal with and that if you heard something that you didn't like, that you would walk out of the room. I heard that you were very defensive, but I haven't noticed that about you at all.

MOTHER: No, I wouldn't say that I'm difficult. But I don't like to be exposed too much. I was always a more private person.

JIM FRAMO: I know. But I thought that I wouldn't be able to talk with you.

MARY FRAMO: I found you very easy to relate to, also. We met before the session[4] and there was no strain at all.

MOTHER: I enjoyed that.

MARY FRAMO: I can understand your need for privacy. Who wants to open up and spill their guts out and stuff like that? But this meeting is not quite like that. It's more dealing with relationships.

MOTHER: That's true, but I never was a complainer or talker.

JIM FRAMO: Well, what do you think can happen between you and Jennifer from now on? The past is the past.

MOTHER: That's right.

JIM FRAMO: It's over.

MOTHER: That's right.

JIM FRAMO: But you've got today. What can it be like from now on?

---

[4]*Editor's note:* While Jim Framo was interviewing the couple, Mary Framo waited with Jennifer's family in another room.

MOTHER: Well, I think we both can work better now that we know.

JIM FRAMO: Um hum. I think she [Jennifer] still has a lot on her mind.

MOTHER: Yeah, yeah.

JIM FRAMO: And I think there are still some things she wants to tell you, but not here. At another time, when you're alone perhaps.

MOTHER: Yes. That's right.

JIM FRAMO: If you could listen, and if Dad could listen instead of going off on his tangents . . . We fathers have trouble listening. We give speeches. I think Jennifer, and perhaps Beth too, have a lot on their minds that they haven't said. I strongly advise that at some point you [Jennifer] sit down with your mom in a safe setting and you talk. Clear up all those old misunderstandings. A lot of them are misunderstandings, in my judgment.

MOTHER: I really think so, yes.

JENNIFER: I think you're negating the feelings.

JIM FRAMO: I'm not negating them. I know they're very real to you. You have a lot of anger and a lot of hurt.

MARY FRAMO: I think what would be helpful . . . some of the things you were saying were true. Mother did the best she could in the only way she knew how at the time. This does not invalidate anything you said. It's saying that this is the perspective from the other side and some reasons for it. Look at it as if you could put her shoes on for a short time and see it from her point of view. She had to pull herself up by her bootstraps. She never had a model. I don't know your mother well enough to know all that she had to deal with.

JIM FRAMO: I have this sense of what Jennifer's struggling with right now. Correct me if I'm wrong, Jennifer, you feel that somehow or other we seem to be too supportive of Mom and are excusing her when you've got all those angry, negative feelings. You feel as if we're not recognizing those feelings enough, especially your sense of devastation when you were younger.

JENNIFER: I think so . . . yeah . . . that's very true.

JIM FRAMO: You are experiencing that?

JENNIFER: Yeah. And I think that what you're doing is justifying what happened.

JIM FRAMO: Justifying?

MARY FRAMO: Not justifying, but trying to explain, maybe.

MOTHER: But Jennifer, didn't you used to exaggerate things and always magnify them when you talked to me? I mean you blew it up more.

JENNIFER: I don't think so. It's just me . . . that's something that you never accepted. That's just how *I* feel. Maybe to you it's an overreaction because you don't feel that way.

MOTHER: No, not this one. I mean all the other things you used to exaggerate so.

JENNIFER: Well, I think that I exaggerated a lot of things because I was displacing a lot of my feelings onto something else. Like if a dog died, I'd go into mourning for five months. Remember that time? It's probably because I was going into mourning, maybe for a lost childhood or something like that.

FATHER: Well, don't consider the dog. It's just an animal.

JENNIFER: Dad, just listen to what I said. I said it's displaced feeling.

JIM FRAMO: You were an unhappy kid. You felt you never had a childhood and you felt unwanted, like you were extra baggage in that family.

JENNIFER: Uh huh, yup. (*Jennifer fights to hold back tears.*)

JIM FRAMO: And what you've heard today doesn't take it away.

JENNIFER: No, it doesn't take it away, but it probably helps.

JIM FRAMO: Does it help explain it? That your mom . . .

JENNIFER: It helps explain it . . . yeah.

JIM FRAMO: That your mom's difficulty in relating to you really, basically, didn't have much to do with you. She had no model.

JENNIFER: Well . . . I understand that.

JIM FRAMO: But if you really understood it, Jennifer, you would get to the point where you would say to yourself, "I'm OK . . ."

JENNIFER: Yes, I think it takes time.

JIM FRAMO: ". . . there's no basic deficiency in me. It isn't that I was just a rotten kid." (*Pause*) That will take time.

SISTER: You don't have to prove anything any more.

JIM FRAMO: And you don't have to be perfect, and you don't have to say, "I apologize for living." And you don't have to give in to Larry, or anybody else you're related to because you always feel like you're in the wrong.

In the following segment Jennifer and her mother continued to try to work out an understanding of each other. Father's participation in the session appeared disruptive to Jennifer rather than helpful. It is unfortunate that Mary and I did not have the time to understand what he was trying to say. We could sense that he meant well.

FATHER: I think we had a happy life. Is that right or wrong? (*asking Suzanne*) You can tell. Maybe I'm lying. . . . (*Smiles*)

MOTHER: We're still together, right?

FATHER: Well, yeah.

JIM FRAMO: Peter, you were crying before, when you saw your two daughters hugging each other. What did that mean to you?

FATHER: Well . . . (*He begins to cry again*) Well, because it seems like there was a strange feeling between them. It hurt me and my wife that they didn't act close like two sisters who understood each other. But, I think Jennifer had something on her mind, a quality, bothering her, that never came out . . . but she'll stay with us for three or four days and then we can talk and get some of that stuff out that she's got in her. Because I know she's got some certain problems buried in her mind that bother her.

JIM FRAMO: You always knew that?

FATHER: I feel that. I felt that.

JIM FRAMO: (*To Mother*) Did you feel that, or were you shocked and surprised by what you heard today?

MOTHER: No, I felt there was a certain distance.

JIM FRAMO: Uh huh.

MOTHER: I felt that she was fighting more and more to stay away and I had thought I was very close to Jennifer.

JIM FRAMO: Uh huh.

MOTHER: I got letters when she was in college in the beginning and everything was very close. I knew everything and she would always write and call. But all of a sudden it stopped.

JIM FRAMO: Did you know she was harboring all these resentments toward you?

MOTHER: No. I felt like there was more and more distance. She was fighting something to get away, and the more she was getting away the more miserable she got.

JIM FRAMO: You thought it was her relationship with Larry that . . . did it [made her distance herself]?

MOTHER: It seemed that way to me, yes.

JIM FRAMO: But it wasn't. The feelings she had, she had long before she met Larry.

MOTHER: But she was very close to me before she met Larry.

JENNIFER: On a superficial level, perhaps.

MOTHER: Yeah, but see, that I didn't know. She was very close . . . but later . . .

JENNIFER: I used to be a good daughter.

MOTHER: I took everything . . . it was very difficult.

JIM FRAMO: Well, I'll tell you, this is more *real*. It's painful, but it's more real. Neither one of you has to play a game anymore. You, Jennifer, don't have to play the "perfect" role. You, Mom, might find that uncomfortable for a while when she starts telling you the truth.

MOTHER: That's right.

JIM FRAMO: (*To Mother*) But that's the way it's going to have to be. It will be a more real relationship. It's more risky . . .

MOTHER: Yeah.

JIM FRAMO: . . . and it's more painful, but at least you're not acting and she won't have to act.

MOTHER: That's right.

MARY FRAMO: Also, it's better to get it out than to not see each other and to be distant.

MOTHER: That's true.

MARY FRAMO: Jennifer will no longer have to say, "The best way I can handle my mother is by not seeing her," because a lot of people do that. They say, "My mother and father are the way I see them." That's too painful for parents; it really is. It's better that she should say whatever she's feeling. At least you have her there. And you can deal with her. You have something solid there.

MOTHER: And open, yeah.

JENNIFER: (*To Mother*) It was always hard for me to get angry at you, because I always felt that no matter what I said you would turn it around. My feelings weren't my feelings any more, and so I felt like I never had any feelings.

JIM FRAMO: Do you think she will listen more now?

JENNIFER: Uh huh.

JIM FRAMO: Is she hearing you today?

MOTHER: I think so, yes.

FATHER: Whatever your problem is, Jennifer, please let us know . . . we can . . . we can understand very much.

JENNIFER: You have to understand it's not just my problem, OK?

FATHER: Well, the only way we can understand . . .

JENNIFER: In the last five minutes, you just blamed me for my lack of relationship with Beth. Again, I'm the scapegoat of the family (*laughs*).

JIM FRAMO: Well, a couple of times you were a little angry at Beth. Was that right?

JENNIFER: Yeah, I thought she was angry at me.

FATHER: I really didn't know what it was because you didn't tell me.

JENNIFER: Sometimes I wasn't angry at her. I just didn't feel close to her. I didn't feel like I could talk to her about certain things.

FATHER: Well, sometimes you can't . . . you both . . . we were very proud of you. You were great in school and were model students, right or wrong . . .

JIM FRAMO: Peter, Peter . . .

FATHER: You accomplished quite a lot.

JIM FRAMO: Peter, excuse me, we only have a couple of minutes.

FATHER: OK.

JIM FRAMO: Jennifer, what do you feel, how do you feel overall about what happened today?

JENNIFER: I don't know. I think it's a good . . .

JIM FRAMO: Is it a beginning?

JENNIFER: It's a beginning, yes.

JIM FRAMO: It's not the end. It's the beginning. It's not even the middle.

JENNIFER: It's scratching the surface.

JIM FRAMO: Right.

MOTHER: Right.

JENNIFER: That's about it.

JIM FRAMO: All right. Can you continue some of this on your own?

JENNIFER: I think so.

JIM FRAMO: I hope so.

MOTHER: I think so.

JIM FRAMO: Because I just started the ball rolling here. I just got it started.

JENNIFER: That's the hardest part.

JIM FRAMO: Yes. How do you feel overall about what happened today (*to Mother*)?

MOTHER: Well, I'm glad that I heard everything.

JIM FRAMO: But it wasn't easy to hear, was it?

MOTHER: No, it was not. No.

JIM FRAMO: Peter, how do you feel?

FATHER: Well, I was glad that these things started off, because it bothered me and my wife that . . . maybe more me because maybe I'm more sensitive than my wife is. That there's something blocking Jennifer's mind. There's something that bothers her and therefore we try to help you straighten her out.

JENNIFER: You're off to a very bad start, Dad.

FATHER: Huh?

JENNIFER: It's *my* problem again.

FATHER: No, no, that's . . . Jennifer . . . I . . .

JENNIFER: You had no role in any of this, right? (*She fights tears.*) I'm like this because of some cosmic force in the universe.

FATHER: Well, we try to help you, Jennifer, if we can. It's just a matter of telling us what the problem is.

JIM FRAMO: See, Jennifer, he can only understand it the way he can see it right now, at this point.

Following this conference I received from Jennifer the following two letters. The first one was a copy of a letter her mother had sent to Jennifer, and the second was from Jennifer to Mary and me.

Monday, January 23, 1983
11:00 P.M.

Dear Jennifer:

It was so nice to talk to you on the phone. You don't know how much you were on my mind day and night. Oh, how much I cried, but it was more of a relief cry. I can't explain. Something opened up and I think the same was for you. It felt like my deep inner feelings came to the surface. Deep down in my heart I *always* felt very close to you and somewhere we both closed up and built a wall. I'm really honestly happy. I thank God that you had the courage and showed me how to open up and deal with my hurt feelings, from childhood. I know we have a lot to talk about, and you will understand much better and so will I. With Dad you have to realize his age and then he said he was also kind of upset. He never dealt with inner feelings like we did; he was always more open and blunt. I hope Larry didn't mind my misunderstanding; it shows how quick we come to a wrong conclusion, by not feeling open and honest. It's so much easier to blame the other. Good luck with your papers and you will be happy when February 15 is here. Hopefully you can relax then. Write when you can. Our love to Larry. Take care, with love,

Mom & Dad

January 31, 1983

Dear Jim and Mary:

I want to thank you for all your help in establishing some form of communication between the members of my family again. It was *largely* through your patience, kindness, understanding, and *empathy* (I can't stress how important that is) that the two of you were able to break through some rather difficult and seemingly impervious barriers which evolved over the last 25 years or so when Beth and I were growing up. This might have never happened without your gentle encouragement, sincerity, and strong conviction that the experience would undoubtedly be a very positive one.

I must admit that I was so *terrified* that I actually thought I was going to faint just prior to the "interview" with my family. I thought that all my *fears regarding the past* would be realized during this re-enactment of the past (i.e., that I would tell my parents how I really felt and that they would interpret my feelings or pass them off as though they didn't matter and I had no right having them in the first place; and in the process, I would feel like the vulnerable, powerless, troublesome five-year-old all over again, who was always in the way. Some of those old feelings did indeed come up along with many others (anger, frustration, etc.), but the feelings which *dominated and prevailed* were those of sympathy for my mother and her own difficult plight. Forgiveness will hopefully come once a lot of my anger is reconciled. In addition, I felt much *freer* with my feelings *in general*, as though I had finally acquired a "license" to have these feelings (especially with Larry).

I called my mother the next day (after the session); we both cried and were so much more open with one another than before. (Larry actually thought that I was talking to one of my close girlfriends in N.Y.C. and couldn't believe my mother was on the other end.) She expressed how very happy she was for this much needed, much overdue, cathartic experience. I feel that at least my mother and I have a *beginning* for establishing a relationship. I enclose a copy of a letter she recently wrote to me which evoked so much emotion that I'd like very much to share it with you.

I was disappointed with my sister, however, as I thought that she was denying or mollifying a lot of the anger she so *strongly* voiced *so many times* to me towards my parents. Also for anger she felt towards me for having to mother me when she herself was only a little child and for having been my "father's favorite." My mother, father, and I were all crying, and Beth looked so calm, detached, and unaffected by this great emotional release. I can't help but wonder if she ever really allowed herself to feel. I feel somewhat sad for her now, even though during the "interview" I was hurt and confused by her unexpected reaction and lack of support. Before the interview, she appeared quite anxious to give a full rendition of her "traumatic childhood." I suspect that some of the anxiety she expressed to you regarding my "mother's psychotic reaction" (i.e., her running out of the room) may have been a projection of her own anxiety stemming from certain *unresolved conflicts in her past?!?* But perhaps with time, honesty, along with serious commitment and a willingness to trust on *both* our parts, we will hopefully be able to work something out.

> With deep appreciation and fondness,
> Jennifer

(Card enclosed said, "'And you shall know the truth and the truth shall make you free.' – Somewhere in the Bible.")

I responded to Jennifer's letter with the following note:

Dear Jennifer:

Thank you for sharing with me and Mary your thoughts about the sessions and also what has happened since then. I'm not only glad you had the courage to do it, but hope the gains will accrue as time goes by. I was curious, by the way, about your reaction to the presentation at the conference. I do believe you are not the same person you were before starting the whole venture. Furthermore, who knows, some day you and your family may want another session.

Please give my regards to Larry and I wish you the best.

> Warmly,
> James L. Framo

In my intergenerational book (Framo, 1991), I have spelled out in much detail the method of family of origin consultation that was approximated in this brief intervention. In that book I have included a section entitled "Difficulties, Limitations, Pitfalls, and Contraindications" of this inter-generational method. I have called family of origin work the major surgery of psychotherapy, and, as in major surgery, there can be side effects. The family is the place where, as Carl Whitaker (1989) put it, there are "life and death voltages," and those who deal with the vital issues that they had with parents and siblings run the risk of re-arousing old, primitive terrors of engulfment, abandonment, obliteration, and being unwanted. The fears, as illustrated by Jennifer, can become intense as they deal with loaded topics and anticipate rejection and invalidation. Some people do not experience these intense fears and use the family of origin sessions as an opportunity to reconnect with parents and siblings, to explore new ways of relating. For them the consultation is a liberating experience. But a certain proportion of clients are very anxious and fearful; why should they go ahead and have these sessions anyway? The major reason is that the basic, positive changes which can ensue are worth the risks and pain. Changes in several areas are possible: the intrapsychic level (raising of self-worth, lessening of narcissism); changes in the couple relationship (reduction in closeness–distance conflicts and control issues; less use of projective identification); and changes in the family of origin itself (more openness and trust among family members—neither fused nor alienated). Those people who have been unable to make a commitment to an intimate relationship are usually better able to do so once they have reordered their deep, inner commitment to their family of origin.

However, this potent method, which shakes the roots of the family, requires certain conditions of preparation and follow-up that the format of this conference did not include. If I had seen Jennifer and Larry conjointly in my own private practice I would not only have worked with their marital issues, but would have spent many sessions preparing them for the family of origin sessions. In addition, following the family of origin sessions I would have continued the therapy so that the experiences of those sessions could have been integrated with the individual and marital problems. Unfortunately, the format of the four interventions did not include a provision for follow-up sessions by the four interviewers.

Some of my regular clients have gone into individual therapy with me or someone else following the family of origin sessions. The success of this further therapy by a different therapist usually depends on the orientation of the individual therapist. If that therapist is a systems therapist then the gains of the family of origin sessions can be consolidated or the information from the sessions can be tied in with the internal conflicts. On the other hand, some therapists' orientation is to ignore, discount, or even denigrate family of origin sessions. Still other individual therapists regard their task as saving their clients from their "crazy" families and they may even discourage their clients from having any contact with family members. I have conducted family of origin sessions for clients who are in ongoing therapy with individual therapists who are systems-oriented; the clients are returned to the therapists following the consultation. These therapists report that the length of psychotherapy with these clients is shortened considerably, because the clients have had the opportunity to reconcile the inner images of their parents with the present-day realities.

In sum, I do believe that the intergenerational encounter can serve as a significant resource for meaningful change in the individual, marital, and family systems. These goals are best accomplished by adequate preparation and follow-up with therapy that is systems-oriented, on either an individual or a family basis. The family of origin sessions themselves, which are not without risk or pain, are but the beginning of a process that will continue throughout the life cycle of each individual and family.

REFERENCES

Dicks, H.V. (1967). *Marital tensions.* New York: Basic Books.

Fairbairn, W.R.D. (1954). *An object-relations theory of the personality.* New York: Basic Books.

Fogarty, T. (1979). The distancer and the pursuer. *The Family, 7,* 11–16.

Framo, J.L. (1970). Symptoms from a family transactional viewpoint. In N.W. Ackerman (Ed.), *Family therapy in transition.* Boston: Little, Brown.

Framo, J.L. (1976). Family of origin as a therapeutic resource for adults in marital and family therapy: You can and should go home again. *Family Process, 15,* 193–210.

Framo, J.L. (1982). *Explorations in marital and family therapy: Selected papers of James L. Framo.* New York: Springer.

Framo, J.L. (1991). *Family of origin consultations: An intergenerational approach.* New York: Brunner/Mazel.

Framo, J.L., Weber, T.T., & Levine, F.B. (in press). *Coming home again: A full length family of origin consultation.* New York: Basic Books.

Guntrip, H. (1952). A study of Fairbairn's theory of schizoid reactions. *British Journal of Medical Psychology, 25,* 86–103.

Napier, A. (1978). The rejection–intrusion pattern: A central family dynamic. *Journal of Marriage and Family Counseling, 4,* 5–12.

Whitaker, C.A. (1989). *Midnight musings of a family therapist.* New York: Norton.

5

Enhancing Empathy in Couples:
A Transgenerational Approach

NORMAN L. PAUL with BETTY BYFIELD PAUL

Success in couple therapy depends upon the development of a quality between the partners that I call "empathy." Perhaps because this phenomenon defies precise description, it has been relegated to the realms of poetry and the theatre, and infrequently finds its way into the scientific literature. Harry Stack Sullivan wrote about the reluctance of professionals to deal with this fundamental aspect of human experience (1953, pp. 41–42):

> I have had a good deal of trouble at times with people of a certain type of educational history; since they cannot refer empathy to vision, hearing, or some other special sense receptor, and since they do not know whether it is transmitted by ether waves or air waves or what not, they find it hard to accept the idea of empathy . . . although empathy may sound mysterious, remember that there is so much that sounds mysterious in the universe, only you have got used to it; and perhaps you will get used to empathy.

Despite its ineffability, it is crucial that therapists explore and assess empathy because of its vital importance in human experience and development (see Givelber, Chapter 9, this volume). It is, in short, what is *right* about human relationships when they are healthy, and what we must strive to engender in clients when something is painfully *wrong* in their relationships. In the clinical literature, much is written about pathology, about what goes wrong. In this chapter I begin with a consideration of what can be right in a couple's relationship; then I hypothesize about what obstacles typically present themselves and discuss ways in which I help couples to remove those obstacles. Finally, I illustrate my theoretical approach and techniques using material from the session I conducted with Larry and Jennifer.

EMPATHIC CONNECTIONS

Empathy is, in essence, a nonverbal, interpersonal phenomenon (Katz, 1963; Paul, 1967, 1970, 1975, 1980; Stewart, 1954, 1955). Although it resists linguistic capture by precise definition, it can be distinguished from sympathy, as Charles Aring does in the following succinct passage (1958, p. 448):

> The act or capacity of entering into or sharing the feelings of another is known as sympathy. Empathy, on the other hand, is not only an identification of sorts, but also connotes an awareness of one's separateness from the observed. One of the most difficult tasks put upon mankind is reflective commitment to another's problems while maintaining his/her identity.

Any human relationship, even that between strangers, can be characterized by the presence or absence of empathy. My particular interest as a therapist is in the empathic connection that unites a healthy, loving couple and in the relation of that connection to its principal forerunner and starting point, the empathic connections between the individual partners and their parents.

The need for such connection does not cease in childhood. In fact, when older parents share their own developmental experiences with their adult children, the children gain a rich perspective on the process of development. Empathy, expressed in this way, enriches children's lives and reinforces their self-esteem. They receive comfort from the notion that certain challenges and changes are common to all human beings; they see that they are not unique in their struggles and feelings of inadequacy. A strong experience of empathy with one's parents creates a potential for empathy (marital or otherwise) in one's own adult relationships.

The forgotten pasts of parents too often become invisible burdens for their children and grandchildren (see also Framo, Chapter 4, and J. Grunebaum, Chapter 10, this volume). In my work with couples I take a transgenerational approach, helping couples to discover and understand their parents' pasts as they relate to their own current burdens. I hypothesize that clients have been deprived of access to some critical elements of their parents' lives, elements that have helped shape the behavior and personality of the parents *as their children (now adults) experience them*. I must emphasize here that what clients need access to is not an objective or comprehensive rendering of the family's history, but an *empathic connection to their parents' life experience*. To borrow a term from the historian R. G. Collingwood (1956, p. 238), clients need to venture into the "inside" of their family history, experiencing it as it was experienced by the parents.[1] They need to appreciate their parents' existential dilemmas, as well as their own, relating to vulnerability, loss, and isolation (Yalom, 1980).

Sympathy often masquerades as empathy. In order for an empathic connection with the parents' experience to be helpful to clients, the connection must be truly empathic, not sympathetic. The client cannot pass off all responsibility for emotional engagement to the parent (or the therapist) by distancing himself or herself through sympathy. The client must take charge of his or her own self-understanding and growth by making a real connection with a feeling state from the lives of his or her parents, and realizing how it operates in his or her own behavior patterns. The therapist can, however, coach clients through their own educational processes. This is what I do in my transgenerational work with adults and their families of origin. I believe that this work has a reverberating impact beyond the family members in the session, as it promotes the self-understanding required for subsequent empathic connections to spouses and children.

OBSTACLES TO EMPATHY: TWO PARADOXES

> Man will become better only when you make him
> see what he is like.
> —ANTON CHEKHOV

> The past is never dead; it is not even past.
> —WILLIAM FAULKNER

Human beings are ambulatory paradoxes. Two aspects of our paradoxical natures account in part for our empathic deficiencies. One paradox is that we are awake to everyone else, but not to ourselves. The other is

---

[1]In *The Idea of History*, R. G. Collingwood presents a dynamic and revitalized account of the role of the historian. He states that in any investigation of the past, the historian is obliged to discriminate between the "outside" and the "inside" of an event. The outside refers to everything observable about bodies and their movements. The inside refers to the presumed thought of individuals. He elaborates, suggesting that the historian imagine himself or herself as Caesar or Plato. The historian thus discovers the thoughts of the persons under study by "rethinking them in his own mind." For example, when Collingwood reads Plato, he imagines himself writing Plato's works. "The history of thought, and therefore of all history," he writes, "is the reenactment of past thoughts in the historian's own mind" (p. 215). (See also Chasin & Roth, Chapter 7, this volume.)

that we experience ourselves as separate entities living in the present and creating a future from the present, but we cannot see how we are connected to others in the past.

With regard to the first paradox, we commonly acknowledge two aspects of experience: *our inner experience,* consisting of our judgments, perceptions, and feelings, and *our outer experience of others*—how they appear to us. Yet we rarely consider how we appear to them or how they experience us. We see one another, but not ourselves. This creates a serious obstacle to empathy, as each partner in a couple is blind to a major aspect of the other's experience. Each knows his or her inner self and the outer self of the other, but not his or her own *observable self,* the one that the partner lives with, fights with, talks to, and tries to love. Without knowledge of one's own observable self, it is impossible to understand the partner's experience of the relationship on which his or her concerns and judgments are based. Because we are constructed without an organ system permitting us to observe the self as it is observed by others, denial and projection of fantasies and feelings become our primary mechanisms for constructing our self-images.[2]

This brings us to the second paradox. We experience ourselves as separate physical and mental entities, engaged in autonomous activities and developing on our own unique paths, physically, emotionally, and socially. This *apparent separateness* contrasts sharply with our *invisible connectedness* to others from whom we have unconsciously created interiorized images, which profoundly influence our style of relating and acting and are projected by us onto others. We don't notice these images of others in our heads, yet they play a powerful role in our lives; we perceive our current relationships through a lens shaped by earlier experiences, particularly by experiences with our families of origin.

GENERAL APPROACH TO COUPLE THERAPY

My approach and techniques differ markedly from those of therapists who conduct individual therapy. What the client says about past and present relationships is the only truth available to both client and

---

[2]A related problem is that our memory is limited under the best of circumstances. As Harold Pinter (1964) wrote, "Apart from any other consideration, we are faced with the immense difficulty, if not the impossibility, of verifying the past. I don't mean merely years ago, but yesterday, this morning. What took place, what was the nature of what took place, what happened? If one can speak of the difficulty of knowing what in fact took place yesterday, one can, I think, treat the present in the same way. What's happening now? We won't know until tomorrow or in six months time, and we won't know then, we'll have forgotten, or our imagination will have attributed quite false characteristics to today. A moment is sucked away and distorted, often even at the time of its birth." (p. 31)

therapist in individual therapy. In my approach, multiple truths are available from which all participants can construct closer approximations to reality. Previously hidden sources of anger and hurt are brought to the light of day, where their power to distort the present can be diminished. New relationships emerge, based upon an empathic understanding of old injuries and current needs. Both partners in the couple can then bring to the relationship a new understanding of their own observable selves, of their own unconscious desires to repeat or work through their past relationships in their current relationship, and of their partner's inner self as it has been shaped by the past. Past needs, frustration, and anger can then be seen as belonging to the past. The numbness that has resulted from unexpressed anger and grief and from projected feelings and compulsive behaviors is thawed, and empathy can emerge.

The approach that I take with couples is educational and experiential. I provide the couple with a laboratory for learning about the many untested assumptions they have made about themselves and their relationship. I create an environment, with couples and with their families of origin, in which clients can first apprehend and then close the credibility gap between their interiorized images and projections on the one hand, and the way things are and what really happened on the other.

My approach is transgenerational in that I don't see in the couple merely a set of relational patterns between two individuals in the here and now. Rather, I see a set of relational patterns with connections reaching deeply into the past and profoundly shaping the future. For me, transgenerational couple therapy involves the progressive discovery of the sources of each partner's identity formation and fragmentation, and the elucidation of how the presenting relational dysfunction is derived from the family of origin. Finally, it seeks to unlock the hidden hurts and vulnerabilities that serve to freeze the empathic capabilities of one or both partners.

TECHNIQUES FOR CORRECTIVE INTERVENTION

To accomplish these goals, I typically see couples with their families of origin; I utilize audiotape and videotape feedback procedures; and at times I play evocative "enabling tapes" to break through the numbness that so often presents itself as a symptom of unacknowledged self-ignorance. Each of these three aspects of my work is touched upon in the following description of a typical couple session, then further illustrated with the case of Larry and Jennifer.

My usual format is to begin by meeting with the couple. Then couple sessions are alternated with individual sessions with each partner. After an average of two to six months, each partner is seen with members of his or her family of origin. A condensed one-session version of this method was used with Larry and Jennifer and Larry's family of origin. Jim and Mary Framo's interview with Jennifer and her parents and sister (see Chapter 4) represents another kind of family of origin meeting.

To set the stage for the first interview with both partners (sometimes I will see one partner alone if the other partner will not come in), I ask that the couple begin their educational process by preparing some background information. I send each partner a comprehensive question-naire and instructions for completing a three-generation genogram, and ask that they bring these completed materials to the first session. Thus, even before the first session, each partner is invited to become an active participant in his or her own decoding process and to consider family events and behaviors that may be relevant to the present dilemma. The partners often begin to imagine themselves as potential conduits be-tween the past generation and that which is to come.

After the couple is greeted, they are led to my office, which resembles a small television broadcast studio, equipped with video recorders, video camera, audiotape recorders, and microphones. The couple is assured that although the setting obviously looks strange, every piece of equipment they see is designed to provide feedback data for their educational experience. Then I briefly describe the difficulties of knowing one's observable self, adding that in this office, one has the opportunity to become aware of a credibility gap that is characteristic of every human being. Here, the term "credibility gap" refers to the discrepancy between one's inner self-image, including one's presenta-tion and style of posture and speech, and the "observable self" that one does not have access to in the usual course of life. I underline the notion that human beings generally don't like to know how little they know about themselves. I add that, in my experience, the anxiety about the technical equipment is generally short-lived, lasting not more than three to five minutes. Clients and colleagues who have seen my work can testify to the fact that consciousness of the equipment quickly recedes as clients become engaged in the novel process of seeing themselves as they appear to others. Perhaps this represents a paradox of the modern human condition: that the capabilities of high technology can be put so effectively to the service of developing empathic connections.

The couple hands in their questionnaires, genograms, and the blank audiotapes I have requested that they bring for recording the session. While each partner describes the nature of the problem, my mind pursues several tracks. As I listen to the specific complaint, I note with particular interest the remembered time of onset, and I scan the family trees to note whether within one year prior to the development of symptoms there had been a critical loss or an anniversary of a loss (Becker, 1973; Paul, 1975, 1986). I note the timing of earlier losses and closely watch the reactions of each partner as I shift focus from the symptom to the subject of loss. The video camera focuses on each person alternately. I underscore the importance of listening; more often than not, I videotape the listener rather than the speaker.

Taping for Playback

The videotape playback technique helps both partners to become "experts" about themselves through observing their own denial mechanisms and projections, and to see how they allow themselves to be provoked by the other, and in turn how they provoke the other. Videotaped recordings of parts of sessions are also useful for playback to other family members. For example, sessions with a couple may be shown, with permission, to their children or to their parents. Often this showing is best done without the original clients present. Sometimes in a session with a couple, playing back the videotape without sound has an even more penetrating and indelible impact than playing it back with sound, as in the following example.

A couple in their late 40s were referred by the wife's divorce lawyer. They had four grown children. The wife, Alice, had suffered from chronic depression, with an array of physical complaints, for over 22 years. Alice had undergone individual psychotherapy and a three-year course of psychoanalysis, with no resolution of her marital distress. She was unable to induce her husband, an eminent corporate attorney, to become affectionate or to participate in domestic activities. Her recourse for her dissatisfaction was to seek a divorce attorney, a classmate of her husband's, at a competing law firm. Reluctantly, Jack came along for the first time with Alice, who was having her third session with me. Jack's self-image as a husband and father was a most glowing one— including his conviction that he was a most loving and considerate person, and that Alice was incapable of appreciating his (obvious to himself) generous nature. The conversation with them was videotaped. When it was played back later in this first joint session, with the verbal exchanges included, Jack appeared smugly bemused by the procedure. When I replayed the same segment without sound, Jack appeared agitated, and suddenly blurted out, "He looked like 'old stone face'! How could she have lived with me all these years?" Jack, who acted as though he were there alone, was directed to ask Alice that question. She responded with surprise, "With great difficulty!" It was only at that point that Jack experienced the discrepancy between his benevolent inner self-image and that which confronted Alice—now seen by him for the first time. A new ballgame could then begin.

The technique of videotape playback provides clients with new data about their observable selves and thereby promotes an empathic understanding of the partner's experience in the relationship. By contrast, in more traditional therapy, the therapist tries to gain greater and greater access to the inner self or "soul" of the individual—an emphasis that can lead to varying degrees of client dependency or addiction to the therapist/expert, an addiction from which neither client nor therapist can easily escape.

I also make audiotapes of sessions so that the couple can review sessions at home. During the course of ongoing therapy the couple is asked to review audiotapes between sessions, to reinforce the idea that the therapy is a collaborative endeavor between the therapist and the couple, and to minimize expectations that the therapist can magically transform them. When therapy terminates, I suggest to clients that they periodically review the audiotapes to foster an ongoing educational attitude toward their relationship and to thwart regression. In the last session, I play the videotape of the first session (without audio) on a split screen with a recent tape. The contrast is usually quite striking. When asked to guess when the old tape was made, clients often place it much further back into their pasts, indicating that they see themselves as quite distant from their old styles of expression and interaction.

Enabling Tapes

In my first session with a couple, as I listen to them describe their dilemmas and as I scan their genograms, I consider how I can enable each partner to connect with his or her unknown and inaccessible emotions. A basic principle guiding my work is that the sources of their anger and hate are concealed experiences of hurt, fear, terror, and pain. It follows that if a client experiences and then shares such basic hurt, pain, and terror, then his or her current hatred can be defused and empathy generated.

I use an enabling tape, either audio or video, with the couple and/or the family of origin, to sanction and evoke suppressed emotional experiences. Each tape presents a vivid sample of a universal human experience of emotional pain, such as aborted grief, despair in the face of invalidating behaviors by a spouse or parent, or terror at the prospect of a family encounter. The tape serves to transcend the use of words, which too often obscure important feelings of vulnerability. Clients are encouraged to scan their own experience banks to empathize with and then match the experience portrayed by the tape. They are assured that any response is normal, and that the tape is used to enable them to tune in to their own forgotten unpleasant—though important—experiences. The evoked recollections can then be shared with the other family members present. Reactions to the enabling tape are routinely videotaped for later playback. The playback validates that emotional release occurred, and thereby challenges the rigidity of the denial pattern and related numbness.

The Case of Larry and Jennifer

In my interviews with Larry, Jennifer, and Larry's parents, I followed my usual procedure, but in a condensed form. First, I met with the couple. After talking with them for about 45 minutes, I showed them a 10-minute playback of a portion of our session. Then we talked for another 15 minutes. After that I met with Larry and his parents for about 45 minutes, showed them a 10-minute enabling tape, and then talked with them for another 15 minutes. Then Jennifer joined Larry and his parents to watch a playback of the family session and to discuss their reactions. Finally, I spent about 30 minutes with the couple alone.

Because the interviews were conducted for a public purpose, however, it was inappropriate to focus on Larry's and Jennifer's individual sexual histories or their own sexual relationship over the years, especially the changes that occurred subsequent to the amputation of Larry's foot. The need to avoid the sexual realm was understandable but unfortunate, in my view, as even in uncomplicated circumstances a couple's sexual life is generally not given adequate attention by couple therapists.

An early portion of the interview with Larry and Jennifer demonstrated clearly that an oscillation in dependency had occurred about five years prior, at the time of Larry's surgery. I asked Larry about the changes at that time. I wanted to know about his inner experience, but I also wanted him to speculate about the impact his "observable self" had on Jennifer.

PAUL: I'm trying to find out a couple of things. One, what was going on in you, Larry? And secondly, what was going on from Jennifer's point of view, in terms of your relationship?

LARRY: That was a midpoint in the last 10 years. It was five years ago. I mean that's just one point in our relationship.

PAUL: Well, she says it was a critical point.

LARRY: It was one of the critical points. There are a lot of critical points in a relationship between two people that lasts for 10 years. That certainly was a large one.

PAUL: Yeah.

LARRY: I think there was probably a changeover in both our personalities at that point.

PAUL: To what? From what?

LARRY: In some sense in our relationship. When we started I think that she was the one who required more of the help, and after five years, I was sort of the one who required more of the help. We switched roles in that respect.

PAUL: When you say "help," what do you mean?

LARRY: Help in dealing with things in general. With the things that come up in life.

Earlier, I had asked Jennifer about Larry's reaction to his amputation.

JENNIFER: I was alarmed by his coolness, I mean, it seemed unusual, unnatural, very bizarre that he was so cool. He seemed very stoic about the whole thing, very self-sufficient, and extremely unaffected by something this traumatic. It seemed very strange to me. I didn't know quite how to react to it. I made a few attempts to get something out of him.

PAUL: Like what?

JENNIFER: Like what he was feeling. And usually he would just be very irritated that I would even try to probe and try to get something from him.

PAUL: He felt you were intruding?

JENNIFER: (Sighing) Well, I felt that he felt that I was intruding.

LARRY: Well, I guess the opinion that I have of this, how I handle something like this, is you have to do it for yourself first. I mean, she wasn't around every minute of the day, and my parents weren't around. I was the one who had to get up on the crutches and take one step, and then with the prosthesis—painful as it was—take the other step. No one is going to take my foot and move it for me.

PAUL: That's true.

LARRY: So the theory I had at the time was to get through this first step on my own, because in the end it's the only way it can be lasting.

PAUL: Right.

LARRY: If you depend on someone else for your happiness or support, and if that someone else is not there for some reason or other, then you are back where you started. So I felt that I had to pick myself up by the bootstraps first, then I'd be able to interact with others.

PAUL: And that's what happened? He would then interact and let you know what he experienced, or he didn't?

JENNIFER: It seemed like he really didn't. I mean I didn't feel it.

PAUL: Well, it's important what you feel.

LARRY: Yeah.

JENNIFER: I mean, he might have felt that, but then again the message maybe wasn't communicated to me.

Larry, like most of us, is subject to varying degrees of denial and numbness, yet can present plausible rationalizations for the inability to experience and share pain. I have yet to hear anyone acknowledge at first blush that he or she may have been "numbed out" for some period of time. When I met with Larry and his parents, Al and Evelyn, I decided to pursue the theme of numbness with Larry's parents, Al and Evelyn. I asked Larry about his father's family. I could have asked his father directly, but then I would have known only one person's perspective about the family. I sought each person's point of view. Additionally, I wanted to see whether Larry had the sort of knowledge and understanding of his father's family that would enable him to make an empathic connection to his father.

PAUL: What do you know about your father's background, about his family? How would you describe them?

LARRY: I know more about some of his family than others, for a variety of reasons.

PAUL: Go ahead.

LARRY: Both his parents were dead by the time I was born. And I have never seen some of his brothers and sisters.

PAUL: Do they live in the New York area?

LARRY: They used to. A number have died.

PAUL: Yeah?

LARRY: Of those I haven't seen, some live in New York and some don't.

PAUL: Yeah?

LARRY: And that's essentially it.

PAUL: From your point of view, what are the factors that accounted for the remoteness between you and his family?

LARRY: Just between my parents and his family. I mean, it had nothing to do with me.

PAUL: OK, between your parents and his family. Why did that arise?

PAUL: Yeah.

LARRY: Well, I think they're just very different people.

PAUL: In what sense?

LARRY: Their . . . I don't know, their opinions about things.

PAUL: Give me an example.

LARRY: I know so little about them, it's hard to say, but obviously they are not the kind of people that my parents would want to interact with.

PAUL: What would you say, Al, about your family?

AL: My parents . . . you have to keep in mind I'm the youngest and my family are old, most of them are very old people.

PAUL: Yeah.

AL: I am close with one of my brothers who lives in the city, and I'm sure that Lawrence has seen him pretty often. He's one of the few that he does see pretty often. The others he doesn't. I have one other brother here in the city, but I don't bother with him too much— neither one of us does, even though he's only three years older than I am.

PAUL: Why is that?

AL: We had some kind of problem between us that was really minor, but he's very self-centered, he thinks of himself.

Al presented himself as disconnected from his large family of origin, a state of affairs that Larry seemed to accept as a simple fact of life requiring no explanation. Larry's mother's family, in contrast, was seen as close and expressive. I gathered this from reading the couple's case report (Chapter 2). I wanted to hear about Al's experience of loss, but I began by asking Evelyn about hers, expecting that she would have less difficulty exploring this realm of experience. I asked her about the death of her mother.

PAUL: How did you take your mother's death? Do you remember?

EVELYN: I think very badly.

PAUL: What did she die of?

EVELYN: Leukemia. She died within six weeks.

PAUL: She did?

EVELYN: Yeah, she had polycythemia for about 10 years. As a matter of fact, she was used as a guinea pig at New York Hospital, because at that time they didn't know much about it. Not every doctor could diagnose it. It was an old European disease at the time.

PAUL: Um hm.

EVELYN: She used to go every month to the hospital, but one month she didn't go because my sister had given birth.

PAUL: Oh yeah?

EVELYN: And the next month she went and they discovered leukemia and within six weeks she was dead. She had acute blood leukemia.

PAUL: And this was within six weeks?

EVELYN: After they diagnosed it.

PAUL: Did she know she was dying?

EVELYN: I think so.

PAUL: Did you ever talk to her about that or did she talk to you?

EVELYN: No, but I remember one time while riding in the car to go to my uncle's house—I don't know why this stays in my memory—she said, "Make sure I'm dead when you bury me." (*Evelyn laughs*).

PAUL: Make sure I'm dead?

EVELYN: Yeah, "I don't want to be buried alive," or something to that effect. But this was before they diagnosed her as having leukemia.

At this point, I tried to direct Evelyn to describe her experience of the loss of her mother. She told me about her last visit to see her mother at the hospital, but with some reserve. Such reserve was not what one might expect from this jovial, talkative, self-described "Jewish mother."

PAUL: Was she in the hospital when she died?

EVELYN: Yes.

PAUL: Were you there with her when she died?

EVELYN: No. What happened was, we used to get there every day at 2:00. This was up in Manhattan, because my sister had a little baby and my cousin used to come over and watch the baby, but this time the baby was sick and we were delayed about 10 or 15 minutes.

PAUL: I see.

EVELYN: When we got there, it was about ten after two and she had died at 2:00. The nurses and doctors were waiting outside because they knew we would come, and she had just passed away 10 minutes before. And we had come to tell her that my brother's wife had had a baby two hours prior. He was my mother's favorite, my brother and his wife. I said to the doctor, "We came to tell her that Sammy's wife just had a baby." And the doctor said, "Well, don't you think she knew? That's why she hung on this long." She knew and then she went.

PAUL: Do you remember how you felt when you were told that she was dead?

EVELYN: Oh yeah. Well, then we were let into her room and we were all there, my other two sisters and myself.

PAUL: Do you remember what thoughts you had? Was she laid out on the bed?

EVELYN: Yeah, she was still in the bed.

PAUL: And as you were looking at her, what was your experience inside? Do you remember?

EVELYN: I remember kissing her finger.

PAUL: You do?

EVELYN: Yeah. We were all crying, hysterical, sad, of course, sad.

PAUL: Yeah, any other thoughts occur to you?

EVELYN: I don't remember. What are you trying to . . .

PAUL: I just want to know if you recall the experience of the event.

EVELYN: Yeah, I recall . . . I recall it vividly. But I remember we were let into the room and we saw her. We were all crying. My sister had to be taken out of the room. I kissed her finger. And we were all crying.

PAUL: Was it an open casket when she was buried?

EVELYN: No, no.

PAUL: Do you remember how Al took that event?

EVELYN: As he does everything.

PAUL: Which is?

EVELYN: Very calmly, you know.

PAUL: Yeah.

EVELYN: You know he doesn't show his emotions very . . .

PAUL: Do you remember, Al, how you took it?

AL: Yeah, I was saddened because I was very close to her mother and father.

PAUL: Were you reminded of your own mother?

When I asked Al this question, I hoped that his experience of listening to his wife describe her loss (albeit without abundant emotion) would have had a facilitating effect on his own expressions of feelings of loss. This was too much to hope for; apparently, Al's response to loss was to become numb. His answer to my question demonstrated his strong preference for attending to the lighter side of life:

AL: Well, they were two different kinds of people. Actually, the two mothers were somewhat similar because they both always cared about the family and they liked to make a lot of food and have the family eat there. My mother was just like hers in that way, but primarily, they were two different types.[3] Her mother enjoyed card games, which my mother did. She [Al's mother] liked dances and enjoyed music. She [Evelyn's mother] was somewhat like that too. There was one instance I remember, my wife told me about it, I wasn't there at the time, but I really got hysterical about it. Her mother was listening to the radio and she was making noises like a sheep. My wife came running into the house. Even the neighbor thought she [his wife's mother] was sick, and her mother was doing an impersonation because someone on the radio had said, "How do you make a noise like a sheep or a cow?" and she was making the noise. My mother was somewhat like that. She tried to be very happy and jokey, so I did like her mother and father very much.

EVELYN: My mother was like an amateur actress and she liked to go places and do things and she liked to play games. We all do that, too.

PAUL: Um hm.

---

[3]Notice that Al says that the two mothers are different from one another, but then describes only the shared upbeat characteristics of both.

EVELYN: My father was a card player and everybody . . . we liked the good times.

Clearly, Evelyn and Al sought out the "good times" at the expense of experiencing a full range of emotions. Al's attraction to Evelyn's "happy and jokey" family was understandable, given his own difficult childhood. The acting ability he admired in his mother-in-law probably seemed to him to be a valuable life skill. In fact, over the years the ability to put on an act seemed to have served him as a primary means of coping with adversity and pain; he seemed to have forgotten how to feel pain. When I inquired about his mother's death, Al told me that she had been diagnosed with cancer of the pancreas "too late." She died at home only weeks later. I asked him if he cried when he heard the news that she had died.

AL: I guess inwardly I did. Like my wife said, I'm not very emotional. Internally I am, but not externally. You don't usually see it on me. (*Larry's mother nods.*) It does work on me inside.

PAUL: It does?

AL: Yeah.

PAUL: Was there ever a time when you were able to show emotion externally? (*Evelyn immediately shakes her head with an expression of certainty and sadness.*)

AL: Not before people.

PAUL: Never in your whole life? (*Evelyn continues shaking her head.*)

AL: Not that I remember.

PAUL: Do you remember your father's death?

AL: I was four years old. That's the only thing I do remember.

PAUL: What?

AL: We lived in a two-family house and we had an apartment below us. I remember I was playing and I heard my father coughing. And then I saw a lot of commotion. My mother ran in and screamed, "Get the doctor!" and I remember that they called the doctor. That's all I remember. I know that they took him away and someone told me that he died. But I was never that close to my father. I didn't know him. I really didn't know him.

PAUL: Not that you remember.

AL: I don't remember.

PAUL: Did you dream of him afterwards? Do you remember?

AL: Well I'd dream of him every once in a while, but only because of a picture. I didn't even remember him. It's a face. My sister had a picture of him. She showed me the picture. Then I was able to picture him. That's all. I never really remember him as a person.

It seemed to me that Larry's denial of postoperative distress paralleled his father Al's general denial of personal anguish. Denial abetted by numbness seemed to be operating powerfully in the relationships of both father and son. During the interview with Larry and his parents, I played an enabling tape that presents the powerfully evocative experience of a father of three, Jeff, who is catapulted back in memory to an incident of intense fear and loneliness in a hospital corridor when, at eight years of age, he learned of his mother's death from cancer. The explosive catharsis that follows usually stimulates the listener to recall and recount a similar experience of early and intense unshared grief. My hypothesis was that Al's inability to recall any living images of his father was an expression of his rage at his father (Larry's grandfather) for dying when he was four. Al, fatherless himself, then became a numbed father who was both there and not there. Al responded sympathetically to Jeff's lostness and distress about his mother's death; however, his own denial and numbness remained largely impenetrable, a strong model for Larry, who unwittingly behaves in a similar manner.

PAUL: What do you think about in reference to this [enabling tape] here, Evelyn?

EVELYN: Well, I think that it's my husband that can't show his emotions. He portrayed [is like] the man [on the tape, Jeff]. He felt ashamed to show any emotion.

PAUL: Hurt.

EVELYN: Hurt. Yeah. To show any hurt. He thought it's a shame.

PAUL: You can show hurt?

EVELYN: Oh yeah. I show all kinds of emotions. (*Larry smiles slightly.*)

PAUL: You do?

EVELYN: Oh yeah.

PAUL: And?

EVELYN: You see, he's . . .

AL: (*At the same time*) I was a little confused.

EVELYN: Just let me say this, he's at this level (*gesturing to show a great difference in emotionality between herself and her husband*). I'm this way.

PAUL: OK.

AL: I was confused in the beginning. I was under the impression that the reason why he [Jeff] wasn't comfortable in the office was that he was a farmer. We owned a farm when I was a child. My father and mother owned a farm up in Albany.

PAUL: Oh, really?

AL: Yeah. I guess I always liked the outside. Spaces. I like big openings, big spaces. As a matter of fact, even when we got our home, we made sure we were unattached. We didn't want our house to be attached, no way, to any other home. We had a nice back yard so we could sit outside. That's the impression I was given, that he [Jeff] wasn't comfortable in an enclosure where he couldn't see out and see the trees or grass. I mean, he was a farmer. But then as I was listening, I began to realize what had happened. I have to agree that what was happening was that he was picturing how he felt that day when his mother was dying. He was sitting in the hall and those things that he saw affected him. He felt no one loved him, like his father was only thinking of the mother and no one thought of him. He felt like he was lost. He had no one to fall back on. I feel that's why he got so upset and threw up, because he felt there was no love there. At that time his father couldn't give him the love.

PAUL: Does it remind you of anything? Any pictures come to mind of your own experience?

AL: Well, we never really had that much. My mother always looked at me as the favorite. As a matter of fact, they always used to call me the baby in the family—because I was the youngest in the family. My mother never showed that much favoritism. She liked us all. I mean, she treated us as children.

PAUL: Any piece of the experience of your father's death come to mind hearing this?

AL: No. I knew my father very little.

PAUL: Do you know where he's buried?

AL: Yeah, sure, we visit. We go to see his stone. He's buried in the next town from me, actually.

PAUL: Where's that?

AL: He's in Beth Abraham Cemetery. Oh, I'm sorry. He's in the old cemetery . . . my mother's in Beth Abraham.

PAUL: When you moved, you lived on a farm near Albany?

AL: When I was a child I lived there.

PAUL: Until when?

AL: I lived there in the summers.

PAUL: I see.

AL: When school was out, we lived there. I lived there until I was almost seven or eight years old.

PAUL: And would you do things with your dad, there on the farm?

AL: I didn't know my father.

PAUL: Well, you knew him up until he died.

AL: I don't remember.

PAUL: You don't remember.

AL: I really don't. I don't remember anything about my father, except the day he died.

EVELYN: I . . .

PAUL: Go ahead.

EVELYN: I think that his feelings were always suppressed because he was the youngest and all the others overcame him. He was the baby. He was like the forgotten child, and then when his mother remarried she married a man that I call a male counterpart of Cinderella's wicked stepmother. He was the wicked stepfather. Al had to do his homework out the window [on the fire escape] because his stepfather wouldn't let him put on the light, and I feel that he couldn't express his feelings at that time.

PAUL: Yeah.

EVELYN: I just feel that he was very suppressed because of that. He had a mean stepfather.

During most of the interview, Larry's mother was expressive and caring, particularly when relating to or talking about others, especially Larry. She described Larry's illness as "the big traumatic experience of our lives." Al agreed. Larry said, not in this interview, but in the follow-up interview (see Chapter 18), that he was not surprised that his mother would say this, but that "it never occurred to me that [it] was the worst thing that happened to him [Al]." In Larry's mind, family emotions and expressiveness resided fully and exclusively in his mother; it was her department, not his father's. What surprised Larry most during this interview was that his mother too had pockets of numbness. These became apparent in the interview when she dealt with her own disappointed or bitter feelings, which she attempted to avoid or discussed in a flat, repressed way.

After seeing the videotape playback of this interview, Jennifer was able to empathize somewhat with Larry's parents and recognize that Larry, by some curious, unconscious osmotic process, had acquired habits of denial and numbness from both of his parents. She also affirmed for herself that she was not responsible for Larry's inability to have or to express his own feelings of vulnerability. She no longer felt obliged to "read Larry's mind."

JENNIFER: I noticed a lot of things that I didn't notice before. A few things were new.

PAUL: Like what?

JENNIFER: Like I didn't know about Larry's father's mother and how she died. I knew it was very sad, or suspected it was, but I didn't know the whole story, and that was very moving and very sad for me to hear. I can empathize and I can imagine what it felt like.

PAUL: For him?

JENNIFER: For him. Also seeing Larry's reaction when his father spoke about his mother's death was very interesting.

PAUL: What did you see?

JENNIFER: It was sort of typical of what he does when we talk about something very emotionally provocative. He blinks his eyes a lot and looks annoyed. He looks very irritated, like he wants to get it over with. He doesn't want to deal with it for too long.

PAUL: Is that what you're seeing here now?

JENNIFER: Yup, he has that look, sort of looking into outer space, like "When is this going to be over?" or "I don't want to deal with this," or "Why do we have to talk about this?" He has that same look in other situations when we talk about something sad, or emotionally very moving. He has that same expression.

PAUL: How does that affect you?

JENNIFER: It makes me feel sort of bad because I feel like he's putting up a wall between us, or between himself and his own feelings. He's not allowing himself to feel. I feel sad, in a way, that he can't or doesn't want to allow himself to feel. I also feel frustrated because so often I feel impotent in terms of getting him to feel certain things.

PAUL: Do you feel it's your job to get him to feel?

JENNIFER: A lot less now than I used to.

After Larry watched the videotape playback, he was able to see similarities between himself and his father.

LARRY: Well, as I said, I'm glad my parents were able to come. I think it's always good to exchange more information. I heard a few stories from my father that I hadn't heard before.

PAUL: Which ones?

LARRY: When his mother was dying. I always realized that I was like my father, but maybe the similarity is more that I had realized.

JENNIFER: You always thought that you were more like your mother?

LARRY: Well, I think I'm more like my mother in nonpersonal interactions, with people I see every day. I was always the life of the party. I always had lots of friends and I still do. In that sense I'm more like my mother, in my interactions with others. My interactions with Jennifer probably put me closer to my father.

PAUL: Mm hmm.

JENNIFER: It's interesting. I learned something today. I think your mother, though, when she's confronted with something very personal, is not that open, contrary to what I thought before. So you might be like her in that respect too. I mean she can be friendly, and overtly emotional to people she doesn't know that well, but when you ask her something about *her* past, like her mother's death, she becomes very quiet and reluctant to talk about it and to feel it, actually.

At this point Larry seemed to acknowledge that, as Jennifer observed, neither of his parents had provided models of emotional openness and vulnerability. His initial reaction to this realization was somewhat defensive, but openness gradually emerged, particularly when I challenged him to seek fun and joy, not just "comfort" in his relationship with Jennifer.

LARRY: Well, what are you trying to optimize? Happiness and contentment in your life? What else is really important? If I am less "emotional," quote, unquote, and I think that I am, I have learned to deal with life in a way that could be better for me. I could have evolved this way for a reason.

PAUL: Yeah . . .

LARRY: Then again, I could have gone down the wrong trail. I mean, maybe I could have been happier if I were more emotional, externally. So you have to make the argument that . . .

PAUL: The problem is, in a marriage or something that approximates a marriage, which is what you two have, how do you make it work so that you both feel not only comfortable, but that it's fun and joyful to be together? It's a challenge.

LARRY: Well, that's right. The point I was trying to get at is what's optimal for me, individually, might not be optimal for us as a couple. (*Jennifer nods. She appears pained, near tears.*)

PAUL: Right.

LARRY: But it could be that the compromises we both make won't affect us individually very much, and could make our relationship better.

PAUL: That depends whether the compromises are such that one is willing to make them out of choice rather than feeling compelled by the other's nagging. (*Jennifer nods.*)

LARRY: That's right.

JENNIFER: That's an important point.

PAUL: That's critical.

LARRY: So I have to be convinced that it's worth changing what I've evolved as some mechanism for going through life in order to make our relationship better.

PAUL: Yeah.

LARRY: And, you know, I'm getting convinced of that.

After some discussion of the decision to enter couple therapy, Jennifer asked about Larry's emerging willingness to change.

JENNIFER: Who are you doing it for is the question. For you, me, or for us?

LARRY: (*Quietly, to Jennifer*) All three.

JENNIFER: (*Sighs and laughs*) OK.

PAUL: Who's number one?

LARRY: (*Pause*) They're all equal.

PAUL: No. (*Laughing*) That's a weaseling kind of answer.

LARRY: I think for both of us. I mean, for me I'm number one and for her she has to be number one.

PAUL: That's right.

LARRY: That's right.

PAUL: You've got to do it for yourself, because if you're doing it for the other guy, or for the relationship principally, over time it can't work. (*Larry nods.*)

JENNIFER: That's right.

In this single session, Larry's empathic connection to his parents allowed him to gain insight into his own numbness and the limitations it put on his relationship with Jennifer. He saw his father's numbness with fresh eyes, and recognized for the first time that his affable mother was in fact quite unexpressive of emotion in her closest relationships. Thus one aspect of Larry's credibility gap was closed. Both Larry and Jennifer developed a heightened awareness of the invisible connections that Larry had to his parents and the ways in which his interiorized images appeared in his relationship with Jennifer, with whom he reacted much like his emotionally suppressed parents. This freed Jennifer to take a less blaming stance toward Larry. She recognized that he did not invent his numbness to push her away; in fact, it had little to do with her. Jennifer also realized that Larry must decide for himself how much he was willing to change. If he were to change for her or even "for the relationship," the change would not be lasting.

REFERENCES

Aring, C. (1958). Sympathy and empathy. *Journal of the American Medical Association, 167,* 448–452.

Becker, E. (1973). *The denial of death.* New York: Free Press.

Collingwood, R.G. (1956). *The idea of history.* New York: Oxford University Press.

Katz, R. (1963). *Empathy.* London: Free Press.

Paul, N.L. (1967). The use of empathy in the resolution of grief. *Perspectives in Biology and Medicine, 11*(1), 153–169.

Paul, N.L. (1970). Parental empathy. In E.J. Anthony & T. Benedek (Eds.), *Parenthood.* Boston: Little, Brown.

Paul, N.L. (1975). The role of mourning and empathy in conjoint marital therapy. In G. H. Zuk & I. Boszormenyi-Nagy (Eds.), *Family therapy and disturbed families.* Palo Alto, CA: Science and Behavior Books.

Paul, N.L. (1980). Now and the past: Transgenerational analysis. *International Journal of Family Psychiatry, 1*(2), 235–248.

Paul, N.L. (1986). The paradoxical nature of the grief experience. *Contemporary Family Therapy, 8*(1), 5–19.

Pinter, H. (1964). Writing for the theatre. *Evergreen Review,* Winter, *8,* 30–32.

Stewart, D. (1954). The psychogenesis of empathy. *Psychoanalytic Review, 41,* 216–228

Stewart, D. (1955). Empathy: Common ground of ethics and personality. *Psychoanalytic Review, 42,* 131–141.

Sullivan, H.S. (1953). *The interpersonal theory of psychiatry.* New York: Norton.

Yalom, I. D. (1980). *Existential psychotherapy.* New York: Basic Books.

6

Systemic Blueprints in a Therapeutic Conversation

CARLOS E. SLUZKI

Conducting therapy with couples entails more complex dilemmas and difficulties for the therapist than a similar undertaking with larger families. There may be good reasons for this counterintuitive observation. In our culture, couples hold standards for their relationship that are difficult, if not impossible, to achieve. For example, they hold to a romantic ideal of fusion—"we two are one"—while at the same time striving toward another deeply ingrained American ideal, that of fulfilling one's individual destiny. They enter marriage with the words " 'til death do us part" in a society with a divorce rate of over 40%. To further complicate the matter, couples' expectations regarding their abilities and wishes to nurture each other and the social roles they play in relation to each other (who does what for whom) vary dramatically throughout life, *while the binding agreement does not.* The explicit as well as the implicit letter of the marital contract is immutable rather than revised on an ongoing, pragmatic basis. Given such a rigid contract, it is not surprising that individual changes are dreaded as a threat to the relationship, and that any attempt at differentiation, or even the proposal of bartering *different* reciprocal goods, is somehow experienced as a betrayal of the original agreement. Ultimately, couples cannot help but fall short of expectations, and partners perceive themselves—or each other—as failures when the unavoidable vicissitudes of life highlight the gap between myths carved in stone and the actual flow of reality.

The oppressive load of these unstated (and often contradictory) cultural expectations and the added weight of everyday life struggles are often experienced in isolation from extended family networks, given the present trend toward geographic mobility and intergenerational distancing. The frequent lack of social support, family or otherwise, increases the tendency of partners to expect their mates to be available and capable of serving as catch-all resources. Thus, it is not infrequent that members of a couple dump on each other their frustrations and dissatisfactions with other things in life, and then bemoan the other's inability to solve what they themselves were unable to solve. This leads to complaints that are perceived by members as unfair and by therapists as unoperationalizable and therefore clinically slippery.

When, for whatever reason, a separation is considered by one of the partners, couples find themselves in another complex quagmire: Social mores tend to stigmatize the partner who wants out of the relationship. As a result, it happens quite frequently that the one who wants out wants the other also to want out, in order to spread the load of the "victimizer" label and gain some of the benefits of the "victim" position, including the sympathy and support of the shared network. Caught on this seesaw of desirable and undesirable positions, both partners frequently lock each other in a tug of war for the establishment and maintenance of alliances or coalitions with third parties, including the therapist. Due to their own ideological dilemmas surrounding these issues, some therapists find it difficult to avoid advocacy and to maintain a position of noncommitment, regardless of how crucial this neutrality may be to reestablish in the couple a sense of responsibility for their relationship.

When asked to describe their dilemmas, partners frequently engage in endless discussions that entail alternative punctuations of the sequence of events (e.g., "I withdraw because you nag" vs. "I nag because you withdraw"). Each member of the couple defines himself or herself as reacting to the other, and each perceives the other as starting the spiral of "games without end." (See Watzlawick, Weakland, & Fisch, 1974.)

In a clinical setting, patterns of interaction are more difficult to detect in couples than in a larger system. In a couple, codes and clues are usually subtle and rather idiosyncratic, and thus easily missed by third parties. From the observer's perspective—therapists included—pieces seem to be missing from the interactional chain. For instance, a member of the couple may read a subtle wrinkling of the forehead in his or her partner as a very important statement and respond to it with a slight lowering of the voice pitch. This, in turn, may trigger an outburst, which for the observer will seem totally unwarranted. The patterned nature of sequences is thus missed.

Concurrently, a structural representation of patterns is also more difficult to determine in couples than in larger systems. A dyad is a minimal system. And even a triad, such as a system constituted by the couple and the therapist, allows for a map with very few permutations. How many possible variations can we conceive in the structural map portrayed, for instance, by the sitting arrangements of the couple and the therapist in the consultation room? How many possible alternative coalitions, how many maps? In comparison, consider the number of potentially meaningful structural alternatives that can be displayed by the initial sitting arrangement of a family of five. Consider the information provided by the mere fact that the father and mother sit, for instance, with their offspring in between them, or flank the identified patient and place the rest of the children on the mother's or father's side. The data are extremely rich, precisely because of the great variety of alternatives. (It should also be noted that there are many possible interpretations for each alternative configuration.)

We may cry and moan that couples are difficult to work with, but we work with couples fairly frequently, and sometimes we succeed in dislodging symptom-maintaining patterns and introducing meaningful changes. Let us examine now the context and text of the interview that I conducted with Larry and Jennifer.

THE INTERVIEW

I was invited to participate in this conference as a representative of the line of thought known as the interactional view, an approach developed chiefly at the Mental Research Institute in Palo Alto. This view emphasizes the importance of detecting and ultimately disrupting interpersonal patterns that contribute to the maintenance of symptomatic/problematic behaviors.[1] By the time of the conference, I was also becoming interested in new ways of talking about therapeutic processes that center in the construction of alternative realities—constructions that differ from those anchoring symptomatic behavior. (See Chasin & Roth, Chapter 7, and Weingarten, Chapter 8, this volume.) In my consultation with this couple, as well as in my discussion about it, those two conceptual discourses, the interactional and the constructivist view, intertwine.

I interviewed Larry and Jennifer last in the sequence of the four interviewers. The interview took a total of one hour and 10 minutes. I was keenly aware that the whole process would be affected by the fact that I would only consult with this couple once, as one of several therapists, and would do it in a context defined as a teaching experience and not as therapy proper. Thus, from the very beginning, my goal was, at the most, to participate with them in a conversation that would offer

---

[1]It is beyond the scope of this chapter to discuss the interactional approach, a school that influenced the very development of the field of family therapy and had as early contributors authors of the magnitude of Don D. Jackson, Jay Haley, Virginia Satir, Paul Watzlawick, and John H. Weakland.

them some new views of their dilemmas and, at the least, to do no harm (which, in fact, may not differ much from my usual clinical goals).

I should add that I chose not to read the background information about the couple provided by the organizers of the conference. When I begin to work with couples or families, I prefer to start the first interview with very little prior information. I especially avoid information offered by previous providers, in order to reduce the chances of distorting my own perceptions/constructions with all the preconceptions embedded in material collected by other parties. A good illustration of the pros and cons of this policy appeared in the course of this interview. As readers will recall from the chapter on the history of the members of this couple, Larry has an artificial foot. In 1977, his foot was amputated due to a rare type of bone cancer. If I had read the couple's file before the interview, I doubt that I would have been able to consider that information as background, because dramatic information tends to float naturally to the foreground. I would have held this information as central, focusing attention on it and thereby *creating* an issue that the couple may themselves hold as old history. The medical information appeared quite late in the course of this interview, when, during a short technical break in the session, I noticed Larry's minor limp and asked him, "What's up with your foot?" He brought up the cancer in a matter-of-fact style, and we exchanged comments about the type of cancer it was, when it took place, and where he was on the curve of danger (the chances of survival increase exponentially with time). Finally, I explored the timing between the diagnosis of the ailment and the couple's moving in together. They informed me that they began living together several months before he experienced any kind of disturbance. I commented that the very basis of the relationship would have been very different if it had happened that they moved in together *because* of the amputation, or even *in spite* of it. They concurred with the observation, and the theme was dropped. Thus, this information, introduced late into the interview, retained a quality of social exchange and could be kept in the background.

A final comment before proceeding to the interview. What has been transcribed here is an edited version. Of the 70 minutes that the interview lasted, I have selected, for purposes of illustration, a sequence of fragments totaling half that time. I caution the reader to be on guard whenever this or any other edited tape or transcript is presented. Therapy sessions are a mixture of good moments and bad moments, of interesting fragments and dull fragments, of pearls and mud. The process of editing consists in extracting the pearls from the mud and organizing them into a string, in order to fulfill certain educational objectives. However, that artifact may create the illusion that the session (and ultimately the therapist) didn't have dull, flat, and uninspiring moments. That is seldom the case. (See Appendix, this volume.)

After greetings and pleasantries, the interview began.

SLUZKI: You've been doing a lot of work around this, for you and for us, and I want to start by telling you that I haven't read any material . . .

JENNIFER: Uh huh.

SLUZKI: . . . on purpose. Mainly because, in general, I don't obtain much information before a first interview. I get overloaded with information and I don't understand most of it. So, my ignorance should not be taken as a lack of interest or lack of respect for your previous work . . .

JENNIFER: Uh huh.

SLUZKI: . . . but to be consistent with my own order of things, yeah? So, I know very little about you. My first question would be, in addition to your contribution to *our* endeavor, what brought you to the consultation to start with?

JENNIFER: To the couples therapy?

SLUZKI: Yeah.

JENNIFER: Well, we were having problems in our relationship, and the nature of the problems revolved around a sort of lack of communication, an inability to interact with one another. I felt the need for more interaction and I was hoping that we would learn how to interact better. I felt that we had been living sort of parallel lifestyles in the sense that we weren't really interacting and communicating with one another. I felt like we had become just roommates, rather than partners or friends or comrades, or, you know, people that we could share our emotions with, that could actually exchange ideas and feelings with one another.

SLUZKI: Uh huh.

JENNIFER: I would say that that's probably the nuts and bolts of the real problem. We were hoping to see whether we could improve that.

SLUZKI: Uh huh. (*To Larry*) And what brought you . . .

LARRY: Well, I agreed that there was something that could be improved in our relationship and one of the things was why the interaction between us wasn't what Jennifer thought it should be, and what I thought it should be, and also how our long history together affected the interaction now, and to try and get a grip on how we can improve our relationship, possibly by understanding what went on in the past and what's happening in the present with some objective help.

SLUZKI: (*To Jennifer*) You were mentioning communication. What does it mean? What were you talking about?

JENNIFER: Well, when I say "communication," I mean an exchange of feelings and ideas and thoughts, you know, a sharing of these things. I mean exposing one's vulnerabilities and feeling that it's safe to do so. And my feeling is that if you can do that with somebody, you establish a closer relationship with that person.

SLUZKI: That makes sense.

JENNIFER: And, uh, that's what I mean by communication. And, also, not being afraid to show these feelings is important. I think that's the first step in realizing that it's OK or it's safe to have these feelings and to show them to the other person.

SLUZKI: Are you talking about yourself, or are you . . . (*Sluzki indicates "gotcha" by making a stabbing gesture toward Larry and simultaneously emitting a short, humorous noise.*)

JENNIFER: Oh, I'm talking more about Larry. I mean . . .

SLUZKI: You know, that's what I've sensed. (*To Larry*) I was afraid she was . . . (*Makes the gesture and noise again. Both Larry and Jennifer laugh.*)

JENNIFER: I think, in the past, I've been a lot less open with my feelings. But I've been in therapy now for a while, and . . .

SLUZKI: For a while? For how long?

JENNIFER: For about a year and a half.

SLUZKI: That's sweet of you! (*Jennifer and Larry laugh.*) No, no, it's great! You know, frequently what happens with people in individual therapy, they end up doing their own stuff and they leave their partners on another point in the planet.

JENNIFER: Uh huh.

SLUZKI: So, you are now trying to bring him up to a point, to a mode or language that you have developed since then. That's very sweet of you and (*to Larry*) of you indeed to follow suit. Are you in therapy yourself?

LARRY: No.

SLUZKI: No, of course not.

JENNIFER: I wish he were.

SLUZKI: (*Makes the noise again. Jennifer and Larry laugh.*) (*To Larry*) So, you are the one who needs to soften up. Apparently, secretly, the couples therapy is for you.

LARRY: What? What was the question? I'm sorry . . .

SLUZKI: I made a statement. I have the impression that secretly the couples therapy is for you.

LARRY: Yeah, in her mind I would say it's more . . .

SLUZKI: Yes . . .

From the very beginning, just by means of the seating arrangements, this couple (any couple, any family) provides me with considerable information. I have already mentioned that this information is less abundant with a couple than with a larger group. But it is there. With this couple, their choice of seating arrangement put Jennifer in a powerful intermediary position between Larry and myself. We were seated on an L-shaped sofa; Jennifer was seated in the juncture, leaning forward toward me, while Larry was sitting to the side, leaning backward. In addition to that, during my opening statement, Jennifer uttered several overlapping "uh huhs" of agreement. In any group exchange, the speaker tends to look at and address more frequently the person who signals reception cues, such as Jennifer did in this case. In this context (and perhaps in other social exchanges) Jennifer was, so to speak, the go-between, the expert. She used the language of feelings and emotions, the official jargon of therapy. Concurrently, Larry yielded the floor to her, and nodded in accord when she spoke. It was tempting for me to follow the socially acceptable behavior of going along with their own definition of the situation; it would have been easy to continue the dialogue mainly with her. However, in order to reach a position in which I could acknowledge competence equally to both, I returned to point zero and asked Larry, "And what brought you [to the consultation]?" The language with which he responded was dramatically different from hers. He spoke more hesitantly, less fluently, and less technically. I had already perceived by this point that the therapeutic situation ran the risk of being mystified. It was important to avoid adopting the hidden assumption that she was a healthy individual or the expert in therapy who brought him to couples therapy, actually to "couples therapy *for him*." Accepting this ploy would imply a relationship of inclusion—a coalition—between the therapist and her, and one of exclusion with him (Sluzki, 1975). To neutralize this situation, I decided not only to make this ploy explicit in a nonjudgmental way, but, more importantly, to utilize their differential traits of codes and styles and to speak more in his language than in hers, signaling to both of them my refusal to align with her. In making the issue explicit, however, I did not wish to alienate myself from her but to attain an equidistant, neutral position. Thus, I chose to define her role from a positive stance, describing it as an attempt on her part to teach him a new language. This positive connotation, even though carried on *ad absurdum* by me in the previous fragment, ultimately shows its power: The subsequent description of issues by the couple contains a new evenness.

SLUZKI: So, if I understand correctly, your individual therapy created some problems in the couple that you're trying to solve, reasonably so, by means of bringing Larry into couples therapy, in which case both of you can tune up a bit.

JENNIFER: Uh huh.

LARRY: I don't think individual therapy *created* problems between us.

JENNIFER: It didn't. It didn't create the problems, but it just made me more aware of problems. The problems were already there, so they weren't created, but . . .

SLUZKI: What kind of problems were there?

JENNIFER: What I said originally, just this inability to communicate, feeling like we were living in separate houses and that we weren't really working as a couple. I mean, I felt that if things happened to Larry, he couldn't talk to me about them.

SLUZKI: He didn't talk to you about them?

JENNIFER: No, he's very, very introverted and very private . . .

SLUZKI: Uh huh.

JENNIFER: . . . and he doesn't seem . . .

SLUZKI: And, when things happen to you, what . . .

JENNIFER: When things happen to me, now with therapy, it's easier for me to talk. I *want* to talk about things. I mean, my feelings are more on the surface and I have a need to . . .

LARRY: I think it's not therapy, I think it's just her personality.

JENNIFER: But therapy certainly brought a lot of it out.

LARRY: Could be.

JENNIFER: I mean, I feel more comfortable about talking about my feelings and expressing them.

LARRY: We're different in that way. When she has a problem, she *likes* to talk about it, and reiterate on it a number of times, a large number of times, in my opinion. So, on that issue, if there is an objective way to look at it, I think she probably overdoes the talking about problems and I tend to undertalk about them, and I think the balance between us is about right.

SLUZKI: Uh huh.

JENNIFER: Well, I'm not so sure that I overdo it, though, because I talk to other people about problems and they seem to have similar reactions. When they have a problem they seem to talk to me about it just the way I talk to them about it . . . so I don't feel like I'm overly reactive or anything like that. I mean, that is very subjective.

SLUZKI: Absolutely.

JENNIFER: The way somebody else would look at it, they might even think I'm *under*reacting to certain problems, so it's again very subjective.

SLUZKI: Um hum. In addition, this is an old discussion between you two.

JENNIFER: An old one?

LARRY: Yes.

JENNIFER: Yeah, definitely an old one.

In the course of attempting to produce a joint description of the nature of their problem, each of them tried to pull me to his or her own side of the description. My response, one that in fact broke up their display, was to depart from the level of the content and to comment on the discussion itself. When I used as referent "the discussion," I was not specifically referring to either of them. This disengaged me from the tug of war and put me in a neutral position. The couple turned to each other:

LARRY: You know, obviously you don't believe you overdo problems, otherwise you wouldn't do it. I mean . . .

JENNIFER: Right.

LARRY: . . . what I'm saying is, you obviously don't think you do it incorrectly, otherwise you would change it, and I don't think I do it incorrectly, otherwise I would change it, but I think what's happening is that we both have a different idea about the correct way to handle problems.

SLUZKI: One way or another, you are involved in a very particular ritual: the ritual of couples therapy. It is a ritual of commitment to the relationship and a statement to each other that you do want *in* somehow, because if not, you wouldn't be exposed to all these stresses and strains, yeah?

JENNIFER: Uh huh.

SLUZKI: Perhaps the ritual of therapy in itself is a very important statement . . . a token of love. If that is the case, it is satisfied by the mere fact that you are in therapy, yeah?

JENNIFER: Yeah (*Both nod assent.*)

SLUZKI: The risk of any change is that you may leave therapy and, if therapy in itself is a ritual, then it doesn't make sense for you to change too much . . . because you have to leave therapy, and therapy in itself is a very important expression of appreciation and love for each other.

LARRY: The real purpose of therapy is to get out of therapy as soon as possible in a way that you would feel happier. I mean, what is the end point? . . . I think one of the problems with therapy is that people do get caught up in the ritual, and so it perpetuates itself. The goals aren't attained because if they are attained, then you leave therapy, by definition. And that's the problem, you know?

SLUZKI: Uh huh.

LARRY: It's a paradox . . .

SLUZKI: There is another risk, and it is that if you (*to Jennifer*) are an advocate of therapy, in the sense of wanting to remain in therapy, and you (*to Larry*) are an advocate of finishing therapy and being able to go on, you are caught in a struggle with therapy, the struggle of "I want more/I want less." That reproduces indeed what may be a stylistic issue in your relationship . . .

JENNIFER: Yeah.

SLUZKI: It sounds like you (*to Jennifer*) are one of those fanatics that jump onto any bandwagon with all her soul, and you (*to Larry*) say, "Hey, wait a minute, reality testing, one, two, three . . ." (*Jennifer and Larry laugh.*) You (*to Jennifer*) would be like a balloon shooting into space if it weren't for the weight. And you (*to Larry*) would in turn remain down there, on flatland, if it weren't for the balloon.

The definition of therapy as a "ritual of love and commitment" led naturally to the recommendation that they shouldn't change. Citing the inconvenience of change and performing the restraining, conservative intervention, which prescribes the problem rather than advocating its demise, have an important freeing effect in the therapeutic relationship that has been abundantly discussed in the literature (e.g. Fisch, Weakland, & Segal, 1982; Haley, 1976; Papp, 1983; Watzlawick et al., 1974). In fact, that prescription prompted Larry's attempt to convince *me* about the advantages of considering therapy, at its best, as an avenue for quick, efficient change and not as an endless ritual. Even if valid, Larry's statement seemed so congruent with my apparent beliefs that it risked putting him too much on my side, and consequently alienating Jennifer. That prompted my next intervention, in which I related the pattern of the discussion to a characteristic previously mentioned by them as intrinsic to the couple—namely, her being expansive and him restrained. I defined this distinction not as a conflict but as a difference of *style*. This way of describing the issue eliminated any critical value judgment on my part. In fact, it was positive, or at least neutral, in connotation, thus countering anyone's attempt to attribute negative intentions to any behavior. At the end of the fragment, I introduced an encompassing metaphor that contained the essence of a new description of the relationship, one in which the complementarity of their reciprocal stances was described as mutually beneficial in spite of the different-ness. This theme was maintained through the rest of the interview.

Throughout the interview, I introduced new (but not *too* new) views while maintaining a one-down, nonauthoritative, conversational tone. These new views were usually delivered as if they were a mere redescription of the couple's own views. In that way, the process of consensual validation in the therapeutic conversation was enhanced, allowing for a smooth introduction of alternative descriptions. The alteration and transformation of the shared frame are central features of any therapeutic endeavor: We introduce a disturbance in the construc-tion of reality proposed by the patients and we ride along with the consequences. If the result has promise, we reinforce it; if it doesn't, we don't. Needless to say, we do not introduce random disturbance; rather, we try to select those disturbances that might alter the frames or world views proposed by the patients that contribute to the maintenance of their symptomatic/problematic patterns (Sluzki, 1983). It should be added that the one-down modality not only favors the joining process, but constitutes a no-lose situation: if the couple resonates and concurs with the new view, they can own it, as we have seemingly only described something already perceived, uttered, or performed by them. If, on the contrary, they do not resonate, we can always treat our position as a misunderstanding and correct it.

It may be noticed that I avoided using the third person when referring to Larry and Jennifer ("When you [*to Larry*] do this to you [*to Jennifer*], then you [*to Larry*] . . ." as opposed to "When you [*to Larry*] do this to her, then she. . . .").[2] The rationale for this, as discussed in more detail elsewhere (Sluzki, 1978), is to define everybody in the session as equal participants, particularly when one of the members of a couple or family has been identified as a patient. Identified patients are frequently "talked about" in the third person ("He looks depressed, Doctor") rather than "talked to" in the second person ("You look depressed"), as if the subject were absent or an object. The effect is, of course, alienation or defensiveness.

JENNIFER: So he's a stable, anchoring force of . . .

---

[2]Needless to say, in the course of the interaction I look at the person to which my statement is addressed, which allows for few misunderstandings.

SLUZKI: That's the way it looks now.

JENNIFER: Yeah, actually that's quite true in many ways. I mean, I have my tendencies to be very emotional about things and fly off the handle sometimes. I wouldn't say I overreact, but I'm just an emotional person. And Larry is just the opposite. I mean, it's like the Odd Couple here.

SLUZKI: Yes, but I insist that it makes for the balance of the couple.

JENNIFER: Um hm.

SLUZKI: So, don't spit on your blessings.

LARRY: Yeah, right. There is some point where you can always want better. I think we should always want better, but if you don't have the ability to be happy, or at least to be content with what you have, you'll never be content. So there has to be some jumping-off point where you can say, "OK, I found at least the minimal answers to my problems. I can be at least content with them and try in the future to work on it." It's in that point that we probably differ.

JENNIFER: I have a response to that. I don't think that I'm planning to stay in therapy for any extended period of time. My feeling is really to learn something . . . or benefit from the therapy so that you'll be in a position to be better able to deal with these problems, because you become more aware of them.

SLUZKI: At the same time, if this complementarity that we were discussing is useful for the balance of the relationship, you shouldn't change it too much.

JENNIFER: Well . . .

SLUZKI: Because if it happened that either you convince him that he should be like you, or you convince her that she should be like you, you are going to find either two balloons drifting in the wind or two rocks there at the bottom of the lake. Yeah? And, up to a point, the differentness between the two of you is something that would be worthwhile respecting, in spite of the fact that on the surface it looks a bit like a conflict.

The logical consequence of this positive description of their conflict in terms of balancing complementarities was to assume a position of restraint (i.e., recommending no change). Larry and Jennifer responded to this position with a new round of their traditional attempt to define it as conflict. Once again I introduced the "balloon and rock" metaphor, enhanced by a description of what would happen if things changed, which led to new restraining recommendations.

The following fragment took place some five minutes later:

SLUZKI: You (*to Jennifer*) mentioned at the beginning of the interview that he is *afraid* [of expressing emotions]. Is that a feeling that fits your (*to Larry*) own perception, that when you don't share your feelings it is because you feel frightened?

LARRY: No.

SLUZKI: No. Then, if I were you, I would object to the statement that you are afraid. Not that you don't express feelings, because I believe that you agree with that. But, the question of being afraid is something that makes me feel a bit uncomfortable.

LARRY: Yeah, I don't agree with that.

SLUZKI: You don't?

LARRY: It's not fear in expressing my feelings. In other situations, I get angry and show my anger easily. I get happy, and I think I show my happiness easily. I'm not afraid to show emotion . . .

JENNIFER: You are with me. You don't do it as much with me as you do with other people.

LARRY: Right, so it's not fear. It might be lack of trust, but it's not fear.

SLUZKI: Uh, lack of trust means the ways in which you worry she may be handling those feelings?

LARRY: Yes. Very good.

Mind reading—that is, the attribution of feelings or intentions to the other—is based on the assumption that one has the power to know the feelings or intentions of the other better than the other. This imposition of supposed omniscience ("You don't really mean what you say"), frequent as it appears in child rearing ("Put on a sweater, you're cold"), can become a rather devastating, disqualifying move. As one partner becomes increasingly expert about the other, the other is deprived of his or her own self (cf. Sluzki, 1978). The statement "he is afraid . . ." was made by Jennifer at the very beginning of the session. I thought that it should be dealt with as soon as feasible; otherwise it would remain a debilitating factor for him in the definition of the relationship. Needless to say, the beginning of the interview would have been an inappropriate time to raise the issue. So I chose to bring it out in the open once I sensed that our relationship was established on a more solid ground. The opening up of this theme led to an equally debilitating counterstatement, this time from him: "I mistrust her." Once again, I resorted to rephrasing that statement into one that was more workable—namely, "You worry about the way she handles your feelings," which acknowledged his being sensitive while defining the problem in pragmatic terms ("handling") rather than in terms of more immutable feelings, carved in historical stone. This formulation permitted a reduction in the intensity and a change in the punctuation of the sequence; if there was something in the way she handled his feelings that he didn't like, he could ask for changes.

JENNIFER: Um hm. Just like with his mother. (*Laughter*)

SLUZKI: (*Whispers*) How psychoanalytic!

LARRY: That's right.

SLUZKI: Terrible! (*continued whisper*) They shoot you with interpretations one after the other . . .

LARRY: In general categories . . . (*Laughter*)

SLUZKI: God! (*To Jennifer, laughing*) You are fantastic! You sound as if you have graduated already.

JENNIFER: Of course (*laughing*).

SLUZKI: How nice! OK, leaving aside your mother for a moment (*laughter*), where were we?

LARRY: We were talking . . .

JENNIFER: . . . fear . . .

LARRY: . . . that maybe I mistrust how she's going to handle . . .

SLUZKI: Yeah, would you mind describing that a bit? What is your experience of her handling your feelings?

LARRY: Well, in the first number of years we were in a stage that I think was fairly different. We were younger and I think she was a different person, and I was a different person in the sense that our values were different and our internal . . . (*he gestures*) whatever drives us, I think, was slightly different. Things have happened to us since then, things that happen to everyone. But in those years, I would express a lot of emotion: "Why are you going out with those other men? Why don't you just stay with me?" "Why don't you move up to Boston?" At the time, she was staying in Pennsylvania for college and she wouldn't move up. She kept a boyfriend, a number of boyfriends, and so there was this triangle for most of those early years. There were a lot of emotions. I would wait by the phone for her to call, and she'd always be late, or not call at all. And I would tell her how distressed I was, you know, "Why didn't you call? I was waiting," and I would show all my emotions. And at that time they weren't handled in a way that made me the happiest, let's put it that way. . . . But I think I would handle that particular situation differently now and I wouldn't be so unhappy as I was then. So, I guess what I'm saying is that you can't just look at what happened last week.

SLUZKI: Well, you can't. But let's try just the same. In the sense that, OK, you do have a reasonable way of explaining why, but I was just being more pedestrian in my question than your sophisticated answer. I mainly want to know what is going on in your experience in terms of how Jennifer handles your emotions, as opposed to the way you would like her to handle your emotions. I know it's a vague question, but I'm talking about very vague issues, so try to be as concrete as you can possibly be.

LARRY: Well, I mean, I always felt that she had enough of her own problems, that adding mine to them wasn't the best thing in the world.

SLUZKI: That's still not getting into the question that I'm asking.

LARRY: Well, that she wouldn't be as interested in my problems as maybe she could be.

SLUZKI: (To Jennifer) Does it fit?

JENNIFER: No, I don't think that's true and I think maybe he's saying that as a way to justify his not being able to talk to me about his problems. He's saying, "Oh, she's not interested anyway, or she has enough of her own problems."

SLUZKI: Do you know what my own fantasy is, of all this?

JENNIFER: No.

SLUZKI: If I may share it with you, it is quite to the contrary of the way you describe the situation, and I already know you for half an hour (laughter). My fantasy is that you (to Larry) express whatever sensible, sensitive emotion, not anger but some tender part, and you (to Jennifer) who are very hungry for that kind of exchange (makes eating noise) . . .

JENNIFER: Devour it . . .

SLUZKI: . . . go for it, and start to feed from it, drink it, want more and more of the same and magnify it, or take it all at full value. And that is a factor that inhibits you (to Larry). But that is only my own fantasy, my educated guess, let's say.

Near the beginning of this segment, Larry adopted a historical description of the relationship that lodged him in the stronger position of victim. In this description, the relationship was composed of fixed events, immutable sequences, and unavoidable consequences. I insisted on an ahistorical perspective, which is less fatalistic and more amenable to a nonjudgmental description of patterns.

When Larry introduced a "mind-reading" statement ("She is not interested in my problems"), I repeated the move made previously, this time in the opposite direction: I described Jennifer as the expert on herself rather than Larry as the expert on her. Then I proposed another construct, building further on the notion of complementarity. I did this by describing/transforming what they defined as a conflict into a mechanism that served to balance their relationship. This description not only legitimized each of their personal styles; it also defined the reaction of each to the other's style as only natural. In subsequent fragments, the nonblaming nature of this description allowed for some constructive, practical suggestions that only reconfirmed the description. This appeared a few minutes later in the course of the interview.

SLUZKI: If that happens to be the case, then there is one rule of thumb that you can apply. If you (*to Jennifer*) want to meet his needs, whenever he expresses emotion you have to listen and do nothing about it. And for you (*to Larry*), when you listen to her expressing emotions, you may have to act amplifying rather than damping. Otherwise, you two are talking different languages. The languages of amplification and of damping are very different. You (*to Jennifer*) can experience him as emotionless, and you (*to Larry*) can experience her as overemotional. Hmm?

LARRY: She *does* complain that I minimize problems, her problems.

JENNIFER: Your problems . . .

LARRY: Or my problems.

JENNIFER: Anybody's problems.

LARRY: Maybe it's intentional. . . . I think that if she has a problem, and there's no one around to dampen it, then it'll blow up. My function is to provide the damping.

SLUZKI: But, you see, each one of you is patronizing the other, up to a point. If you (*to Larry*) are saying, "I'm doing it because otherwise she gets crazy with emotions," and you (*to Jennifer*) say, "I'm doing it for him because otherwise he becomes a block of ice," then you are patronizing each other. You're saying, "I am doing it for you, baby," when it may not be the case at all. It may be simpler that each of you has a different style in one aspect, and the interaction between the two of you may generate the misunderstanding that the other one should be like you. (*Laughter*) If you want to interact more successfully and happily, you have to be more like the other when you're with the other. When you're with yourself, you can be yourself! But when you (*to Larry*) are with her, unless you amplify a bit, she feels that she's throwing fire and getting nothing. In turn, when you are opening up what for you is an intense emotion, for her it is minimal. A "technique" of getting in touch with his emotions may be for you (*to Jennifer*) to just listen and not react. I know, it's easy for me to say. I'm an outsider. I'm not involved in an intense relationship like the two of you are. But that would be, in my view, an important way of doing something for each other.

By means of these rather practical recommendations, I reinforced my proposal of an alternative description of their predicament, this time through the language of action. Larry once again attempted to define himself as the reactor rather than an actor, and I insisted once again on the reciprocal nature of the pattern. After this fragment there followed a lively dialogue, not transcribed here. At one point Jennifer asked me, jokingly, whether I had a degree in engineering because of my use of "amplification" and "damping" as part of the metaphor. In turn, I promised her that I would introduce more "psychoanalese" in my discourse. During a short intermission, I asked Larry what the problem was with his foot, and the dialogue summarized earlier in this chapter ensued. The information about that period in their lives was incorporated into the general design of the newly proposed description/intervention shortly afterwards.

SLUZKI: If what we were discussing before makes any sense at all, putting myself in your place, during the period around the amputation, emotions must have been very intense for both of you—the amount of fear, pain, self-doubt, in addition to stubbornness and joys, etc. So, if you (*to Larry*), in your inner world, had emotions at maximum intensity, what you needed was somebody to dampen them and not to . . .

JENNIFER: Augment?

SLUZKI: . . . augment them. Regardless of the fact that for you (*to Jennifer*), it isn't augmentation. For you it's just . . .

JENNIFER: Natural . . .

SLUZKI: . . . a natural way of dealing, in which case it makes sense that in moments of maximum intensity, you (*to Larry*) would close up in order to reduce the resonance, and I assume that in turn, you (*to Jennifer*) felt starved for emotional contact. Whenever he would throw a small drop of something, you would make it a major thing to meet your needs. And so, it is an interesting vicious cycle in which you (*to both*) have been caught. Up to a point, it also shows how wise you were to have decided to make some moves in order to break that cycle.

Jennifer and Larry, through nodding, tracking, and adding new information, participated actively in fitting the new proposal to their experience of that period of their past, and to their present. A new description with retrospective and prospective value was being built, which entailed both a new definition of the goals of their therapy, and perhaps its termination.

A few minutes later all three of us exchanged body signals indicating that the session was in the process of closing.

SLUZKI: You know, in the contact right now . . .

JENNIFER: Uh huh.

SLUZKI: . . . I have experienced you (*to Jennifer*) as more (*gestures: guarded*) and you (*to Larry*) as (*gestures: expressive*).

LARRY: I think that's a pretty good assessment of . . .

JENNIFER: Why?

LARRY: Uh, I think I tend to . . .

JENNIFER: I think it's the way I'm sitting . . . how's that? (*She shifts in her seat, sitting now facing Larry and equidistant from Sluzki and Larry. Larry, in turn, has accommodated to leave space for her by him.*)

SLUZKI: All right! (*Laughter*)

The spontaneous shift in Jennifer's position and the corresponding accommodation by Larry, stemming from a seemingly unrelated comment by the therapist, once again highlights the isomorphism between structural arrangements and the definition of the nature of the relationship. That is, a change in their perception/description of their relationship led them to find their previous physical arrangement to be dissonant. They sought consonance through a new arrangement. Their more equidistant arrangement crowned my effort to establish an equal "balance of power." Different views about power between them were proposed and counterproposed, discussed, and renegotiated implicitly by the three of us in the course of the session. Such deliberations contribute to the central work of all therapy—namely, the construction of alternative realities.

The dialogue continued.

LARRY: So you think I tend to deal with things a little bit more straightforwardly. Well, that's not better or worse, it's just that you (*to Jennifer*) deal with them a little more roundabout. It's just different styles.

JENNIFER: No, I'm not so sure. I don't think so. I think you deal with things very rationally, and very logically, and systematically, and with the minimum amount of emotion. Maybe because I am more emotional, it seems like it's more roundabout. I don't think it's indirect.

SLUZKI: In fact, in a sort of curious gut reaction, the two of you may have been doing here already what I suggested, or perhaps what I am suggesting is something that you at one level do. That is, you (to Jennifer) have been dampening the contact and you (to Larry) have been maintaining the contact at full range, which is what I was mainly referring to. In fact, it was a curious experience because in your words it was like the opposite.

JENNIFER: So you were really picking up something. . . .

SLUZKI: Maybe *you* are picking up, maybe *I* was picking up something *you* have.

JENNIFER: You are also the first therapist who brought out something positive in our relationship, which is very nice, very interesting. I mean, most people say, "OK, what's the problem? And let's tear apart the problem," instead of looking at what's there.

LARRY: But our couples therapist has brought out positive . . .

JENNIFER: Sure . . .

Perhaps as a result of my effort to realign with the couple by means of developing a stronger coalition with Larry during the first part of the session, when Jennifer was the dominant member, Jennifer became more guarded and Larry more expressive. In order for my new description to fit their (and my) ongoing experience, I indicated that my new view of the relationship may have been a previously unrecognized aspect of what was already taking place. Thus, they had access to both the experiential and the cognitive representation of the proposed design. By the same token, I granted them total ownership of the whole session. The fact that I suggested a therapeutic task to be carried out by them also increased their experience of autonomy and their sense of conjoint responsibility. All this defined them as their own agents of change, rather than claiming that role for myself.

It was my expectation that, by means of this progressive reformulation of their predicament, the overall experience of the interview would convey to the couple the notion that they are stuck in a problem, not that *their relationship* is the problem. It would allow them to experience their strengths as a couple and to regard their differences as stylistic traits, not as acts of ill will or error. By suggesting to them some concrete ways to reduce their entanglement (e.g., respective amplifying and dampening), I further conveyed the idea that whatever is defined as the problem is tangible, limited, and manageable, rather than an overwhelming, incommensurable characteristic of the whole relationship. The frame was shifted by reforming the reason for consultation; ultimately, the essence of their problem was reduced to a managerial issue, and the rest of their presenting complaint to a pseudoproblem, as it consisted simply in the description of normal, complementary styles in each of them.

As the interview closed, they offered me a symbolic flower, while sensitively reassuring their (usual) therapist that she shouldn't feel jealous, that they love her too.

REFERENCES

Fisch, R., Weakland, J. H., & Segal, L. (1982). *The tactics of change*. San Francisco: Jossey-Bass.

Haley, J. (1976). *Problem-solving therapy: New strategies for effective family therapy*. San Francisco: Jossey-Bass.

Sluzki, C. E. (1975). The coalitionary process in initiating family therapy. *Family Process*, 14(1), 67–77.

Sluzki, C. E. (1978). Marital therapy from a systems therapy perspective. In T. J. Paolino & B. S. McCrady (Eds.), *Marriage and marital therapy: Psychoanalytic, behavioral and systems theory perspectives*. New York: Brunner/Mazel.

Sluzki, C. E. (1983). Process, structures and worldviews: Toward an integrated view of systemic models in family therapy. *Family Process*, 22(4), 469–76.

Papp, P. (1983). *The process of change*. New York: Guilford Press.

Watzlawick, P., Weakland, J. H., & Fisch, R. (1974). *Change: Principles of problem formation and problem resolution*. New York: Norton.

PART III

TREATMENT APPROACHES TO COUPLES

7

Future Perfect, Past Perfect:
A Positive Approach to Opening
Couple Therapy

RICHARD CHASIN and SALLYANN ROTH

The four approaches presented in Part II of this volume differ markedly from each other. Even so, all of them place more emphasis on the couple's problems than on their strengths. Here we offer another approach, one that specifically postpones and downplays the discussion of problems, and opens with a discussion of strengths and enactments of visions of an improved future.

Our approach also differs from three of the four demonstration interviews in its heavy reliance on psychodramatic techniques. Papp alone includes them, but our use of fantasy differs from hers. She asks a couple to portray fantasy versions of their ongoing relationship. By contrast, we do not ask clients to enact their current problems in any way. The enactments used in our approach are of the future and the past.

To illustrate our method, we use the device of a hypothetical interview with Jennifer and Larry. In describing the way we might work with this couple, we fully acknowledge the skill and creativity of the therapists who conducted the actual, live interviews. Our alternative "interview" takes place only within these pages, and its beneficial outcome is as imaginary as the therapeutic conversations and enactments that engender it. In plain fact, we cannot predict with certainty how our approach would have worked with this couple. Although we must acknowledge the advantage of having our session develop and end as we wish, we offer it as a credible illustration of this alternative approach.

Therapists and clients ordinarily begin their work with a detailed discussion of problems. Although opening with a problem focus addresses concerns that are usually uppermost in the minds of clients, it also tends to construct a therapeutic reality that is grounded in those problems. This construction, ironically, may reinforce the very problems that bring clients to treatment. Therefore, our model for an opening interview emphasizes strengths rather than problems. This approach also minimizes discussion, the usual form of therapeutic interaction, and relies principally on action techniques to stimulate fresh perspectives.[1]

In using this approach, we first inquire about each partner's individual strengths.[2] Next, we explore the dreams each has for their future as a couple by asking each partner to imagine and enact a detailed scene to illustrate his or her desired future relationship with the other. Third, we invite each partner to dramatize a critical past injury or unmet need that influences his or her future dreams for the couple. We follow that enactment with a "reformed," magically improved version of the painful past scene in which the other partner plays the role of a central healing figure. Finally, we invite the couple to describe briefly their current difficulties, or, if they prefer, to describe them in light of what we have just done. (See Table 7.1.)

Although this sequence of steps does address the couple's difficulty, it does so in a way that enables clients and therapist to avoid becoming mired in the details of the clients' current problem and in the inadequacies the partners repeatedly attribute to themselves and to each other. It is an approach that provides the couple with an evocative shared experience, fertile ground in which the therapeutic process can take root.

As we illustrate this method, we will speculate about how Larry and Jennifer might have responded to it. These speculations are based on what we know about the couple from background material and from presentations by the four therapists who interviewed them. Our speculations are informed by experience in using the method with over 150 couples since it was originated by Chasin in 1982.

DESCRIPTION OF THE METHOD AND ITS HYPOTHETICAL APPLICATION TO THE CASE OF LARRY AND JENNIFER

Larry and Jennifer are bright, articulate, talented, and competent in many areas of their lives, and they are able to discuss the problems in

---

[1]While many family therapists have made substantial use of action techniques (Satir, 1972; Duhl, Kantor, & Duhl, 1973; Papp, 1976; Kantor, 1980; Madanes, 1981; Minuchin & Fishman, 1981; Papp, Chapter 3, this volume), few avoid enacting current problems or work within a Milan-derived systemic frame.

[2]In this chapter we describe the sequence of steps we most commonly follow in using the model with couples. The model also provides for alternative paths when certain conditions prevail. Omitted here for the sake of simplicity, they are described in Chasin, Roth & Bograd (1989).

TABLE 7.1. Outline of the Method of Opening Therapy by Dramatizing Future Goals, Past Injuries, and Reformed Pasts

I. *Making a Contract*	
1. Negotiation of a "safe participation" contract	Therapist and clients negotiate an initial working agreement to promote safe and voluntary participation.
II. *Articulating Strengths and Goals*	
1. Statements of individual strengths	Each client names and describes his or her own strengths.
2. Statements of goals for the relationship	Each client names and describes his or her own goals for their relationship.
III. *Performing Enactments*	
1. Future dreams: enactments of relationship goals	Each client creates a scenario for the relationship, each illustrating his or her goals. Partners participate in enacting each other's scene.
2. Painful past: Enactments of childhood injury that the goals would heal	Each client re-enacts an injurious childhood experience that achieving the goals would heal.
3. Reformed past: Enactments of the past as it "should have been"	Each client enacts a revised scene in which the original injury is averted or healed with the partner playing the protective or healing role.
IV. *Stating Problems*	Each client gives a condensed statement of the relationship problems, speaks of them in light of the enactments, or passes.

their relationship in sophisticated terms. In spite of these strengths, they remained unable to resolve their problems at the time of the conference, and at times they despaired of ever being able to do so. Although they had learned much from Jennifer's two years of individual therapy and their four months of couple therapy, their difficulties persisted. In the six-month follow-up meeting with Chasin and Grunebaum (see Chapter 18), Larry ruefully noted that the therapists who conducted the demonstration interviews did not seem to acknowledge the positive aspects of their relationship and did not even ask if he and Jennifer loved each other. According to Jennifer, she and Larry nonetheless experienced some hope, particularly in those moments when they saw that their roles did not need to be static or fixed.

Using information derived from the presentations, we will illustrate how this method can provide opportunities for couples to break out of the kind of fixed beliefs and positions that Jennifer and Larry described and displayed.

Stage I. Making a Contract

In this first stage, we make an explicit contract with the clients about various aspects of our working together, such as voluntary participation, confidentiality, taping, and the length of the session (usually two hours). Discussing this essential business together, establishes a sense of shared responsibility for the therapy process. Before we start the interview, we always suggest that we adopt an agreement that each person has the right to "pass"[3] during the session. The pass agreement gives anyone the right to decline to answer any question or follow any suggestion without even giving a reason. One need only say, "Not ready" or "Pass." The pass agreement augments a sense of control and safety, enabling clients to enter quickly and fully into a collaborative therapeutic relationship. The clinical material from the Framos' interview indicates that control of the pace and direction of the therapy session is important to Jennifer.

Stage II. Articulating Strengths and Goals

Step 1. Statements of Individual Strengths

As the next step in this approach, we explain to couples that learning about the skills of both partners is helpful for the present endeavor, and we ask each client to recall, list, and describe his or her own *individual* strengths or valued personal qualities. This activity shifts attention away from supposed weaknesses or deficiencies and onto already available skills and resources which the partners might be able to apply in resolving their current dilemma. From the outset, each individual is viewed and treated as a resourceful and successful person rather than as a patient experiencing failure.

We might introduce our inquiry this way: "Before we go any further, I would like to learn about the important strengths and skills each of you has. Specifically, I invite you each to describe a few of your personal resources, your strengths." Larry, who is characteristically taciturn, might hesitate initially and object to the task, but eventually state that his self-reliance and independence had helped him in his recovery from cancer. Jennifer, who is characteristically self-critical, might interrupt this habit to recall and detail those personal qualities she most values in herself. She might mention the persistence and intelligence that gained her an advanced degree.

We help clients to amplify their descriptions of their strengths and

---

[3]As indicated by Richard Lee (1981), the right to "pass" was originated by James Sacks.

other valued personal characteristics. If they are vague about such traits, we help them to sharpen their descriptions; if they are tentative, we encourage them to make more confident statements. If they speak of their attributes in general terms, we ask for specifics; if they offer only specifics, we ask them to generalize.

Behavioral examples of each skill serve to clarify what the clients mean, remind them of times of successful coping, and may elicit the feeling state that accompanies the exercise of those skills. Conversely, a move from the concrete to the general serves to give the client a sense of how what is seen as a narrowly defined skill may have applicability across contexts. If either partner brings up problems at this stage, we discourage discussion of them, assuring him or her that there will be time to address problems later.

We have noticed that each partner becomes acutely interested in the skills and attributes the other claims to have. The listening partner's stance is usually one of respectful curiosity. Sometimes, one partner starts to prompt the other in naming resources—an impulse toward cooperation and assistance which often appears even when there is great conflict within the couple. Thus, we would not be surprised to hear Larry try to help Jennifer enumerate her strengths and vice versa. We would interrupt such behavior, however, as the goal at this stage is for each partner to claim his or her own resources. In doing so, each partner usually becomes more confident of his or her own individual ability to solve problems.

Step 2. Statements of Goals for the Relationship

At this point, we ask each partner to make a statement about his or her goals for the relationship. This inquiry brings the future into the present: Each becomes engaged in constructing a vision of an improved relationship and becomes less preoccupied with the chronic complaints that may have dominated awareness. Since the affective connections between problems and goals are universally strong, couples usually experience this focus on goals as attentive to their pain.

With Jennifer and Larry, we might open the discussion of future goals by asking, "How would it be between you now if your relationship were already better? Imagine an improved future for your relationship. What would be happening?" We would encourage Larry and Jennifer to muse and follow their own thoughts, providing both of them with time to develop their separate ideas and images before asking either of them to speak.

Jennifer might include "a closer relationship" and "better communication" among her goals. Larry might name "more privacy" and "freedom to watch television without reproach" among his. Clients frequently describe goals in vague generalities, retreat from citing wishful hopes, and begin to recount present annoyances instead. In such cases, we persist in trying to draw out specific, concrete objectives and resist the drift toward a problem focus. For example, if pressed about "better communication" as a goal, Jennifer might initially say that Larry is "sometimes dead silent." But with coaching to be specific and positive, she might ultimately express a wish that Larry "always be willing to spell out how he feels about matters of importance."

The listening partner usually expects criticism or unacceptable demands, and relaxes only as the therapist diligently holds the speaking partner to feasible and constructive images of the future. Larry might worry that Jennifer would cast him in a negative light, but would soon be relieved if Jennifer positively described him in her dreams for the future. He might then show curiosity and even interrupt to "help" with unsolicited amendments. If so, we would respectfully block his suggestions so that Jennifer could proceed to define her own goals without influence or distraction. Larry, in turn, would be asked to articulate his own goals for the relationship. Here, as in every other step in the interview, we strive for symmetry of opportunity and experience.

Stage III. Performing Enactments

Step 1. Future Dreams: Enactments of Relationship Goals

At this point we invite each partner to author and play out a scenario that illustrates how he or she wishes the relationship to be in the future. Over the course of these goal enactments, each partner plays four roles: the roles of self and partner in his or her own future ideal scene, and the roles of self and partner in the partner's dream for the future.

Because it is difficult for most people to fully articulate their goals, the construction of scenes illustrating those goals helps to reduce ambiguity and misunderstanding. We would expect that this exercise in specificity would be helpful to Larry and Jennifer, given their tendency to describe their dilemmas in broad terms such as "difficulty of communication," "lack of closeness," and "not enough privacy." We would also anticipate that they would willingly engage in our enactment task since they both entered readily and playfully into Papp's fantasy exercise.

Jennifer's ideal scene might start with her returning home after working late to find Larry watching television. The minute she comes through the door, he might turn off the television set, get her a cup of tea, and ask her about a conversation she had planned to have with her boss that day. She might say that she has been having difficulty because her boss is a silent, inaccessible person from whom she wants feedback but never gets it. Her scene might show Larry as gently persistent ("I am really interested. I know this problem has been on your mind for weeks"). From the outset we would help her to give her scene a sense of immediacy. For example:

THERAPIST: (*To Jennifer*) When you come home, do you walk in quietly or do you call out?

JENNIFER: I call out.

THERAPIST: Open the door and call out.

JENNIFER: (*Making a gesture*) Hello, Larry, I'm home!

THERAPIST: What are you thinking as you wait for a response?

JENNIFER: He'd better be here. He said he would.

THERAPIST: Remember, this is your ideal scene.

JENNIFER: He said he'd be home. He'll come to the door in a second.

THERAPIST: (*To Jennifer and Larry*) Reverse roles. Larry, be Jennifer standing at the door. Jennifer, you be Larry hearing Jennifer's greeting. As Larry, show us how he reacts in this ideal future relationship.

The enactment would proceed with Jennifer creating each move in the interaction and with Larry assisting her by playing whomever she is not portraying during each step of the developing scene. Jennifer would demonstrate exactly how she wants Larry to act in her ideal future relationship with him by assuming his part, speaking his words, and performing his actions. He would then play himself precisely as Jennifer had modeled him, while Jennifer enacts herself. Finally, when Jennifer is satisfied that they are both demonstrating all the elements of her scene as she desires, they would try to perform it perfectly from beginning to end, each cast in his or her own role. The whole scene would be played and replayed until Jennifer says that all of its elements—the wording, the intonation, the gestures—are exactly as she wishes them to be.

The same care would be taken in enacting Larry's scene as many times as necessary to have it be precisely as he wishes it to be. Larry might create a scene in which, after dinner, he retires to a television room while Jennifer reads elsewhere, protecting him from phone disturbances by telling callers, "I'm sorry, but the championship games are on. Please leave a message or call back later." After fielding a call, she might sit next to him and watch the final game of the season go into overtime. Usually in these future enactments, only a few interchanges (5 to 10) are needed to illustrate clearly the interactional pattern the partner desires.

Enactments of future wishes by the partners often lead to an appreciation of one another's goals and an unsettling of certain fixed and limiting expectations. The dramatization of goals requires cooperation—which may in itself constitute new interactional behavior. For example, cycles of accusation and counteraccusation are interrupted when each partner listens carefully to the other and engages fully in playing out scenes from the other's ideal future. Defensiveness and negative expectations are also lessened as partners become more open and vulnerable in showing and experiencing what each really wants.

Step 2. Enactments of the Painful and the Reformed Past

We would next invite the couple to move directly from enactments of goals to enactments of painful past events. Ordinarily an individual's goals for the future of a relationship feel connected to painful experiences that occurred prior to the formation of the couple, often in childhood. In our hypothetical example, we would ask Jennifer and Larry each to "recall a painful time from the distant past when you wanted something similar to what you realize in your future dream, a time when you yearned for something similar but it simply did not happen. Don't worry about precision. There need not be any obvious connection between your dream for the future and the painful past event."

When enacting the past occurrence, each would play himself or herself as well as the other key roles; however, roles that embody the recalled "source" of pain—the roles of apparently cruel, neglectful, or thoughtless others—would always be played by the therapist, never by the partner. After we had played out one remembered painful scene, we would return to the beginning of that scene and replay it, this time altering its script and perhaps its cast, so that it comes out as the client believes it ideally "should have happened." In this reformed scene, the partner, not the therapist, is cast in the central protective or healing role.

For example, Jennifer might select a painful scene when she was five. Having awakened from a nightmare, she runs to her mother's room for comfort, but her mother scornfully rebuffs her and orders her back to bed. The scene might end as she leaves her mother's bedroom and enters the dark and empty hallway leading to the room she shares with her father. First, Jennifer would perform the scene, playing in turn both herself and her mother. Then she would observe a replay of the scene in which the therapist played her mother and Larry played her child-self.

The therapist would ask her, "What needs to happen here? Show us what should have happened." While Larry played the young Jennifer, Jennifer herself would play her "reformed" mother, one who comforts and protects her. Then they would reverse roles: Jennifer would become her young self, as Larry took the role of the "reformed" mother.

If Jennifer felt that such a revision, although desirable, was simply too unbelievable to have any dramatic impact, we would invite her to reform a scene even further back in the history of her family, perhaps in an unremembered generation. "What would have had to happen in your mother's life," we might ask, "in order for her to be understanding and responsive in this way?"

Jennifer might create a different background for her mother, one in which the runaway grandfather miraculously returns and the grandmother relinquishes her secretive and shadowy ways before the birth of Jennifer's mother. She might then enact another scene in which her unabandoned grandmother (played by Larry) treats Jennifer's mother (played by Jennifer) with great care and tenderness. Following this scene Jennifer would probably find it quite credible for her mother, with this greatly improved childhood, to comfort and protect the terrified, five-year-old Jennifer. She would then be able to enact the final reformed scene in which her mother (played by Larry) comforts her and provides her with her own room so that she does not have to share a room with her father. It is quite unnecessary at this point, unless Jennifer deems it so, to revise and correct other troublesome elements, such as the rift between Jennifer and her sister.

These past scenes are often so charged that they profoundly affect all participants. For example, Larry, usually cool and rational, might be moved to tears watching and playing Jennifer as a hurt and helpless child.

Next, Larry would be invited to create enactments of his painful and reformed past. He might choose a moment when he felt his mother was exclusively occupied with him and his father did not notice either Larry's distress with his mother or his growing interest in sports. At first, Larry would play himself and both parents. Then the full painful past scene would be replayed with Jennifer taking Larry's role while the therapist played both the father and the mother. In this scene his mother might be interrupting Larry as he was mending his baseball mitt. Larry might silently look toward his father for help. His father might peer up from a newspaper, glance at his wife and son, and then continue reading.

At the end of the painful scene, the therapist and Larry would then set the stage for the reformed scene. It might proceed this way:

THERAPIST: (*To Larry*) What needs to happen here?

LARRY: Dad needs to show his appreciation of my mother and maybe even get a little romantic with her. He definitely needs to encourage his son's interest in sports.

THERAPIST: Would you be willing to play your father and show us what he would do?

LARRY: (*As father, addressing mother, played by the therapist*) You handle everything so beautifully. But you have much too much to do. You need some time off. Let's go out tonight, by ourselves, to that restaurant we went to on our anniversary.

LARRY: (*As father, addressing the childhood Larry, who is still played by Jennifer*) Your baseball glove is torn apart and it's much too small for you. Tomorrow, let's get you one that fits—maybe one of those new ones that will make you look like Joe DiMaggio.

Larry would then be invited to play himself as the child in the scene he scripted. If he agreed, Jennifer would play the reformed father, and the therapist would be the mother.

If he felt unable to enact the reformed scene, saying that it seemed too implausible, we would invite him to invent and enact a different life story for his father, one that would make his father's behavior in the reformed scene more credible. Larry might then imagine a new childhood for his father, one in which Larry's grandfather does not die when his father is four, but instead lives a long life. Larry might construct a simple scene in which his grandfather and father wander out into a field with each other and pick flowers for his grandmother's birthday. In the enactment, Jennifer would play Larry's grandfather and Larry would play his father as a young boy. Following this brief dramatization, Larry might feel ready to enact the reformed version of his painful childhood scene, feeling his father's transformed behavior in that scene to be a natural consequence of his father's new history.

In each reformed scene, it is important that the partner be cast in the central protective or healing role, be it in recent, historical, or mythic time. In group psychodrama, the protective or healing role is called the "reformed auxiliary" (Sacks, 1978). The reforming process is the psychodramatic equivalent of Milton Erickson's hypnotic incorporation of a healing person into the client's memory, which enables the client to move to a future that seemed unachievable before this new experience (Erickson, 1954; Haley, 1973). When used in a couple session, the experience of enacting a reformed past derives additional power from reverberations between the partners. When one partner takes the role of a protective or healing person in the other partner's past, the climate of their relationship is significantly affected. The "healing one" has an experience of effectiveness that may have been missing for him or her in the relationship. The "healed one" leaves with a precise memory of gratification to replace a vague sense of what a better past might have been—one which may alter fixed images of the partner as frustrator. In the future, each partner may be able to perceive the other's pain in new ways and may have access to a greater range of responses.[4]

---

[4]The developments suggested here are not the only possible outcomes. For example, a couple might become clearer through the enactments that their goals are incompatible or

Stage IV. Stating the Problem

Frequently the partners are stimulated, even a bit bemused, by the rapid sequence of brief enactments of the past and present, the real and imaginary, the painful and relieving. They still have not had an opportunity to explicitly describe their difficulty. At this juncture, we invite them to briefly state their problems, or, if they prefer, to refer to them in light of the experiences they have just had, or simply to pass and say nothing at all about them. Sometimes both partners feel hopeful and closer, having just shared emotionally powerful and constructive experiences, and prefer to savor the mood rather than spoil it with an inventory of present complaints. If they do choose to describe their problems, they are likely to present them with less acrimony and despair and with greater softness than they would have prior to the work of this session.

Thus, when asked about problems, Larry might say that he doesn't see any point in mentioning grievances at a time like this. Jennifer might say that although Larry can be uncommunicative, he has been different during this session.

We would close the interview by eliciting Jennifer and Larry's thoughts about whether we should meet again, and, if so, how soon. We would expect that following this session, Jennifer and Larry could do a great deal of their therapeutic work on their own and would select a longer than usual interval between meetings.

USES AND LIMITATIONS OF THE METHOD

The method we have outlined here can be used with clients in any long-term committed relationship: a couple; a parent and a child; two siblings; or, in an adapted version, whole families or even workers in an organization. When used in couple therapy, it is immaterial whether the couple is heterosexual or homosexual, married or unmarried.

What is important is that both partners are willing and able to experience the high levels of exposure that the method entails. Their readiness can be gauged at the beginning, in the stage of identifying their strengths. The therapist/consultant also draws on information gleaned from the clients' initial phone call and/or the referral.

This method probably should not be used with recent difficulties (where simpler methods may suffice) or in crises (where additional

---

that commitment is no longer present and choose to separate. Such a decision might be a positive step.

affect and confusion may make matters worse), but rather where there are chronic, grinding problems that persist despite apparent mutual investment in the relationship. We tend to use this approach in the first interview with couples who have been unsuccessful in prior therapy.

The model may be used by therapists, in a kind of self-consultation, to get fresh perspectives on ongoing work with their own clients. It may also be used in consultation on therapies that are bogged down (Chasin, Roth, & Bograd, 1989), and, with some variations, in interviewing families with young children (Chasin & White, 1989). When used in consultation with a couple in ongoing treatment with another therapist, it has been most productive when the couple is generally satisfied with a therapist who ordinarily does not work with action techniques. We make available to the therapist, if the clients permit, a videotape of the session.

Initially, we expected that few couples would be able to carry out the enactments, but we have found that most couples perform them with ease. Action-oriented people have less difficulty with them than with verbal methods, and people who intellectualize do better than we (or they!) expected. In our experience, the method appears to have the greatest impact on individuals of intellectual bent, perhaps because the very act of engaging in these unfamiliar psychodramatic processes constitutes a significant departure from their normal patterns.

We have not been able to judge the long-term effectiveness of the method, since there are few instances in which it has been the only interview and we have not studied its use under controlled conditions. In the short run, however, couples typically take from the experience of the enactments fresh perspectives, a sense of motion in the relationship, and a richer view of the possibilities for its evolution.

We have often been asked what the therapist should do after using this technique. We respond that the therapist should simply follow sound clinical practice based on feedback from the clients.

As for contraindications, we have avoided use of the method in crises, as mentioned above, or when there is a high level of denial or deliberate lying, as in many cases of substance abuse. Furthermore, since the method can bring complex and intense emotions to the fore, we have not used it when either partner has difficulty with reality testing or is very suspicious of professionals. Of course, not only clients but therapists, too, need to feel comfortable. Although the method does not require sophistication with action techniques, the therapist needs to feel confident using them.

SOME REMARKS ON THEORY

We offer this method as an illustration of the general approach of incorporating action techniques into the systemic frame. It is not a definitive prescription for how to begin therapy, but rather part of an evolving set of techniques being adapted to a theory base which is also evolving. The theoretical base on which we rely is that of Milan-derived systemic thinking (Hoffman, 1988). With others who subscribe to these ideas, we share the belief that an objective of the therapist is to evoke "the new" rather than prescribe it—that is, to participate with the clients in its evolution, and to behave in a way that is respectful of the clients' ability to design their own future.

We also see the therapist's job as taking part in and facilitating a "conversation" that allows for the beliefs and behaviors of clients and therapist to shift and expand (Anderson & Goolishian, 1988). We have found that our method promotes in clients an expanded range of affects, ideas, perspectives, and behavior, enhancing their abilities to find their own solutions. As therapists, we have experienced significant expansion of our own beliefs, viewpoints, and range of behaviors from participating with clients in this work.

Generally, therapists relying on this theoretical base have also relied primarily on client–therapist discussion and avoided action methods out of concern that directing clients' actions might function to impose the therapist's ideas and values on the family (Selvini-Palazzoli, Boscolo, Cecchin, & Prata, 1980; Penn, 1982, 1985; Andersen, 1987; Tomm, 1987). Yet we have found that our action methods can also effectively serve the objectives of this theoretical framework. The model uses action co-created by clients and therapist and draws its material from the clients' own experience, perceptions, and longings. In guiding the sequenced enactments, we avoid imposing interpretations on the clients' beliefs or experience, but instead try to provide an evocative context in which the clients can develop, and experiment with, their own new ideas, perceptions, and feelings.

As we have noted, this approach differs markedly from the usual practice of beginning the first interview with a problem focus.[5] Its opening emphasis on resources and goals, in combination with the particular arrangement of dramatic enactments, helps therapist and clients to bring forth novel ideas, novel behaviors, and strong and varied affect, generating many new and different elements from which the couple can construct their own solutions.

Finally, we have used the model in consultation with therapists subscribing to other theory bases. They and their clients have found it very helpful. Just as we have discovered that a structured action sequence not normally associated with our theoretical frame can enhance our effectiveness within that frame, so other therapists may find

---

[5]Notable exceptions include the work of Steve de Shazer (1985), Eve Lipchik (Lipchik & de Shazer, 1986), and Michael White (1988a, 1988b).

that this or other action sequences can enhance their effectiveness within their own theoretical frames.

ACHIEVING MOVEMENT

We can arbitrarily group the new elements commonly generated in the context of our method as occurring in three domains of experience:

1. *Affect.* Between the partners, the climate generally becomes warmer, judgments are softened, hope increases, empathy is stimulated, expectations are aroused, and openness and vulnerability expand as defensiveness is reduced.

2. *Behavior.* The partners may come to the interview accustomed to ignoring, undermining, and attacking each other for past failures, current frustrations, and hopelessness about the future. Our objective in using this method is to provide a context in which clients can interrupt chronically frustrating behavioral patterns—a context that is conducive to their developing and trying out new realities and interactional patterns. In this session, the partners may experience attentiveness, cooperation, and support. The scenes they play out may have a kind of rehearsal value. While they are unlikely simply to repeat them at home, clients often report that their subsequent interactions include analogues of their enactments or changes that appear "out of the blue."

3. *Cognition.* The focus shifts away from entrenchment in difficulties. Those clients who attribute all problems to the partner "who will never change" have food for thought in the material of the enactments. The presence of the desired behavior and the absence of the problem behavior provoke each partner to ponder what it would be like not to respond in the habitual way. When habitual reactions are excluded, partners may realize that their usual responses are not compelled by the other partner. They develop other possibilities, other ideas about their own and their partner's behavior.

Moreover, the role reversals employed in these specific enactments provide alternative perspectives from which each client can experience and view a given interaction. Empathic understanding can be called into play where before there was defensiveness or blame.

The specific enactments and sequencing used in the model can provide a safe context in which participants can experiment with different constructions of the past, present, and future, and this, we believe, may be the model's central value. It allows clients and therapist to defy the convention that the past is immutable. While the "objective" events of the past may not change, the way we construct them can and does change. The enactments can free the client from the "illusion" of a fixed past, and open the way for fresh constructions about the past and all that follows it. Furthermore, the enactments stimulate clients to develop new and vivid images, which can enrich and enliven their vision of the future and disrupt the sense they may have of simple linear continuity from past to present to future.

The enactments in multiple time frames are compressed into a very short period of time. The juxtaposition of experiences in all time frames with rapid role reversals and intense affect fosters an enrichment of clients' and therapist's ideas about what is, what was, what is desired, and what role each partner plays in the couple's developing partnership. The partners are not simply victims of past and present tribulations, nor is each destined to continue disappointing the other in the future. The confusion of time, place, and person unsettles the static images each partner has held of the self, the other, and the relationship, allowing new visions of the future to form.

Acknowledgment

We thank Michele Bograd for her invaluable contributions to the conceptualization of this chapter.

REFERENCES

Andersen, T. (1987). The reflecting team: Dialogue and metadialogue in clinical work. *Family Process 26*(4), 415–428.

Anderson, H., & Goolishian, H.A. (1988). Human systems as linguistic systems: Some preliminary and evolving ideas about the implications for clinical theory. *Family Process, 27*(4), 371–393.

Chasin, R., Roth, S., & Bograd, M. (1989). Action methods in systemic therapy: Dramatizing ideal futures and reformed pasts with couples. *Family Process, 28*(1), 121–136.

Chasin, R. & White, T. (1988). The child in family therapy: Guidelines for active engagement across the age span. In L. Combrinck-Graham (Ed.), *Children in family contexts: Perspectives on treatment.* New York: Guilford Press.

de Shazer, S. (1985). *Keys to solution in brief therapy.* New York: Norton.

Duhl, F.J., Kantor, D., & Duhl, B.S. (1973). Learning, space, and action in family therapy: A primer of sculpture therapy. In D.A. Bloch (Ed.), *Techniques of family psychotherapy: A primer.* New York: Grune & Stratton.

Erickson, M.H. (1954). Pseudo-orientation in time as a hypnotherapeutic procedure. *Journal of Clinical and Experimental Hypnosis, 2,* 261–283. Reprinted in J.Haley (1967) (Ed.), *Advanced techniques of hypnosis and therapy: Selected papers of Milton H. Erickson, M.D.* New York: Grune & Stratton.

Haley, J. (1973). *Uncommon therapy: The psychiatric techniques of Milton H. Erickson, M.D.* New York: Norton.

Hoffman, L. (1988). A constructivist position for family therapy. *Irish Journal of Psychology, 9,* 110–129.

Kantor, D. (1980). Critical identity image: A concept linking individual, couple, and family development. In J. K. Pearce & L. J. Friedman (Eds.), *Family therapy: Combining psychodynamic and family systems approaches.* New York: Grune & Stratton.

Lee, R. (1981). Video as adjunct to psychodrama and role-playing. In J. L. Fryrear & R. Fleshman (Eds.), *Videotherapy and mental health.* Springfield, IL: Charles C Thomas.

Lipchik, E., & de Shazer, S. (1986). The purposeful interview. *Journal of Strategic and Systemic Therapies, 5,* 88–89.

Madanes, C. (1981). *Strategic family therapy.* San Francisco: Jossey-Bass.

Minuchin, S., & Fishman, H. C. (1981). *Family therapy techniques.* Cambridge, MA: Harvard University Press.

Papp, P. (1976). Family choreography. In P.J. Guerin (Ed.), *Family therapy: Theory and practice.* New York: Gardner Press.

Penn, P. (1982). Circular questioning. *Family Process, 21*(3), 267–280.

Penn, P. (1985). Feed-forward: Future questions, future maps. *Family Process, 24*(3), 299–310.

Sacks, J. (1978). The reformed auxiliary ego technique: A psychodramatic rekindling of hope. *Group Psychotherapy and Psychodrama, 23,* 118–121.

Satir, V. (1972). *Peoplemaking.* Palo Alto, CA: Science and Behavior Books.

Selvini-Palazzoli, M., Boscolo, L., Cecchin, G., & Prata, G. (1980). Hypothesizing–circularity–neutrality: Three guidelines for the conductor of the session. *Family Process, 19*(1), 3–12.

Tomm, K. (1987). Interventive interviewing: Part II. Reflexive questioning as a means to enable self-healing. *Family Process, 26*(2), 167–183.

White, M. (1988a). Assumptions and therapy. *Dulwich Centre Newsletter,* Autumn, 7–8.

White, M. (1988b). The process of questioning: A therapy of literary merit? *Dulwich Centre Newsletter,* Winter, 8–14.

8

A Systemic Perspective on the Opening of a Therapeutic Encounter

KATHY WEINGARTEN

INTRODUCTION: A SYSTEMIC APPROACH

In this volume we are shown four actual approaches to one couple, Larry and Jennifer, and we are shown how several other therapists would have approached the case had they had the opportunity. Since none of the therapists represented here was in a position to conduct long-term therapy with the couple, the focus of this volume is on approach—that is, on theoretical orientation, problem definition, and initial therapeutic hypotheses and maneuvers. In this chapter, I will use systemic thinking in approaching this case. Specifically, I will discuss how I, as a systemic therapist, would have identified the meaningful system, defined the problem, and selected for myself the therapeutic position in which I would be least likely to become a part of the problem. I will begin by outlining some of the core concepts of systemic theory; then I will apply those ideas to assessment; and, finally, I will suggest how a systemic assessment of the case of Larry and Jennifer might have proceeded.

The meaning of the word "systemic," as I intend it, goes beyond two common uses of the term. I am not using the word "systemic" simply to signify the gestalt notion that the whole (e.g., a family or system) is greater than the sum of its parts (the individual members), though I would certainly agree with this idea. Nor am I using the word "systemic" to connote an adherence to general systems theory (von Bertalanffy, 1968), although aspects of general systems theory are incorporated into systemic work. Rather, I am using "systemic" to refer to a type of clinical thought and action that has been developed by therapists who put into practice a cluster of theoretical ideas that include (1) second-order cybernetics or the cybernetics of observing systems (Hoffman, 1985); (2) circular epistemology (Auerswald, 1985; Bateson, 1979); (3) the social construction of meaning (Maturana & Varela, 1987; Watzlawick, 1984); and (4) discontinuous change (Prigogine & Stengers, 1984). (For a discussion of these ideas, see Weingarten, 1988.)

One clinical team, known as the Milan Associates (Selvini-Palazzoli, Cecchin, Prata, & Boscolo, 1978, 1980a, 1980b), has played a pioneering role in applying these ideas to treatment. Drawing heavily upon the works of Gregory Bateson and Paul Watzlawick, they developed a clinical method that was presented and published in the late 1970s and early 1980s. At the time of the Harvard Couple Therapy Conference in 1983, my own thinking and clinical work were highly influenced by and congruent with the work of the Milan Associates. Now, in late 1987, as I set myself the task of making a book chapter out of my presentation at the conference, I see more clearly the theoretical lens I was using at the time. It was a systemic lens, but even at that time, it was not the only systemic lens being used by therapists. Nor does it adequately reflect my current systemic thinking. I have chosen not to rewrite my presentation for this volume, but rather to footnote those places where my current thinking is substantively different. My current amendments carry numbered footnotes. The footnotes that appeared in the paper I originally presented in 1983 are indicated with asterisks. In addition, I have modified the text where I believe my current thinking allows me to more clearly convey my earlier ideas. Although this format is less than ideal, I trust that the reader will appreciate the dual purpose this chapter now serves; it is a commentary both on the Harvard Couple Therapy Conference of 1983 and on the subsequent evolution of thought of one systemic thinker.

In what follows, I discuss how I think about the beginning of any therapeutic encounter. In many respects a systemic approach is more a manner of thinking than a method of doing. Although there is a great deal to learn in order to work systemically, novices are often startled to realize that there is no array of techniques to master. Rather, a systemic approach is a way of thinking about any situation that involves living beings, whether they are individuals, or they comprise a couple, a family, a community, an agency, or a government. The characteristics that distinguish these groups from one another are not necessarily significant to a systemic analysis; a systemic analysis would approach the problems of a couple in much the same way it would approach the difficulties of a community. Consequently, I will not comment in this chapter on the peculiar properties of couples in general; rather, I will concentrate on the specific patterns revealed by the way this particular couple, Jennifer and Larry, related, not only with each other, but with other people and events.

I will preface my discussion by presenting briefly four Batesonian constructs that are fundamental to the kind of systemic work that I do. Note that these constructs are not separable from one another, but are completely interwoven.

Circularity

When trying to understand how and why events occur and how and why we experience what we do, people often take a kind of "mental shortcut," making simple explanations about short sequences of events and identifying one event in the sequence as the "cause" and another as the "effect." This way of thinking is called lineal. By contrast, a circular way of thinking emphasizes large, holistic patterns among events. Consider the classic examples: The wife nags/the husband withdraws or the husband withdraws/the wife nags. Each spouse is likely to view the interaction in a lineal fashion, attributing blame to the other: "He (or she) starts it, then I react." The systemic therapist begins with the notion that each of these sequences of behavior represents only a fragment of the complex patterns of interaction between the husband and wife. The therapist would immediately attempt to broaden the domain of explanation, to search for regularities in larger patterns of interaction that include more people, more time, and more settings. He or she would view the simple lineal explanations offered by the husband and wife not as incorrect, but as incomplete and, ultimately, as unhelpful to the couple. The couple's search for simple attributions of blame—their insistence on "punctuating" their cycle with simple attributions of cause and effect—mires them in a limited understanding of their problems and of their needs, expectations, and capabilities.

Information

Bateson viewed information as the "receipt of news of difference." What we can know is limited by our perceiving apparatus: "Differences that are too slight or too slowly presented are not perceivable. They are not food for perception" (1979, p. 32). New information, however, need not involve a new current perception of an external reality. For example, the lack of a behavior where one might be expected (e.g., a "thank you") provides new information: The difference between the nonevent and an expectation provides information. The same nonevent would provide different information to an observer with different expectations: "zero, *in context*, can be meaningful: and it is the recipient of the message who creates the context" (1979, p. 51). Thus, the information received by an individual witnessing an event or an utterance (or even the lack thereof) is relative to that individual's beliefs.

A therapist may utter a single sentence to a couple in a session. Each member of the couple will interact with the sentence differently in accordance with his or her own beliefs and experiences, and thus each will receive different information from the therapist. The systemic therapist will seek to bring such differences of perception, and the premises on which they are based, to the surface.[1]

To illustrate this concept with an example close to home, if I tell my daughter that I am really enjoying her company today, I have in mind a comparison, a Batesonian "difference." She may understand that difference to be between how we are getting along today and how we didn't get along yesterday. My son may hear the same utterance and walk away with different information. He may construe the "difference" as between my enjoyment of my daughter and my enjoyment of him. If his mistaken assumption about my intention is not revealed and corrected, his later anger or sulkiness will seem unprovoked.

Pattern

Patterns involve relationships among bits of information about beliefs, actions, and the like. In a simple sequence such as AABBAABB, the pattern cannot be located in the A's or in the B's, but rather in the relationships among them—relationships that can be described but not quantified. According to the Batesonian view, the bringing forth of pattern is always an observer-dependent process. In perceiving a pattern, one must make a selection. The basis for that selection reveals as much about the person selecting as about that which is perceived. An observer can never be outside of, or separate from, that which he or she observes.

Context

Every event—every behavior, feeling, perception, or utterance—is embedded in multiple contexts: historical, political, cultural, interpersonal, personal, and so on. For example, a single act can be construed as a

---

[1] In recent years I have been influenced by the writings of Humberto Maturana and Francisco Varela (1980, 1987), who assert that the idea of information transfer, what they call "instructive interaction," is misguided. Rather, they believe that all systems are "information tight," since there is no interpretation-free transfer process from person to person, and thus, the only "meaning" is that which is specified by the system interacting with information (See also Dell, 1985.) The therapeutic activity I propose for Larry and Jennifer is not intended to "put in" specific ideas, but rather to create a context in which new ideas can be experienced.

personal rebuff, a political statement, an act of revenge, a cry for help, or a culturally defined expression of maturity. The meaning one constructs is inseparable from the contexts one attends to. One of the contexts that therapists may neglect to examine is that of the therapeutic context itself (i.e., the context in which the therapist is not an outside observer, but a full participant). As I will discuss in this chapter, I have found it helpful in my clinical work to examine that context very carefully for themes in it that are analogous to recurring themes in the client's life as revealed in other contexts.

CREATING THE OPENING OF A THERAPEUTIC ENCOUNTER

Assessment, as I view it in my work, is a process through which I try to understand as fully as possible the situation with which I have been asked to work. Assessment *is* intervention. In fact, no clinical session can provide the therapist with ideas about the situation without simultaneously influencing the situation. The therapist assesses and thereby influences (1) the client group; (2) the therapist's own position in the group; and (3) the problem. This process involves many activities designed to elucidate the situation, including, for example, questioning, listening, describing out loud, and offering possible distinctions. For the purpose of this discussion, I will present three different focal areas of assessment. As many writers have observed (Auerswald, 1971; Keeney, 1983), communication of systemic ideas might be greatly enhanced if people could write and read on spheres. But, limited as we are to writing line after straight line, it is necessary for me to present the three interconnected assessment activities sequentially rather than simultaneously, which is how they really occur in clinical thought and practice. Each assessment activity applies one or more of the Batesonian constructs I have described earlier.

Identifying the Meaningful System

Systemic therapists have always understood the importance of including nonfamily members as part of the treatment unit (Goolishian & Anderson, 1981; Hoffman & Long, 1969). By doing so, they tend to generate a more comprehensive definition of the problem than the clients alone are able to articulate. Recently, Evan Imber-Black used the term "meaningful system" to describe "that configuration of relationships and beliefs in which the family's problems and issues make sense" (Imber-Black, 1986, p. 2; see also Imber-Coppersmith, 1983). The meaningful system can include, besides nuclear family members, extended family, neighbors, members of the clergy, health care providers, previous and current mental health professionals, law officers, and agencies or institutions themselves. In short, any person, group, or institution with which people can have significant interactions may become part of a "meaningful system" at any point in time.

There is a theoretical rationale for including any involved person or agency in the meaningful system. Bateson (1972) has described a species as "coevolving" with its environment; that is, as the species evolves with the environment, the environment also evolves in response to changes in the species. The idea of coevolution has been used to explain many aspects of problem formation, maintenance, and change: A symptom is said to coevolve together with a pattern of relationships; a therapeutic team coevolves with the clients they are treating; and, as applied to the idea of a meaningful system, a problem can coevolve with any person or group that tries to understand or solve it. Thus, to work systemically, a clinician needs to embrace as much of the relevant field as possible. To be complete, the clinician will also have to include himself or herself, the "observer," in this meaningful system, as a tricky but necessary step to working systemically—that is, working in a way that respects the importance of circularity and context.

Identification of the meaningful system influences another activity: assessment of the problem. When the meaningful system is identified in one way, one definition of the problem emerges. When it is identified in another, a quite different definition of the problem emerges.[2] The reader will appreciate the central significance of identifying the meaningful system when they contrast my approach to the case of Larry and Jennifer with those presented in other chapters. Although Larry and Jennifer, as participants in a Harvard Couple Therapy Conference, may be in a unique situation, I hope to show that the process of identifying the meaningful system is critical to all cases.

Adopting a Therapeutic Position

A clinical encounter is most often initiated by a family member, therapist, or agency worker who asks for help from a clinician, either as a therapist or a consultant. In most instances, an individual or several individuals have already offered help or suggestions, and this help or

---

[2]Recently, faculty from the Galveston Family Institute have proposed an alternative conceptual framework for understanding problem formation. They suggest that problems exist when people communicate with each other in a way that reveals that they strongly agree or disagree with each other that there is a problem. From their point of view, "the problem to be diagnosed and treated, and the membership of the problem system, is determined by those in active communication regarding the problem" (Anderson, Goolishian, & Winderman, 1986, p. 7).

advice has proven ineffective in resolving the problem. In some cases, the very help or advice itself, or the way it has been offered, has inadvertently contributed to or exacerbated the problem. A clinician, of course, always wants to avoid becoming part of the problem. In fact, the "position" the clinician takes may directly influence whether the therapeutic encounter releases or hinders a process of positive change. "Positioning" refers here to the way a clinician acts with and is perceived by the members of the meaningful system. In thinking about positioning, therapists are applying ideas of context and pattern. How a clinician positions himself or herself will vary with each clinical situation, but there is one guiding principle: The positioning of the clinician should promote new openings for thought, feeling, and action, rather than closing off or entrenching current thought, feeling, or action. There are several therapeutic positions that can operationalize this principle. I will discuss two: neutrality and acceptance.

"Neutrality" refers to the capacity and activity of the clinician to remain unaligned with persons, ideas, values, and the process and outcome of the therapeutic encounter itself. By holding a position that is as neutral as possible, the therapist promotes the capacity to change, but does not foster any *particular* change or outcome. One way of adopting this stance is to accept everything that is said at one level through listening, but, at another level, through the challenging nature of the questions asked, to reject everything that is said. (See Part II of Tomm, 1984.)

Another approach to therapeutic positioning can be termed "acceptance." The clinician behaves in such a way that all members of the meaningful system feel that their beliefs are taken seriously and are understood. By not directly or indirectly challenging anyone's belief system, the therapist may also promote an especially self-revealing type of conversation.

Neutrality and acceptance are useful in guiding the clinician's positioning, in that they help the clinician to think differently from any one member of the meaningful system. However, the experience of the clients will obviously be quite different, depending on which way the clinician positions himself or herself. The clinician must make a quick assessment of the problem and what has maintained it in order to determine what he or she needs to consider in adopting a position. The rule of thumb, in general, is to avoid doing "more of the same" (Watzlawick, 1978). "More of the same" often entails appearing to ally with one subfaction against another, which tends to happen when members of the second subfaction (e.g., family members or agency representatives) are not included and cannot give their ideas about the nature of the problem or its possible solution. "More of the same" in some cases entails repeating the type of behavior of people who were involved with the problem earlier on, such as offering help from the stance of an "expert."

While systemic clinicians are deciding on the specific position they need to take, their behavior should express lively interest and concern. Once the clinician has identified the specific position required, holding it should enable members of the meaningful system to behave and feel and think differently from before. Thus, the position one holds is a form of therapeutic activity that influences the subsequent interactions.

Identifying the Stuck Place

Systems, in my view, are evolving rather than stable.* Thus, a system— for example, a family—cannot be slowly and predictably shaped into a more harmonious configuration by a therapist with clear ideas about how the family "should" be. Rather, the systemic clinician searches for those few aspects of the system in which fluctuation has slowed, where natural evolution seems stuck (Tomm, 1984), and an effort is made to cocreate new openings in meaning where no options seemed possible. It is common that the stuckness we observe is associated with beliefs that seem to us inadequate to guide current action productively. Often these beliefs involve holding a rigid duality or polarity (e.g., he is weak, she is strong) rather than embracing a more multifaceted view (e.g., he is weak in this situation but not in that one). When old beliefs that fit former circumstances guide current behavior in new circumstances, stuckness can develop. Obviously, identifying signs of stuckness is no easy task, it requires skill. Lynn Hoffman notes that "the family gives up to the therapist a little part of its 'truth' in any one session. And this 'truth' keeps changing. For example, it is constantly being modified or even created by the encounter with the therapist. It takes hard work, observation, and intuition to get a 'fix' on a family. . . ." (Hoffman, 1983, p. 49).

Though I may be stretching the metaphor of "stuckness" too far, I have found it useful to imagine that those parts of a system in

---

*My view of a system derives from a number of sources, including Gregory Bateson's work (1972, 1979); the applications of Bateson's theory to family systems by the Milan Associates (Selvini-Palazzoli et al., 1978, 1980a, 1980b); the work of Ilya Prigogine in physics (Prigogine & Stengers, 1984); Humberto Maturana's work in biology (Maturana & Varela, 1980); and the application of these theories to family systems made by Karl Tomm (1984) and Bradford Keeney (1983). A system maintains equilibrium through continuous fluctuations. Precisely because of these continuous fluctuations, a system can potentially make a change in its pattern, a change that seems to an observer to be rapid and discontinuous with everything that has existed before. This idea of rapid, discontinuous change contrasts sharply with the view derived from general system theory that a system is stably organized, and that change is gradual and continuous.

fluctuation seem to vary so much that one cannot even perceive a pattern to describe. Only those aspects that are stuck, are slowed down, and show minimal fluctuation can be perceived as a describable pattern. To identify stuckness, the clinician must consider all levels of data, from content and process to overall (meta)patterns based on both. The clinician will search for redundancies, for bits of content, process, and pattern that reappear across contexts and over time. In this view, such redundancies provide clues to the stuck place insofar as they direct the therapist's attention to those constraints in a system that limit its capacity to evolve. For example, in a family in which both parents believe that men must always be strong, the father may feel constrained from showing tenderness toward his young son who cries when he is hurt or distressed. If the parents are trying to establish more equal child care roles by increasing involvement of the father with the son, their belief about "male strength" may not serve them well and could influence the development of repetitive, frustrating exchanges between the father and son and between the parents — a stuckness that surfaces in the context of decisions about child care.

Lynn Hoffman (1983) has developed what she calls a "metaphoric scaffold" to help organize the wealth of data the clinician collects. She calls this scaffold a "Time Cable" (see Figure 8.1). It has three concentric rings: The inner ring, Ring 1, is where the therapist puts data related to family dynamics; in Ring 2, the therapist stores data related to the family–therapist or family–team interactions; and, in Ring 3, the therapist puts data related to the referring context, or, as I would modify it, data related to any members of the meaningful system (e.g., school-teachers) who are not part of the family or team. Each of the three rings stretches forward and backward through time, in periods Hoffman has labeled Future or Hypothetical Time, Present Time, Onset Time, Historical Time, and Mythic Time. Virtually any datum can be located on the Time Cable, which then serves as a template for mapping information and making redundancies stand out in bold relief.

Other Therapeutic Activities as Part of the Opening of the Therapeutic Encounter

A number of therapeutic activities[3] (some already described as assessments) appear to "release" constraints within complex systems and

---

[3]In my earlier draft of this chapter, I used the word "intervention" instead of the phrase "therapeutic activity." As indicated in footnote 1, I am uncomfortable with the instrumentality implied by intervention, to the extent that it implies that information from outside a system (individual, couple, family, etc.) can be simply "put in" to it. Rather, conversation and similar therapeutic activities can help open individuals to what they already know or can accept.

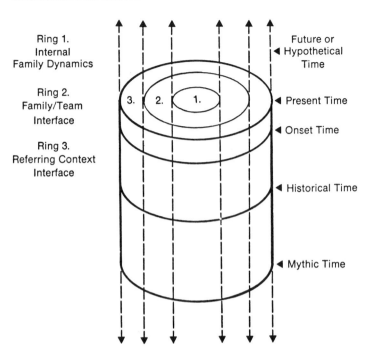

Ring 1.
Internal
Family Dynamics

Ring 2.
Family/Team
Interface

Ring 3.
Referring Context
Interface

3.   2.   1.

Future or
◄ Hypothetical
Time

◄ Present Time

◄ Onset Time

◄ Historical Time

◄ Mythic Time

FIGURE 8.1.   The Time Cable. From "A Co-Evolutionary Framework" (p. 42) by L. Hoffman, 1983, in B. Keeney (Ed.), *Diagnosis and Assessment in Family Therapy.* Rockville, MD: Aspen. Copyright 1983 by Aspen Systems Corporation. Reprinted by permission.

permit or activate changes in behavior. Also of importance is the attitude of the systemic therapist. In accordance with systemic ideas, he or she must avoid the temptation to import "better" solutions into the system. Stuckness is not conceptualized as a system's using an inadequate solution which will be replaced when "better" solutions are offered; rather, useful change can take place when the therapist helps make "room" for new thinking by the clients. A systemic therapist, using neutrality or acceptance as positioning principles, does not struggle over whose solutions are better.

In the designing of questions, the clinician has an opportunity to put systemic constructs into practice. Questioning is a primary therapeutic activity. Questions that encourage *new connections* are useful in stimulating new thinking. For example, "Did the school guidance counselor change his level of involvement with Karen at any point in the fall? What else was going on at the time?" Such questions might prompt the family to consider the connection between events they previously treated as unrelated. They will be more receptive to connections that they have made for themselves than those "put to them" by an "expert" outsider.

A second form of useful question is one that specifically asks about *differences*, whether they are differences over time (e.g., "What was the family like when Joe was at home?") or differences between relationships (e.g., "Do you agree more with your father or with your mother about how the problem affects Carol?"). These questions, called "circular questions" (Penn, 1982; Tomm, 1984), are a technique for provoking system members to realize and express what they already know, and learn what others know. They don't impose solutions. These questions also emphasize that there are specific contexts for specific behaviors and that there is a relationship between one person's behavior, thoughts, or actions and those of another. Ultimately, they bring to the surface information that may stimulate family members to let go of outmoded beliefs and construct new ones.

A third type of question, the reflexive question (Tomm, 1985), promotes *self-awareness* by purposefully activating the "reflexivity" that exists among meanings within an individual's own belief system. This complex concept is best conveyed by examples. If a couple describes a fight as taking place within the ongoing context of a generally loving relationship, a reflexive question such as, "When you are fighting, do you feel more loving or less loving?" might startle the couple and produce sudden shifts in thinking.

In another form of therapeutic activity, the therapist introduces a slightly different view that does not violate the current views of anyone present. When individuals simultaneously consider their original view and a new one that is slightly different, they may experience a new level of awareness—what Bateson likens to the bonus of binocular vision, depth perception (Bateson, 1979; de Shazer, 1982). Reframing messages and suggesting rituals (Imber-Black, Roberts, & Whiting, 1988) are two examples of therapeutic activity that can offer a view just different enough to trigger such a new depth of awareness.

Many people are familiar with one type of reframing message, in which the therapist connects the presenting problem with a wide array of "positively connoted" family behavior. The therapist presents all family behavior connected to the problem as somehow desirable. It then seems reasonable for the therapist to suggest that the family temporarily restrain itself from changing the problem behavior, since that behavior is inextricably tied to valuable family practices. The message that the family should restrain change is not what directly makes the difference. Rather, it is the new thinking triggered in the family as they grapple with the distinction between their original "negatively connoted" frame for the problem and the new, also tolerable, "positively connoted" frame for it.

Working with a broadly defined meaningful system is another systemic practice that facilitates change. When one enlarges everyone's field of vision to include all relevant contexts, circularity or "holistic patterns" may be realized. This is one reason it is useful to include all those people and agencies that contribute to the maintenance of the problem (even though these same people and agencies may be trying to solve the problem).

I have described some forms that therapeutic activity can take at the opening of a therapeutic encounter. These activities are also useful at later stages of therapy. The content of these activities is, of course, determined on a case-by-case basis, and is guided by the conceptual activity of hypothesizing. Although all therapeutic activity is guided by hypothesizing, the hypothesizing that I refer to here is a deliberate part of a carefully tracked, continuous feedback loop between therapist and members of the meaningful system. The object of the therapeutic activity is to loosen constraints in thinking and permit the coevolution of meaning to occur. Using the case of Larry and Jennifer, I will illustrate one therapeutic activity that could have enabled new meanings to evolve, creating openings for new thinking, feeling, and behaving for me and the conference participants.

To summarize, the systemic therapist's task in the beginning of the therapeutic encounter is to simultaneously engage in three interconnected activities: to determine who and what contributes to the pattern that maintains the current problem; to work on a definition of the problem that can make sense of the widest number of significant contexts in which the problem exists; and to consider what position the therapist will take in interacting with the diverse elements of the meaningful system so as not to become caught up in the problematic pattern, or stuck place. By carefully exploring the situation at hand, the clinician begins to interact with system members in a way that frees up the system's own inherent capacity to find alternatives.

THE HARVARD COUPLE THERAPY CONFERENCE AS A THERAPEUTIC ENCOUNTER

Although the efforts of a great many people contributed to the Harvard Couple Therapy Conference, chief among them were those of the couple themselves, Jennifer and Larry. Their generosity in sharing their stories with strangers is rare and wonderful. If in this chapter I focus "analytically" on this quality, I in no way wish to diminish their contribution.

Jennifer and Larry are both articulate, bright, caring, and loving people whose relationship has seen rough times and good times. Through the 10 years of their relationship up to 1982, they had—in a sense—grown up together, and had also weathered a significant crisis.

In 1982, with the crisis seemingly behind them, they turned from matters of survival to matters of happiness. Neither was as happy as he or she would have liked. They attributed their unhappiness to their "relationship." They could have become resigned, had affairs, or separated. Instead, they turned to couple therapy as a possible vehicle through which they could learn enough, and change enough, to find happiness with each other.

Assessment of the Meaningful System and My Position

As a workshop leader for the conference, I received the case report presented in Chapter 2 of this volume, which was written by the psychiatric resident who had been seeing Larry and Jennifer in couple therapy. My analysis of the case is based solely on this case report, which was the only information I had about the couple prior to the conference. The couple's therapist had collected information about those people she believed contributed to problem formation in the couple— namely, Jennifer, Larry, their parents, and members of their families. In one paragraph she describes tasks she assigned to the couple. This material suggests that she confined the treatment unit to Jennifer and Larry. Although one might be able draw some inferences from that material about the therapist–couple dynamic, we are presented mostly with the "problem" as something that is in the relationship or in Jennifer (and her history) or in Larry (and his history). There is little evidence that the therapist locates any problems in the therapy itself, or in any other configuration of relationships.

From my theoretical orientation, the meaningful system in this case would be more inclusive. I would highlight parts of the report that are mentioned only in passing and also examine the context of the report itself. The report mentions Larry's mother, father, brother, and cousins; Jennifer's mother, father, sister, brother-in-law, nephews, and niece; Jennifer's individual therapist; and the friends and work colleagues of Larry and Jennifer. Any or all of these people could have been part of the meaningful system. To find out whether they are, I would ask the couple a series of questions, such as these:

- What are your parents' explanations for the difficulties the two of you have?
- What kind of advice, if any, do they give you?
- Did you discuss coming to treatment together as a couple with your therapist, Jennifer?
- What were your therapist's thoughts about the couple treatment?
- Was seeing your therapist jointly ever a possibility?
- Of the people who know about the problems you have with each

other, who is most optimistic (pessimistic) about your future together?

• How would you describe your relationship to your physician, Larry?

• Do your work colleagues share with you their opinions about your relationship?

The answers to these questions would yield information about the extent to which any of these people should be considered part of the meaningful system; or, put another way, they would reveal to me which people communicate with Jennifer and/or Larry about their relationship, and define it as "problematic" or "not problematic." (See footnote 2.)

I would also consider the context within which the couple were selected and the report was written. As I tried to reconstruct the conference history, I would imagine that its leaders circulated a memo to family therapy supervisors and trainees asking them to consider whether any couple they had in treatment might be an appropriate "case" for the conference. The supervisor and psychiatric resident involved in Jennifer's and Larry's treatment obviously felt that they were a suitable couple, and, I trust, discussion followed about how to present the possibility to them. I am guessing that once the therapist accepted the idea that Jennifer and Larry might participate in the conference, her relationship to them shifted, as did theirs to her. At that point, the therapist (and, I presume, the supervisor and conference leaders) had a different stake in the couple. The therapist could no longer feel detached from the couple's feelings and decisions regarding their part in the conference. She and her teachers were no longer solely providing psychotherapeutic services for the couple, but were asking the couple to go through an extraordinary process for the educational benefit of others as well as themselves. If this description is roughly accurate, then a curious shift in the therapeutic relationship may have occurred. Jennifer and Larry were empowered, since the conference was dependent on their cooperation; but they were simultaneously disempowered, since the people who would attend the conference would regard them as objects of scrutiny. This created an incongruous hierarchy (Madanes, 1981) between the couple on the one hand, and their therapist, the conference personnel, and the audience on the other. An incongruous hierarchy is said to be created when the same action(s) confers superiority and inferiority relative to others.[4] The incongruous hierarchy in

---

[4]Since the time of my original writing, I am less comfortable asserting that hierarchy is created. Rather, I am more comfortable thinking that "perceiving" hierarchy is one way that observers/participants describe patterns of interactions to themselves. That is, hierarchy doesn't objectively exist in this situation, but may be brought forth by

this situation is associated with an extreme "complementary" relation-ship, a type of relationship I will discuss at length in a few pages. One would expect that the couple was not impervious to their simultaneous empowerment and disempowerment. This would make the conference situation a part of their lives, a part of their meaningful system.

Assessment of a Position

Once the meaningful system is defined as including (at least) Jennifer, Larry, their relatives, the therapist, supervisor, and conference leaders, certain therapeutic positions would be untenable if I were to conduct a systemic session with the couple only. I couldn't position myself as a therapist or a consultant, because then I would become a simple addition to the existing system. I would need to find a position that enabled me to operate respectfully toward everyone without a trace of my being hierarchically above or below anyone else (i.e., without contributing to the incongruous hierarchy that I felt had developed). Using my given role as a workshop leader, however, I could position myself outside the hierarchical pattern. I could take the stance of "doing my homework so I can lead a productive workshop"; I could ask for additional information, perhaps even convene a short meeting of the meaningful system, without immediately becoming part of what may have become a stuck place for this group.

Assessment of the Meaningful System's Stuckness

After having defined the meaningful system more broadly, I would look for "stuckness" in interactions in that system. Unfortunately for my purposes, the report does not give me what I need because the original therapist's lens is set differently from mine. She includes some data that are not particularly relevant within my theoretical framework, and she does not include other data that would be useful to me, such as detailed information about the therapy itself and the negotiation with the couple to participate in the conference. Upon these points, I am forced to speculate. Putting speculation aside for the moment, I will look for stuckness in the data given in her report. If there is stuckness there it will appear as redundancies across Rings 1, 2, and 3, and it will appear over time. The majority of the data the therapist has collected can be located in Ring 1 (the family) and in Present, Onset, and Historical Time.

---

participants or observers by the way they communicate with each other about this situation. Clearly, I brought forth "hierarchy," and this idea organizes much of my subsequent thinking about the couple and this conference.

The description of the therapist's task assignments can be located in Ring 2 (family–therapist interaction) and in Present Time.

Searching for redundant elements involves a tracking process, which is sometimes easy and sometimes laborious. In my review of the materials, I perceived at least two redundant elements, potential indicators of stuckness, appearing across contexts and over time.[5]

The first redundant element appears in Jennifer's and Larry's families' backgrounds, their personal histories, the history of their relationships, and in recent interactions. It consists of themes of paired opposites: open–closed, intimacy–distance, and intrusion–separateness.* (Later in the discussion, I will refer to the three paired opposites using the single term "open–closed.") Because examples of these paired opposites are so numerous in the report, I will comment on representative samples starting with Ring 1, hoping that the reader will then be able to locate others.

The cursory facts Jennifer highlights about her parents' histories can be labeled using one of the paired opposites. Jennifer's father was an "adventurous type"** (open to new experience), but her mother's history is "dark with secrets" (closed). Growing up, Jennifer says, feelings could not be discussed (distance, separateness, closed), yet her body was regularly invaded by enemas and her phone calls were monitored (intimacy, intrusion, openness).

Larry's background contains a similar mixture of the three paired opposites. Although they came from a religious and ethnic tradition that values closeness, Larry's father's sisters quarreled and several didn't speak to each other for years (closed, separate, distant). His mother's family had much intimate contact with each other (open), but his mother restricted what Larry could tell them (closed, separateness). Curiously, for such a friendly, intimate family, Larry reports that only at his brother's wedding, when his brother was leaving home, did he feel he "was introduced" to him. In a family with open doors, open refrigerator policies, and TVs on, Larry had to "closet" himself to get breathing space.

Open–closed is a theme that is present in all families' histories and interactions, and is not necessarily connected to a belief system that has outlived its usefulness. Jennifer and Larry, though, appear to have

---

[5]The fact that I perceive two redundant elements doesn't make them useful theoretical constructs. I remain skeptical about my own cognitive processing at this point, knowing that when I begin interacting with the other members of the conference this perception may be useless.

*I am assuming that this redundant element "exists" independently of the therapist's cognitive schema that led her to write about the data she collected in a particular way.

**From this point forward, all quotes not attributed to other sources have been taken from the therapist's written report (see Chapter 2, this volume).

submerged, de-emphasized, or overlooked examples of their families' behavior that do not fit with their characterization of Jennifer's family as "closed" and Larry's as "open." Thus, we seem to have evidence that they hold distorted beliefs about their own and each other's families. They have created, probably cocreated with each other and their families, a polarity, such that there is "openness" on the one side and "closedness" on the other. Finally, when they entered couple therapy they indicated that they value "openness" more than they value "closedness"; they expressed a shared desire "to improve communication."

Obviously, the situation cannot be adequately described by these simple characterizations. I would say that each grew up in (and continues to create in the present) an environment in which each of the polar opposite dimensions contextualizes the other: Intimacy existed in the context of distance (e.g., Jennifer dated other men while still very much involved with Larry; Jennifer's mother conducted "night inspections" that left Jennifer feeling more and more alienated—separateness in the context of intrusion). Openness existed in the context of closedness (e.g., when Larry's mother insisted that he include his shyer cousin in his play, reinforcing the idea that Larry could be involved with outsiders *only* if an insider, a relative, were part of the group). I could also give examples of the opposite (i.e., distance in the context of intimacy, etc.).

I am not certain that Jennifer and Larry are doing justice to their total experience when they suggest that they value openness over closedness. I think their behavior shows that they feel some conflict both individually and as a couple as to whether it is better to live in an "open" or "closed" way. Since they conceptualize the two as pure types, with no shades in between, it is certainly easy to understand why conflict would arise.

The second redundant element I noticed, again locating it first in Ring 1, appears in the form of the relationships Jennifer and Larry have developed with many of the significant figures in their lives. Gregory Bateson, in *Naven* (Bateson, 1958), proposed that there are two basic forms relationships can take.[6] In the complementary form, one person's behavior fits another's behavior but is essentially different from it. In the symmetrical form, one person's behavior provokes the same kind of behavior in another person. There are many types of complementary

---

[6]I used to find it very helpful to order my observations about relationships by using Bateson's schema. His descriptions still seem valid to me, but I rarely order my observations using this paradigm. In effect, the terms summarize complex interactions. I prefer to think about the complexities of the interactions, rather than working with a summarizing label.

relationship: for example, master–slave, expert–novice, abuser–victim, caretaker–dependent, to name a few. Usually one role is believed to be hierarchically superior to the other. Jennifer and Larry seem to engage in complementary behavior, especially of the caretaker–dependent sort. Historically, both were in such complementary relationships with their opposite-sex parents. Jennifer shared a bed with her father until age six and "felt responsible for his survival." Larry's mother was an all-nurturing woman who, even now, brings chickens in her suitcase when she visits.

With their parents they were in complementary relationships of the caretaker–dependent sort, and they formed this type of relationship with each other as well, but adopted reverse roles. Jennifer, who felt she had to take care of her father, saw Larry for the first five years as "someone she relied on"; she could count on his consistent presence. Larry, who was nurtured by his mother, took the nurturing role with Jennifer, who he thought was "mixed up and needed to be taken care of."

Jennifer and Larry believed that their behaviors—Jennifer's dependence and Larry's caretaking—were characterologic features intrinsic to each of them. From a systemic perspective, these "characteristics" would be described as repeated patterns of transaction between people in certain contexts, patterns that will change if the circumstances change, (Bateson, 1979). This is precisely what seems to have happened after Larry developed cancer. Jennifer took care of him when he seemed to be the one more needy of help—physically and emotionally. Thus the complementary pattern of caretaker–dependent one remained stable, but the assignment of roles switched.

The two redundant elements in Ring 1 are that Jennifer and Larry (1) have the following thematic elements in many of their experiences: open–closed, intrusion–separateness, and intimacy–distance; and (2) form complementary relationships. These two elements were also present in the traumatic situation of Larry's cancer. Larry's cancer posed the threat of death, a threat that created the possibility of ultimate distance/closed/separateness. Whatever the quality of Larry and Jennifer's daily transactions, they were then contextualized or framed by the specter of death. If once Jennifer's affairs and separations contextualized their intimacy and closeness and introduced distance and separateness, later the possibility of Larry's death did this too.

I think that cancer almost always places those who get it into complementary relationships. They are described as "victims" of cancer, which is the "attacker." Chemotherapy, radiotherapy, megavitamins—all "counterattacks"—are compensatory symmetrical challenges in this grim complementary game. Although there may be many explanations for Larry's refusal to endure the chemotherapy any longer, one consequence of his decision is that it will be harder to predict how successful his "fight" against the cancer will be. His decision freed him from the tyranny of chemotherapy, while at the same time it intensified his complementary relationship with the cancer, since his survival is less certain than if he had continued with treatment. Only time will tell.

It is noteworthy that Larry and Jennifer sought treatment, another complementary relationship (albeit of a different type: doctor–patient not attacker–victim) just when Larry crossed the five-year cancer survival milestone. With the passage of time, their complementary relationship with cancer has faded. Also, the passage of time, and Larry's continued cancer-free existence within it, have rendered his cancer a less potent symbol of distance/closed/separateness. Now, if the enduring pattern is to be retained (i.e., if intimacy, openness, or even intrusion, is to be contextualized by distance or closedness or separateness), something besides the specter of death will have to provide distance.

Entering couple therapy established another complementary relationship (therapist/expert/caretaker, couple/clients/needy ones); once the therapist included in her work the assignment of tasks that addressed themselves precisely to the issues of intimacy and distance, both redundant elements that I have described as present in Ring 1 became present in Ring 2, the clients–therapist interactions. The therapist assigned Larry and Jennifer the task of spending "four hours together without TV or work." They responded by Jennifer working at home while Larry was studying. The task was reassigned with the "emphasis on no work. Both read. They were surprised to realize they didn't use that time to talk. Distance was maintained."

I would say that in the therapy there was a fit or consonance between the therapist's guiding clinical premise (that this couple needs to be able to experience noninvasive closeness without resorting to distancing mechanisms like TV watching or studying) and the couple's outmoded* belief (that one should seek openness, intimacy, and separateness and avoid their respective polar opposites: closedness, distance, and intrusion). To the extent that the therapy amplified the outmoded belief—to the extent that the couple perceived the therapist to be endorsing "openness"—their stuckness was not loosened.

At about this time, the therapist began negotiating with Jennifer and Larry to participate in the Harvard Couple Therapy Conference. They were "needed" to put on the conference; the people in need of help (the couple) would be helping the conference staff to help the professionals (the audience). If they agreed, their intimate private lives and therapy would be exposed to hundreds of people. The two redundant elements that appear in Ring 1 (forming complementary relationships and having open–closed, intrusion–separateness, intimacy–distance be the context

---

*It was outmoded because the belief did not adequately represent their full experience.

for each other) now appear also in Ring 3. The conference presented many opportunities to form complementary relationships with conference staff (e.g., with the senior therapists who would interact with them as clients, and with the conference leaders who would need to attend to anxieties in these therapists and the couple). The conference also was a setting in which the three paired elements could contextualize each other in quite a dramatic way. Hundreds of therapists would be learning (intruding on) intimate details of their lives, while remaining fundamentally separate and distant from them. The seeming privacy (closedness) of the interviews with each of the senior therapists would be illusory, since the sessions would be shown on a large screen to the audience (openness). Given my own way of thinking about this clinical situation, I conclude that, unintentionally and unwittingly, the conference may have added to the very stuckness it hoped to diminish. However, since I may be the only conference participant who describes or identifies the stuckness in the way I do, I may be the only one who is troubled by this irony. Now that I have formed this hypothesis, it becomes important for me to enter into conversation with other conference participants so that I can modify or reject the hypothesis through the feedback that will occur. In other words, I must enter into dialogue and leave what has been said above, essentially, a monologue.

Implementing Therapeutic Activity

I will now describe how I, as a systemic therapist, might have implemented therapeutic activity in the relevant systems that included the couple at the time of the conference. Above all else, I would want to avoid contributing to the stuckness that I conjectured had developed in the meaningful system. I would take a position from which I could quickly get a sense of the nature of the problem and the meaningful system within which the problem definition had emerged. From the first time I read the couple's case report I felt that the problem, the "stuckness," existed at many levels, not the least of which was at the level of the entire conference itself. It seemed to me that as a workshop leader I could identify a position from which I could interact with the conference community in a new way, a way that would not establish yet another complementary relationship. I could use my status as a workshop leader to try to introduce a noncomplementary form of relationship to the meaningful system defined as all the conference participants. From my vantage point, I might be able to introduce some new ways to think about the open–closed, intimacy–distance, and intrusion–separateness themes.

My initial hypothesis was simple: Having passed the five-year survival mark, Jennifer and Larry came to couple therapy to improve their relationship. The couple entered a complementary relationship first with the therapy and then with the conference. Additionally, the therapy and the conference were two settings in which intimacy and distance could contextualize each other. Finally, the therapy and the Conference subtly supported the same polarization of open versus closed that characterized Jennifer's, Larry's, and their families' thinking, and indirectly suggested that openness is better than closedness.*

I believe that my hypothesis is systemic, that it describes a holistic pattern across contexts and over time, and that it respects the fundamental systemic principal of circularity. I believe that it could be useful as a springboard to open conversation between me and the conference participants. But I must emphasize that my hypothesis would serve only as a starting point; my mind would remain open, receptive to feedback about it and about other ideas that may develop. The hypothesis must not function like a Procrustean bed on which I must lie because I made it.[7]

In addition to assuming a particular position vis-à-vis the meaningful system (that I have now defined as including the couple, the therapist, the supervisor, the conference leaders, the therapists, and participants), I would also want to behave in such a way that I could influence the beliefs of members of the meaningful system. The beliefs I would want to influence are the ones that are outmoded or that appear to be connected to redundant patterns of behaviors. The polarization of open versus closed, and the associated belief that open is better, seem to represent a source of constraint (stuckness) for Jennifer and Larry; insofar as this belief has been taken up by the conference staff, it represents a source of constraint for them (and us) as well. New thinking and new behavior about openness–closedness can be facilitated by engaging in conversation that stimulates various alternatives (intermediate positions) to the two poles: "open is good" on the one side and "closed is bad" on the other. Conversation that fosters new distinctions about open–closedness (e.g., openness in this context is useful but openness in that context is not) may release the system members to experience and create new meanings for themselves.

When I attempt to identify the meaningful system I prefer to work individually, by phone or in person, with as many potential members of the meaningful system as possible. I find that by doing so there is less

---

*One not so subtle way that this happens is that the conference depends on the liveliness of the couple's interviews with the senior therapists. The less open they are in these interviews, the less rewarding will the conference be for the audience.

[7]Forming a systemic hypothesis at the opening of the therapeutic encounter is not the only way of promoting a circular epistemology in the therapist's thinking. Listening for each person's hypothesis, fresh, without having formulated one of one's own, is another way to promote a circular epistemology (Anderson & Goolishian, 1986, 1988).

likelihood that I will offend significant people, who, if they are offended, may react in ways that would intensify the system's stuckness. I also find that by working with as complete a meaningful system as possible I am less likely to replicate moves already tried by other members of the meaningful system, because I have more information about what these moves have been. In this way I gain insight into how I can avoid contributing to the system's stuckness.

Sometimes my work with a large meaningful system is followed by shifts in the composition of the meaningful system. For example, some people who have been intensely involved bow out—temporarily or permanently. The meaningful system evolves over time. I continue to work as much as I can with the group that continues to be engaged with each other about "the problem." Sometimes, I do end up working with only a couple or an individual.

In the case of Larry and Jennifer, given my particular hypothesis, I could imagine two ways of proceeding that might be useful. I present them in order of preference.

Plan One

I would call the conference leaders and ask if they were going to have a preconference gathering of the central conference group—that is, Jennifer, Larry, their therapist, her supervisor, the senior family therapists, and themselves. If so, I would ask if I could attend the meeting and ask some questions that would help me prepare my workshop. If they were not planning such a meeting, I would request a brief one, and volunteer to coordinate the arrangements for it.

During all contacts with members of the meaningful system, I would position myself as a workshop leader, a committed family therapist, experienced and junior to the conference leaders and senior family therapists. My stance would be sincere but not deferential, curious but not intrusive. I believe that this position would allow me to interact with everyone at the meeting in a noncomplementary way. I think it would introduce an alternative to both complementary and symmetrical modes of behavior and, as such, could be helpful in introducing variety into the behavioral repertoire of the assembled group.*

Many of the questions I would ask would be circular and reflexive. The effect on the people (including myself) of hearing the questions and the answers to them would, I hope, also introduce ideas about relationships that are neither in the complementary nor the symmetrical mode. By asking, for example, about performance anxiety and exposure

---

*I do not mean to suggest that any individual's behavioral repertoire is limited. Rather, in the context of the conference, given this couple's issues, the behavioral options of the group have narrowed.

anxiety, I would not intensify the complementarity roles of therapist–client or leader–participants or caretaker–needy one; noncomplementary patterns would likely emerge.

Additionally, I would hope that the effect of the questions would be to depolarize the ideas of "open is good; closed is bad." The content of the questions might suggest that in some contexts it would be self-protective and wise for the couple and the senior family therapists to behave in a guarded way. Clearly many different questions would be needed to dissolve the polarity, but I think the questions and the process of answering them could set the stage for an expansion of the group's thinking on this matter. It is also likely that the assembled individuals would vary considerably in the way they reacted to the meeting. New experiences with new people around familiar themes by themselves might help free the thinking in the group.

Examples of questions that could be interspersed throughout the general flow of conversation and that, along with others, could help accomplish the goals stated above are the following:

- Who do you think has the most "on the line" at this conference? And then who? Who will be exposing the most and for whom will this matter the most?
- If Jennifer and Larry decide not to participate or to participate less fully, who will be most upset? Least upset? Then who?
- What can Jennifer, Larry, and the senior family therapists do during their interviews to protect their own and each other's interests—to safeguard the couple's right to privacy and to "save face" for the therapists—while promoting everyone's learning? Under what other circumstances would all these people be so cautious about self-disclosure?
- What discussions have taken place about the handling of the videotaping and the editing of the videotapes?
- What do you think will be the most likely/least likely and most optimistic/most pessimistic outcomes of the conference for Jennifer? Larry? their therapist? her supervisor? the senior family therapists? the workshop leaders? the conference leaders? the Cambridge Hospital Department of Psychiatry? Harvard Medical School?
- Six months after the conference what will Jennifer and Larry, their therapist, her supervisor, and so on, be thinking about couple's therapy?
- What do people think can be accomplished by the conference over time that could not be accomplished in any other way?

Plan Two

I would request a brief interview with the supervisor, therapist, Jennifer, and Larry. Again, I would position myself as a workshop leader who, in preparing her presentation, needs some background information about how Jennifer and Larry came to be the conference's featured couple. I would make it clear that I need information, not help, to fill in a small section of my talk; thus I would guard against inadvertently establishing another caretaker–needy one relationship. This position would be both therapeutically useful and intellectually honest. Given my agenda, the therapist, supervisor, Jennifer, and Larry are all equally expert.* This would alter their former complementary relationships to each other. In the process of my questioning, Jennifer and Larry would learn about their therapist's relationship to her supervisor, and the therapist and supervisor would likely hear more about Jennifer's and Larry's early thoughts on the subject of their participation in the conference. This kind of information would also tend to create greater equality within the group and moderate the hierarchical elements that can be schematized as "supervisor > therapist > Jennifer and Larry."

The new context reveals information about what gets shared, by whom, when, and under what circumstances. This information could lead to more distinctions about complexity regarding the three paired opposites. For instance, if conversations between therapist and supervisor are usually concealed from clients (closed) but in the context of this meeting it makes sense to share some of them, then the strict polarization between open and closed will have to be abandoned. Or, put another way, if the therapist acts "as if" the sessions between her and the couple are private (separateness), but in fact they are reported to a supervisor (openness, intrusion), then the meanings and values of separateness, closedness, intrusion, and openness would have to be rethought; opening of sessions to supervisory input is desirable and expected in a training context.

CONCLUSION

I have argued that it is useful to expand one's focus to include all those people, agencies, and contexts that can both hinder and facilitate

---

*I do not want to leave the reader with the impression that in systemic work the clinician never positions himself or herself as an expert. Positioning is always determined on the basis of what the case requires. For example, if two prominent child psychiatrists were to come to me for treatment with their ten-year-old daughter, I would try to identify the problem and the meaningful system. Suppose I learn early in the course of the first sessions that they have seen several psychiatrists, all of whom have been deferential to their esteemed colleagues, and were perceived by the parents as offering little help. I might then position myself as an expert with a set of particular skills and experiences that I can draw upon to help these experts with a problem for which they *want* guidance.

change. The situation of the Harvard Couple Therapy Conference, though unique in some respects, is not at all unique in others. In many ways it is just like that of any training/service institution, only its lifespan is briefer.

Jennifer and Larry, however, are unique. They have courageously faced the crisis of cancer and strengthened their commitment to each other through the ordeal. Participating in the conference is another courageous act. Though I believe the conference contained stresses for their relationship, I am also confident that their resilience, intelligence, and receptivity, combined with the skill of the conference leaders, the senior family therapists, the supervisor, and the therapist, prevented harm and promoted change.

How the elusive "change" would occur is, for me, an unanswerable question, since I deeply believe that change occurs in quirky, unpredictable ways, a belief from which I derive continual exhilaration. If I had implemented either of my two plans, I would have had at least one gauge by which to measure the likelihood that a process of opening up people's thinking was taking place: shifts in my own thinking. The therapist participates in the very processes that are designed to stimulate others. This is one of the reasons systemic work is so exciting.

REFERENCES

Anderson, H., & Goolishian, H. (1986). Systems consultation with agencies dealing with domestic violence. In L. Wynne, S. H. McDaniel, & T. T. Weber (Eds.), *Systems consultation: A new perspective for family therapy.* New York: Guilford Press.

Anderson, H., & Goolishian, H. (1988). Human systems as linguistic systems: Preliminary and evolving ideas about the implications for clinical theory. *Family Process, 27,* 371–393.

Anderson, H., Goolishian, H., & Winderman, L. (1986). Problem determined systems: Towards transformation in family therapy. *Journal of Strategic and Systemic Therapies, 5,* 1–13.

Auerswald, E. H. (1971). Families' changes and the ecological perspective. *Family Process, 10,* 268–280.

Auerswald, E. H. (1985). Thinking about thinking in family therapy. *Family Process, 24,* 1–12.

Bateson, G. (1958). *Naven.* Stanford, CA: Stanford University Press.

Bateson, G. (1972). *Steps to an ecology of mind.* New York: Ballantine Books.

Bateson, G. (1979). *Mind and nature: A necessary unity.* New York: Bantam Books.

Dell, P. (1985). Understanding Bateson and Maturana: Toward a biological foundation for the social sciences. *Journal of Marital and Family Therapy, 11,* 1–20.

de Shazer, S. (1982). *Patterns of brief family therapy: An ecosystem approach.* New York: Guilford Press.

Goolishian, H., & Anderson, H. (1981). Including non-blood related persons in family therapy. In A. Gurman (Ed.), *Questions and answers in the practice of family therapy.* New York: Brunner/Mazel.

Hoffman, L. (1983). A co-evolutionary framework. In B. Keeney (Ed.), *Diagnosis and assessment in family therapy.* Rockville, MD: Aspen.

Hoffman, L. (1985). Beyond power and control: Toward a "second order" family systems therapy. *Family Systems Medicine, 3,* 381–395.

Hoffman, L., & Long, L. (1969). A system's dilemma. *Family Process, 8,* 211–234.

Imber-Black, E. (1986). The systemic consultant and human service provider systems. In L. Wynne, S. H. McDaniel, & T. T. Weber (Eds.), *Systems consultation.* New York: Guilford Press.

Imber-Black, E., Roberts, J., & Whiting, R. (Eds.). (1988). *Rituals in families and family therapy.* New York: Norton.

Imber-Coppersmith, E. (1983). Families and multiple helpers: A systemic perspective. In D. Campbell & R. Draper (Eds.), *Applications of systemic family therapy—The Milan method.* New York: Academic Press.

Keeney, B. (1983). *Aesthetics of change.* New York: Guilford Press.

Madanes, C. (1981). *Strategic family therapy.* San Francisco: Jossey-Bass.

Maturana, H. R., & Varela, F. J. (1980). *Autopoiesis and cognition: The realization of the living.* Boston: Reidel.

Maturana, H. R., & Varela, F. J. (1987). *The tree of knowledge: The biological roots of human understanding.* Boston: New Science Library.

Penn, P. (1982). Circular questioning. *Family Process, 21,* 267–280.

Prigogine, I., & Stengers, I. (1984). *Order out of chaos.* New York: Bantam Books.

Selvini-Palazzoli, M., Cecchin, G., Prata, G., & Boscolo, L. (1978). *Paradox and counterparadox: A new model in the therapy of the family in schizophrenic transaction.* New York: Jason Aronson.

Selvini-Palazzoli, M., Cecchin, G., Prata, G., & Boscolo, L. (1980a). Hypothesizing, circularity, and neutrality: Three guidelines for the conductor of the session. *Family Process, 19,* 3–12.

Selvini-Palazzoli, M., Cecchin, G., Prata, G., & Boscolo, L. (1980b). The problem of the referring person. *Journal of Marital and Family Therapy, 6,* 3–9.

Tomm, K. (1984). One perspective on the Milan systemic approach: Part I and Part II. *Journal of Marital and Family Therapy, 10,* 113–126.

Tomm, K. (1985). Circular interviewing: A multi-faceted clinical tool. In D. Campbell & R. Draper (Eds.), *Applications of systemic family therapy: The Milan approach.* London: Grune & Stratton.

von Bertalanffy, L. (1968). *General systems theory: Foundations, development, applications.* New York: George Braziller.

Watzlawick, P. (1978). *The language of change.* New York: Norton.

Watzlawick, P. (1984). *The invented reality.* New York: Norton.

Weingarten, K. (1988). *What is systemic therapy?* Unpublished manuscript, Family Institute of Cambridge, MA.

9

Object Relations and the Couple:
Separation-Individuation, Intimacy, and Marriage

FRANCES GIVELBER

The basic developmental task of marriage is to learn to resolve conflicts around intimacy. Barnett (1971) refers to this task as the "development and integration of constructive and viable patterns of intimacy" (p. 75). His choice of words suggests that successful intimacy enhances growth ("constructive"), endures over time ("viable"), and can be expressed in a variety of forms ("patterns").

The desire for intimacy is a major motivation for marriage (Feldman, 1979). Intimacy is related to attachment: "a bonding to the other" leading to a feeling that "home is where the other is." In marriage each partner hopes for "a permanently accessible attachment figure" (Weiss, 1975, pp. 39-42). Theorists of diverse orientations emphasize the link between early infantile attachment and later adult love relationships (Bowlby, 1968; Sager, 1976a; Meissner, 1978; Dicks, 1967). An adult's capacity to give and receive love freely is seen as directly related to a successful loving reciprocity with his or her own parents. In the context of a harmonious parent–child dyad, the child develops a core sense of the self as valued, lovable, separate, and competent in relationships, and a sense of the world as good, trustworthy, and responsive to the child's unique self. An adult with this experience desires and can risk intimacy.

Every adult struggles to achieve a balance between a need to be part of something greater than the self and a need to be separate – a balance between mutuality and individuation. Bach (1980) sees the capacity to achieve such balance as directly related to the ability to establish oneself "as a center for action and thought" and to experience oneself "in the context of other selves" in relationships (p. 175). One can pose a developmental question about intimacy as follows: To what extent can one's world of self and one's world of objects be "real, intermingled, and relatively stable?" (p. 179).

In this examination of intimacy in marriage, I will begin by describing five components of viable intimacy: separateness, mutuality, acceptance of self and other, empathy, and collaboration. Then I will discuss barriers to intimacy, different styles of intimacy in marriage, and finally treatment of problems of intimacy, using Jennifer and Larry as a case example.

COMPONENTS OF VIABLE INTIMACY

Separateness

The process of separation–individuation begins in infancy with the parent's recognition and validation of the baby's unique self, expressed in the child's specific preferences for feeding, soothing, and being held. Through locomotion and actual physical separation, this "psychological birth" leads to "the first level of self-identity" (Mahler, 1974, p. 90).

The small child emerges from the mother–infant dyad with a sense of self as separate, as a center for action, feeling, and initiative. But there is a paradox inherent in this process. The child's push toward separation is supported not only by the mother's tolerance for the separateness, but by the mother's availability to the child. The adventuring toddler who can check back with his or her mother and "refuel" learns that separation is manageable, is pleasurable, and does not entail loss of the object. This process leads to the internalization of the mother so that longer periods of separation can be experienced. Separation–individuation is repeated throughout the life cycle: in adolescence, in marriage, and in parenthood.

In marriage each partner has a chance to rework patterns of separation–individuation and adopt either old or new solutions. Marital partners tend to seek in one another a similar degree of individuation. This similarity is often masked by the different defensive organizations or character styles of husband and wife so that one partner may appear quite independent and the other dependent. When both partners are relatively undifferentiated, efforts to individuate are experienced as profound threats to the relationship because differences are perceived as loss. Poorly differentiated couples cannot bear intense emotion easily; emotional flooding is common. Effective communication cannot be achieved because each mate responds with hurt feelings leading to attacks or protective withdrawal. The lack of secure individuation interferes with the assumption of responsibility for one's feelings and inadequacies. The partner is blamed with the conviction that if only he or she were different, one's own suffering would be relieved (Meissner, 1978).

The process of individuation is hampered by unresolved relationships with one's family of origin. A husband or wife who is not well differentiated imports troubled early object relations into the marriage. Dicks (1967) notes that the marital relationship might be the only arena in which these failures show up. Norman Paul (1976; Chapter 5, this volume) writes about how unresolved loss in childhood, real or fantasized, can lead to a choice of a mate who is to play a restitutive role: A person seeks what he or she had and lost or never had. Paul's ideas have their counterpart in Dicks's formulation (1967) that each marital partner seeks and sometimes persecutes in the other the lost (repressed libidinal and aggressive) parts of himself or herself. In a disturbed marriage where the partners are not well differentiated, each is so ambivalent about a conflicted area that once it is located in the partner, it is continuously elicited and criticized.

In a marriage of two reasonably integrated people, differing character styles are complementary to one another and are experienced as pleasurable and valuable. For example, a mildly obsessional man may show obvious delight in his flamboyant wife; his wife feels cared for and grounded by her partner's serious attention and enjoys his mock disapproval of her displays.

Boszormenyi-Nagy and Ulrich (1980) describe a "ledger of unpaid debts" to one's family of origin. This kind of guilt creates an "invisible loyalty" that binds the person to his or her parents so that full investment in the partner is experienced as disloyalty to the parents. Alternatively, a "deprived child" may be collecting from the wrong source, trying to settle an old debt within the marriage (pp. 170–171). (See also J. Grunebaum, Chapter 10, this volume.)

Mutuality

Mutuality implies giving and receiving, a sharing of feelings, and an experience of joint reciprocal endeavor. The capacity for mutuality is rooted in the early mother–child relationship. Dicks (1967) states that if the early dyadic experience is loving and successful, "the first, and perhaps essential step towards a good marriage will have been taken" (p. 37). Good enough mothering leads to a foundation of inner goodness and basic trust. The infant experiences a confidence in engaging the mother that creates an expectation of safety and effectiveness in relationships.

George Klein (1976) has some intriguing ideas about the relationship between individuation and what he calls "affiliation." He criticizes psychoanalytic theory for positing an ideal of autonomy and individuation that is overstated, noting that "distinctions between self-interest and interest in the other are probably less clear-cut than has been assumed in the past." Early mother–infant exchanges in play or vocalizing reveal a pleasure in pleasing the other; one's joy is enhanced if it is shared with an important other. This enables the infant "to proceed from reaction to interaction, into a self that can both affirm and be affirmed by others" (pp. 228–229). Klein believes that one's identity includes the idea of mutuality, of affiliation. He delineates two aspects of the self, the autonomous self "distinct from others . . . a locus of action and decision [and] the self construed as a necessary part of a unit transcending one's autonomous actions." He emphasizes that "'we' identities are also part of the 'self'." A person can be troubled in either or both of these two aspects. One can experience a need to be autonomous and/or a need to be needed (pp. 178–179).

Kohut (1971, 1977) also emphasizes the intrinsic relationship of self to other as part of the human condition. In contrast to some psychoanalytic writers who imply that an autonomous, separated adult does not *need* intimate relationships, but rather *chooses* to be intimate because of pleasure (Binstock, 1973), Kohut (1977) points to the need of even psychologically healthy adults for self-objects (p. 188 n.). What he means is that one's self-esteem and well-being are to some extent derived from and embedded in a relationship. The early need for the affirming echo of the mother's approval is never outgrown, but transformed.

The achievement of intimacy requires the capacity to regress and be dependent. Each partner has to be able to tolerate these states in self and other. Dicks (1967) emphasizes that the mature union is based on the mutual ability to tolerate the infantile needs of one another (p. 117). He calls this "giving over oneself into the keeping of another" (p. 43). Fairbairn uses the term "mature dependence" to describe relationships exercising this capacity (quoted by Karpel, 1976, p. 67); Boszormenyi-Nagy refers to "dependencies which [are] reciprocal" (Boszormenyi-Nagy & Ulrich, 1980, p. 171).

Mutuality requires a secure sense of individuation, so that closeness is not experienced as a dangerous fusion threatening the cohesiveness of the self. Experiences of fusion (when they occur, as in sexual intercourse) are temporary and restorative rather than depleting or frightening. In our culture, the average male client is more menaced by the threat of fusion; in conformity to gender stereotypes, he seeks independence and autonomy. Women generally feel more comfortable with fusion, sometimes to the detriment of their individual development. (See Low, Chapter 12, this volume.)

Jean Baker Miller (1987) describes mutuality in relationships as the exercise of the ability to engage in interactions that foster the psychological development of both people in the relationship. She believes that although this is most characteristic of the mothering role, it is necessary in all successful relationships, creating in each person a capacity to alter destructive cycles and to initiate a more positive progression of events.

Acceptance of Self and Other

The ability to accept oneself and one's partner is related to the degree of acceptance that one has experienced in childhood from one's parents. The adult who has grown up with a secure knowledge that his or her whole self (including impulses and limitations) is lovable and cherished can extend this generous tolerance to his or her mate. The corresponding ability to accept one's parents as whole people whose limitations are acknowledged begins in childhood, as the child confronts the inevitable empathic failures of the parents and the keen disillusionments that characterize both oedipal and adolescent periods. Such disillusionment must be balanced by an overall feeling that one's parents were "good enough"; otherwise, the marriage will be burdened by enormous restitutive efforts that attempt to force the spouse to *make up* for the pain and deprivation of the earlier parent–child interactions. Alternatively, a contrary pattern can prevail in a marriage that replays the old parent–child battles with a new object.

Either way, husband and wife treat one another as if each were the original hurtful object. The partners may become quite regressed, using long-discarded childish patterns for revenge or special favor. A mutual attribution and eliciting of forbidding and rejecting qualities can occur as "'the bad object' is shuttled to and fro in their contest which is indeed the essence of a *collusion*" (Dicks, 1967, p. 58).

Acceptance implies an emotional integration of all aspects of the self: sexual and aggressive drives and narcissistic vulnerabilities or limitations. When earlier structural conflicts or developmental deficits have prevented this degree of integration, the marital partner may be used as an attempted solution, as a carrier of the forbidden impulse, or as a self-object whose job it is to complete the self. It is as if each partner agrees not to be a whole person.

Sometimes it is the relationship itself that extrudes the bad object. Dicks (1967) calls this the "'all-in-all' relationship, in which . . . every cue is taken up in just the way the self wants." He maintains that hate and boredom are not to exist, and each partner is expected to uphold the ideal image. Each agrees, no matter what, that both are perfect. If these idealizations are shared and collusive, they can be quite stable, depending on matching defensive styles and life events. If, instead, each partner maintains idealizations that are contradictory to one another, open conflict can quickly develop (p. 84).

Unresolved hatred toward one's parents is very damaging to the intimacy of the couple. Boszormenyi-Nagy describes the corrosive effects of unresolved hostility on feelings of deep loyalty to the parents. Unresolved hostility drives the old bond underground so that loyalty and full commitment to the new object are invisibly prevented. Through identification with the hated parent, the husband or wife feels a shared badness or inadequacy which interferes with self-acceptance and intimacy. These findings highlight the importance of making peace with one's parents in some fashion. The solution is definitely not to free up one's anger and turn it against its original source but "to exonerate," to see that one's parents were victims too (Boszormenyi-Nagy & Ulrich, 1980, p. 181). (See also Framo, Chapter 4, and Paul, Chapter 5, this volume.)

Dicks (1967) suggests that ultimately the task of acceptance in marriage is "to tolerate, fuse and use ambivalence . . . to contain hate in a framework of love" (p. 31).

Empathy

To feel empathy is, essentially, to feel what the other feels while maintaining psychological separateness (see Paul, Chapter 5, this volume). The capacity for empathy develops early in the mother–child relationship and is mobilized by physical body contact. It is an intimate and nonverbal process (Greenson, 1978). Although empathy involves temporary identification and merger, it can only occur reliably with well-differentiated persons. Otherwise, it slips into a type of identification that obscures the needs and individuality of its object. Such failed empathy easily leads to confusing one's own conflicts and inadequacies with the partner's and to inappropriate responses that can be overly critical or controlling.

> At a party an insecure man hears his wife make a politically naive comment about which she is teased. She flushes. He is consumed by feelings of shame and handles this by berating her for her stupidity.

Because empathy involves immersing oneself in the object's emotional life and temporarily leaving one's own world, it always presents the threat of loss of self to those who are less securely individuated. They avoid it defensively, fearing that paying attention to the feelings of another is equivalent to being forced to submit to the mother. They feel controlled by their partners. If one's sense of identity and autonomy is shaky, feeling another's feelings is tantamount to giving up or discounting one's own feelings and position.

There are other factors that interfere with empathy. For example, competition for nurturing or special handling can consciously or unconsciously disrupt the empathic process.

In a dual-career couple, the husband was fired suddenly. The therapist commented on the wife's lack of involvement in the discussion. She responded, "Why should I get all supportive here? He doesn't do that for me. No one ever did that for me."

Greenson (1978) points out that empathy is a two-way process. Each partner has to want to be understood. One can be afraid of being understood if understanding is equated with being found out, controlled, or taken over. Empathy becomes impossible if the cues that might be helpful to the partner are hidden, or if his or her efforts are rebuffed and no attempt is ever quite right. These rebuffs can also be related to wishes for perfect understanding and an intolerance for anything less. Rather than helping one's mate to understand with clear statements, one takes a dismissive stance, discouraging all efforts.

Collaboration

Collaboration is the act of working together and cooperating in a partnership. It is the only key element contributing to viable intimacy that does not have its primary origins in the early parent–child relationship. Pregenital issues can certainly interfere; one has to be reasonably free of the fear of being controlled and dominated, for example, to be comfortable in a partnership.

The primary origins of the ability to collaborate are found in sibling and peer relationships. Henry Grunebaum (1976; Chapter 15, this volume) emphasizes peer–peer relating as a major determinant of adult heterosexual relating and the ability to establish friendships as basic to marriage. Collaboration requires the ability to work together toward a goal, to share power and decision making, and to invest in an activity or a project. The skills that one acquires in latency seem particularly pertinent here: the ability to team up, to subjugate one's wishes for the success of the group, to identify with a goal of a unit larger than the self, to negotiate, to tolerate losing, to play by the rules, and to be fair. Unresolved sibling issues can easily interfere. One cannot collaborate comfortably if the mate is experienced as a hated rival who always won out, got the mother's attention, and so on.

Collaboration can anchor intimacy by infusing the relationship with aspects of one's identity that are often less conflicted. Successful collaboration contributes to daily problem solving so that a mutually respectful ambiance is nurtured. Dicks (1967) writes about the importance of each partner developing flexible role behaviors in response to the needs of the other. This kind of comfortable exchange of roles applies to leadership, caretaking, aggression, sexuality, activity, and passivity (p. 31).

CLINICAL ISSUES

Barriers to Intimacy

Couples attempt to negotiate a viable level of intimacy. Fogarty (quoted by Karpel, 1976) uses the metaphor of two magnets to describe a couple's efforts to regulate closeness, suggesting that the goal of closeness is to create an "emotional tug without fusing." (p. 68) Similarly, Karpel is intrigued with the model of an optimal point along a continuum. He uses the concept of "dialogue" to characterize the mature intimacy that is experienced by two differentiated people (see also J. Grunebaum, Chapter 10, this volume).

If we consider viable intimacy to be a negotiated balance in the relationship, symptoms are markers of interference with that balance. They represent an attempt to protect against whichever danger is feared: closeness or distance. Symptoms can be thought of as "consequences of, defenses against, or ambivalence over . . . fusion" (Karpel, 1976, p. 67). The symptoms are myriad: fighting, avoidance, difficulties in communication, interactional patterns, sexual problems—particularly disorders of sexual desire. The clinician is alerted to problems in intimacy by these behavioral manifestations of the conflicts.

Intimacy can engender many fears in each partner. These fears can be conscious or unconscious: fear of merger or loss, fear of exposure or shame, fear of attack or of one's own aggression, fear of disappointment, fear of needing the object, or fear of risk. Such fears can derive from preoedipal or oedipal levels of experience. In sexual intimacy, for example, sexual activity can signify loss of the mother, turning toward a forbidden oedipal object, or both. On the deepest level we are social beings and need others desperately. When the normal intensity of this need is coupled with neurotic reactions, we may hate, fear, and envy the very object we turn to.

Pathological interactions are difficult to interrupt since the fears that underlie them are often intense and long-standing. Though the symptoms often function defensively to effectively reduce fears of intimacy, they perpetuate destructive interactive patterns. (See Feldman, 1979, on the role of marital fighting.)

Styles of Marital Relationships

A number of clinicians have examined styles of marital relationships and have concluded that *intensity* of involvement is a major defining parameter. Marriages differ as much in intensity of feeling as they do in direction of feeling: positive or negative (Lieberman, 1976). Marriages are not necessarily categorizable on a continuum of happiness–unhappiness; some unions may be high in happiness *and* unhappiness or low in both states (Bradburn, cited in Lieberman, 1976).

The two models for classifying couples that I will discuss here do not constitute a definitive overview; rather, they illustrate that myriad perspectives on marital relationships can be used to organize interactional data.

Karpel (1976), drawing heavily on the work of psychoanalysts, proposes a classification that charts the degree of individuation of the partners and their mutual freedom to interact in intimate and affirming ways. Most couples seeking treatment are neither extremely fused nor extremely unrelated (schizoid), but in a state of ambivalent fusion. In this transitional stage, the "I" and the "we" are recognized, but each represents a conflicted position. In the "I" position one feels unconnected and unrelated, and in the "we" position one experiences a loss of separate self. This is the least stable form of relationship and the most open to change and growth. The category of ambivalent fusion is broken down into five types: (1) One partner always distances; (2) each partner takes turns; (3) both partners together alternate between fusion and unrelatedness; (4) constant conflict; (5) impairment of one partner, competence in the other. The mature union, in Karpel's schema, is characterized by dialogue, the hallmark of a nonfused, mutually affirming relationship between individuated partners who can tolerate differences.

Clifford Sager (1976a) has delineated seven behavioral profiles and over 20 combinations of behavioral types. His descriptions are wonderfully vivid and detailed, evoking countless associations to friends, patients, and one's own relationships. In contrast to theorists who write from a more traditional psychoanalytic viewpoint, Sager does not emphasize the polarities of individuation and fusion. He draws our attention to the nature of the *contract* between partners as revealed by their mutual transactions. There is no assumption in Sager's clinical descriptions that an ideal of individuation is the *sine qua non* of a stable or satisfying relationship. Rather, it is the *fit* of the partners' contracts that leads to contentment; a unilateral *change* in contract can cause difficulty. Within the profiles of couple types are differences in capacity and desire for intimacy, patterns of control, and degree of regression.

Some combinations are inherently less stable than others. Sager indicates that a range of couples will demonstrate varying combinations of behavioral roles, including (1) equal partners; (2) romantic partners; (3) parental partners; (4) childlike partners; (5) rational partners; (6) companionate partners; and (7) parallel partners. Couple relationships can be based on combinations of two similar behavioral styles (e.g., both may be romantic) or on two styles that are complementary (e.g., equal–romantic or parallel–rational). The paired behavioral roles, whether similar or complementary, will characterize the pattern of the relationship. The amount of flexibility within each partner and the degree of mutual acceptance of the mate as he or she is *now* will determine the viability of the couple's relationship.

Equal partner relationships are closest to the psychoanalytic ideal of two fully individuated people; each person is complete and self-initiating, yet free to be emotionally interdependent. The couple is capable of close sustained intimacy without merger. Romantic partner relationships seem evocative of descriptions of fused couples and of Dicks's "all-in-all" relationships; however, Sager feels that many romantics can feel securely loved. The romantic partnership is characterized by a life-or-death soul-mate quality. It is inherently precarious because the intimacy and passion of the early years may fade, and the loss in intensity can feel unbearable. The basic theme here is that of completing oneself with another. Parental partner couples are usually conflict-ridden, ambivalent, and unstable; they have one "parent" and one "child." A subtype includes an ability to exchange these roles. Mutual rescue operations occur in this category. Sager cautions that unless the "child" is motivated to change, the therapist should not challenge the balance. Childlike partner relationships avoid responsibility and compete around neediness. These are unstable unions unless each can learn to alternate parental roles. Rational partners try to form logical, orderly relationships. Sager has found that "pure" rational partnerships are rare because, typically, the rational partner seeks and finds a complementary partnership (with, e.g., a romantic or childlike partner) to supply the liveliness and emotion that he or she cannot feel. Companionate partners seek friendship, respect, and caring. The emphasis is not on love, but on kindness. The companionate contract is most common among older couples or younger couples defending against sexual feelings. Parallel partnerships can be quite stable and satisfactory, but require a mutual acceptance of their hallmark, a nonintimate relationship. This type of relationship is based on emotional distance and independence.

CONDUCTING THERAPY WITH MARRIED COUPLES

Cautions

It is critical for the therapist to respect the couple's style of relationship, pathological though it may be. It represents their best effort to manage the interlocking intrapsychic conflicts and core vulnerabilities that drew them together at the start. This caution applies especially to work on marital intimacy. Many trainees and therapists have a working model of intimacy that is extraordinarily idealistic and probably reflects better a therapist's wishes for his or her own life than the patients' wishes or capabilities. Treatment must be grounded in an appreciation of the couple's contract around intimacy. The couple's particular style of interaction reflects both their position on the continuum from unrelated to fused positions and their current contractual resolution of issues of intimacy, power, and regression. The treatment plan should reflect each partner's desires and capacities for intimacy. To use Sager's terminology, the therapist shouldn't try to turn a parallel partner relationship into a romantic relationship.

The therapist must also attend to the therapeutic relationship and the therapeutic alliance. In couple therapy as in individual treatment, the therapist needs to nurture the alliance in an active way; it doesn't simply happen. The therapist encourages an identification with a problem-solving approach to conflict. A clear distinction is made between blame and responsibility. Each partner is encouraged to assume responsibility for his or her own thoughts, feelings, and perceptions and to identify personal traits that cause problems.

In treating problems in intimacy, the therapist first identifies which of the five components (separateness, mutuality, acceptance, empathy, and collaboration) need attention. Through careful exploration of thoughts, feelings, and perceptions, the therapist encourages the expression of the specific fears experienced by each partner that interfere with each particular strand of intimacy. For example, deep fears of exposure of one's inadequacies may underlie an isolated stance that prevents mutuality. The therapeutic work traces each partner's vulnerability in the past and present, bringing to light the unconscious identifications, fantasies, and conflicts that are operative. It is the very nature of couples to manage these fears and conflicts in an interactive mode—by projective identification and the resulting polarization of conflict. The therapist must therefore train the couple to think in terms of interactions and behavioral sequences rather than individual behaviors. They need to become sensitized to their intersecting unconscious conflicts and the related shared patterns that perpetuate them.

> Mr. T. complains that his wife is cold, that he needs love and affection to feel secure. After much exploration of mutual feelings and perceptions, the therapist proposes daily homework of five minutes of nonsexual kissing and holding. Mrs. T. looks eager. Her husband puts his hand over his mouth, looking tense. She turns away, joking, "I won't look at him. I'll pretend I can't see his expression." The therapist is aware that each one is afraid of physical intimacy. Mrs. T.'s eagerness is not typical of the couple; it is usually she who avoids intimate contact. Before the underlying fears can be elucidated, the couple must recognize that they take turns saying no to each other. In this

sequence it is Mr. T. who has to see how his nonverbal rebuff discourages the very closeness he so desperately wants.

In therapy each partner has the chance to develop a differentiated self that can now own previously denied and projected parts of the self. The therapist's constant attention to process interrupts and labels the collusive interactions. Each partner learns what he or she misperceives in the other and denies in himself or herself. This leads to a new sense of self and other as whole and safe; if each partner is free to recognize the commonality of needs in the couple and to tolerate the genuine differences, the longed-for intimacy will become less dangerous.

It is the rare couple therapy that doesn't include some work related to the family of origin of each partner. Bowen's (1972) position is that no one is completely differentiated, that everyone is fused with his or her original family to some extent. (See also Paul, Chapter 5, and Framo, Chapter 4, this volume.) His goal is to make his patients aware of the fusion—how it can be concealed by hate or distancing behavior and how to get disentangled from one's family during frequent visits with them. In a disturbed marriage, fusion with one's original family can appear as generalized conflict or as more specific rigidities in role behavior and equally rigid perceptions of the partner's role. Wexler and Steidl (1978) call these distorted perceptions "unsuccessful attempts to change present persons into past persons" (p. 79). To the extent that one can face the loss inherent in separation from one's parents, one becomes free to see and accept one's partner as himself or herself and to negotiate with the partner a comfortable intimacy, one in which both closeness and distance can be tolerated and even enjoyed.

Therapists differ in their conviction as to the locus of the work. Bowen (1972), Boszormenyi-Nagy and Ulrich (1980), Framo (1976; Chapter 4, this volume) and Paul (1985; Chapter 5, this volume) encourage work with the original family members. Boszormenyi-Nagy, Paul, and Framo employ a family therapy format. In Bowen's case, the family work occurs in brief visits that the client makes to his or her family of origin without the therapist. Others emphasize intrapsychic and interpersonal work with the client and family of origin within the therapy hour. Either way, the goal is not to change the parents. The client has no control over his or her parents' interest in or capacity to change. What is critical is the patient's determination to change his or her part in the relationship, whether the attempt is successful or not (Boszormenyi-Nagy & Ulrich, 1980). I would add that this commitment may be to intrapsychic change; the effort can take place solely within one's *internal* relationship to one's parent.

When a couple has major problems with intimacy, their sexual life is usually affected. Either partner may have specific sexual dysfunctions or what Helen Singer Kaplan (1979) has named "disorders of sexual desire": a lack of sexual interest and/or satisfaction. Intimacy problems that manifest themselves in the sexual arena can best be addressed in a flexible, multilevel approach including both psychodynamic and behavioral techniques. Sensate focus exercises without genital stimulation can encourage physical intimacy in a way that allows for tenderness without performance anxiety. These exercises can be used in an evaluative way to highlight specific fears of intimacy and to reveal self-destructive patterns. The couple is helped to identify and "work through hostilities, poor communication, fear of emotional closeness, and difficulty in verbalizing desires [and to experience] a concrete demonstration of the importance of *quid pro quo* maneuvers" (Sager, 1976b, p. 557). On both the behavioral and intrapsychic levels, the work focuses on negotiation, risk taking, and overcoming identifications with the oedipal prohibiting parent, as well as any intrapsychic conflict that makes the experience of sexual pleasure a danger.

The Case of Larry and Jennifer

In the case of Jennifer and Larry, the context for data gathering and intervention is a public one. This setting creates certain goals or aims that may conflict at times with the couple's aims to get help and with the consultant's need for as much openness as possible to grasp the reality of the couple's world. To gauge the extent of these problems is beyond the scope of this chapter. However, the question of the *validity* and *reality* of what we can know clinically is not qualitatively different with this couple than with our own patients.

Jennifer remarks that she and Larry have been "living sort of parallel lifestyles," that they "had become just roommates." Their difficulties in working out a fuller intimacy can be traced by looking at the dimensions of separateness, mutuality, acceptance, empathy, collaboration, and the couple's changed contract.

Separateness

At the time of the conference, Jennifer and Larry showed a similar degree of differentiation from their families of origin. Each was reworking within the couple unresolved relationships with parental figures. Jennifer experienced her family as nonvalidating. They saw her as problematic, an exaggerator of her feelings. In the family session with the Framos, Jennifer's mother comments, "But Jennifer, didn't you used to exaggerate things and always magnify them when you talked to me? I mean you blew it up more." Jennifer lives with a man who obliges her by adopting a similar viewpoint. His statements of reassurance (e.g., "no big deal") are experienced by Jennifer as negating her. Because her self-esteem is not cohesive, she is quite threatened by his efforts and ends up thinking she should not be upset, finally doubting how she does feel. Larry is not comfortably differentiated from his very emotional mother. He must resist Jennifer not just because she threatens his defensive style, but because resisting the woman is his way of defining himself as a man. For each of them, only withdrawal leads to the desired separateness. Although the intimacy patterns of their families of origin are different, both families have difficulty with intimacy, perhaps including sexual intimacy. Jennifer and Larry may each be maintaining their same-sex parent's style of intimacy. Larry is keeping quiet and is nonexpressive of affect like his father. Jennifer may be "dark with secrets" and suspicious of men like her mother. We know that Jennifer had affairs in the early years of her relationship with Larry; in the interview with the Framos she said to Larry, "Don't forget that you are a man. We have secrets from men."

Mutuality

Because individuation is not secure for either Jennifer or Larry, mutuality is experienced as threatening their separateness, as engulfing and potentially destructive. On the surface Jennifer seems more threatened by separateness than fusion, but her workaholic lifestyle and her very choice of Larry speak to her own need for distance. Each holds back from the commitment of marriage. The fantasies that Peggy Papp elicited from them reveal a constant fear that engaging in a joint endeavor involves being controlled. Alone or in nonintimate relationships, each one functions well; it is in the unit of the couple that conflict appears. In his ballgame fantasy, Larry wants Jennifer "on the side," an admirer, not a full partner. Both Jennifer and Larry have mothers who have been controlling and invasive. Their accompanying unresolved fears are played out in their couple relationship. Each is afraid of depending. For Jennifer, who experienced her mother as angry and unnurturing, being given to by Larry leaves her feeling "furious . . . empty and scared as though I've lost something." At such a moment she is flooded by her unmet needs, her long-standing rage, and the terror of giving up a lonely but safe, contained state. Larry is equally afraid to depend; he tells Norman Paul, "If you depend on someone else for your happiness or support, and if that someone else is not there . . . then you are back where you started."

Acceptance

Jennifer never felt cherished or even wanted by her family. She felt that her mother wished her dead. Her development reflects a "false self" identify, one in which superficial compliance and performance (e.g., academic achievement) hide a more authentic self (Winnicott, 1976, pp. 140–152). Although Larry appreciates his lively, warm extended family, he notes that his ambitions and wishes for privacy were not validated by his family. There is a hint that he may not have felt securely loved by his unexpressive father. Because Jennifer feels that her parents failed her so devastatingly, she burdens the couple relationship with restitutive wishes. Each one is trying to remake the other. Larry projects his own neediness (made more acute after his amputation) onto Jennifer, and she projects her own fears of openness onto him. This is especially clear in the follow-up session (see Chapter 18) when she emphasizes her *own* new openness; earlier, with Carlos Sluzki, she had described Larry, not herself, as "very, very introverted and very private."

Empathy

Despite their superficial differences (Jennifer is on the side of expressing feelings, Larry stands for rationality and pragmatism), each one equates empathy and being understood with invasion and control. When Jennifer's parents insisted on a psychiatrist for her during her troubled adolescence, she experienced them not as nurturing but as trying to change her disturbing behavior. Larry and Jennifer actually have a great deal of feeling and sensitivity toward each other, as evidenced by Larry's clear effort to help Jennifer face her family and by Jennifer's fantasy with Peggy Papp of the scared boy "paralyzed with fear." Yet often their expressions of empathy are tinged with projection. They offer empathy as they would like to receive it, rather than trying to match the other's style. Carlos Sluzki picked this up and encouraged each "to be more like the other when you're with the other."

Collaboration

Collaboration is a more successful area. Larry and Jennifer not only came together for therapy, but partook of the ambitious challenge of the conference. Together on a long car trip they conquered Larry's addiction to painkilling medication. However, when competitive issues or control struggles surface, this area can be a source of conflict. Compromise is difficult. When Larry agrees to attend a party at Jennifer's lab, he is resentful and shows it, ruining the effort.

Changes in Contract

Early in their relationship Larry was the pursuer–rescuer, the parental partner; Jennifer was the distancer, the child in need of help. At the time of Larry's illness, the roles switched: Larry needed help. It is not clear if he allowed emotional sustenance, but he did let Jennifer be active and effective, and she responded capably. By the time of the consultations, Jennifer commented that they were living "parallel lifestyles . . . like roommates," with Jennifer pursuing intermittently.

Larry's illness and amputation still figure strongly in their difficulties. Although some consultants suggest that this subject is no longer critical, the references throughout the tapes echo and reecho it, in Peggy Papp's session especially, with such phrases as "paralyzed with fear," the "very frail" and "dying wife," a document that can "stand throughout history," the "requiem mass," and so on. The most significant moment for Larry in his family session was his astonished realization that his illness meant so much to his father.

My hunch is that the amputation continues to be stressful for this couple. I speculate that Larry feels less manly and worries that he is now not enough for Jennifer, now that she can no longer lean on him. His fear would merge with earlier feelings of mistrust during the time of her affairs. An amputation would be especially hard for a man who has so much invested in showing off physically, in testing himself. For Jennifer, her earlier conflicted feelings of overwhelming responsibility for a sick father whose bed she shared would be triggered. The combined scared, guilty, and resentful feelings could lead to avoidance of physical closeness. The sexual life of the couple would require negotiation: Larry would need to learn to ask for help; Jennifer would need to become more active. It is interesting that Larry's first fantasy focuses on age 12 — a highly ambivalent period sexually. Everything is "on the verge." Jennifer's first fantasy is even earlier developmentally — perhaps latency. I sense for both a retreat from sexual issues.

Outcome: The Six-Month Follow-Up Session

This couple illustrates the concept of different styles of intimacy as opposed to an ideal single kind. By the time of the follow-up session (see Chapter 18), the area of intimacy is less conflicted for Jennifer and Larry. They each show more comfort with both separateness and mutuality. Larry is more at ease with the thought of Jennifer's possibly going to Kenya for two months; at the same time, he is withdrawing less and watching less television. They each show more tolerance for their separate emotional styles. Both feel they can talk things out more freely. Their styles have not altered radically. There is not a deep exchange of innermost thoughts (particularly from Larry), but rather a more workable complementarity. Jennifer, having achieved a new understanding and acceptance of her mother, is burdening the relationship less. She no longer "asks" Larry to make up for past hurts; Larry, perhaps feeling a stronger identification with his father, seems more at ease with Jennifer's "female" emotional style (linked unconsciously to his mother's emotional expressiveness); he pushes her away less and can risk agreeing with her a bit more. As a couple, Jennifer and Larry experience more confidence in themselves and in their relationship.

What has helped? The context for change is an unusual and interesting one: a public forum, a large couple therapy conference with a huge video screen. They became a *star* couple. This in itself may have offered certain satisfactions to this couple, whose grandiose ambitions were revealed in their playful fantasies of being Jefferson and Mozart with Peggy Papp. In an intriguing reciprocity, a few carefully selected *star* therapists involved themselves intensely in their situation, offering validation and recognition of their uniqueness as a couple. On the ambivalent side, Larry comments that "we didn't fit in each style [of each therapist] equally well," and Jennifer objected that "nobody really emphasized any of the positive things in our relationship." Larry speculated that "[it's] not to say that we wouldn't have sort of gotten to this point without any conference or couple therapy." They both wish the interviewers had commented on their love for one another. One has the impression that despite Jennifer's insistence on how wonderful it had all been, a subtle repositioning had occurred, with Jennifer and Larry banding together against the therapists and the conference with a newly felt confidence in *themselves* and in *their* own way.

It is difficult to know which clinical interventions or experiences were the most helpful. Perhaps the sheer impact of the amount and intensity of the consultation sessions was transformative. Each partner repaired something in the relationship with the same-sex parent. Jennifer's experience with her mother was the more dramatic, leading to clear, observable changes in the mother–daughter relationship and in Jennifer's perception about her relationship with Larry and the world: "I think I'm a lot more open than I used to be," "I think he's been a lot more open about things," "I feel more open now in general," "that communication with my mother . . . enabled me to just be, feel freer, in general. " Predictably, Larry's observations about his relationship with his father are less clear, and he does not speak at all to a change in their relationship, but to a change in his perceptions. He focuses on his surprise that his illness meant so much to his father and on his new awareness that "there are definite aspects that move me more towards my father." This statement seems to be a condensation of (1) my father loves me; (2) I am a lot like my father (perhaps revealing a fear of being too emotional and womanly); (3) my father now thinks it's OK to express deep feeling. I wonder if this internal shift has freed him to risk more emotional expressiveness, to fend Jennifer off less, to join with her more.

Both Jennifer and Larry valued Carlos Sluzki's attention to the need for acceptance of their very different emotional styles: The rock and balloon each *balance* the relationship. This seems to have helped lead not only to behavioral change—Larry is more likely to join Jennifer emotionally—but also to an inner feeling of both tolerance and freedom for both.

The follow-up session did not explore changes in the sexual aspect of their relationship; presumably, the public aspect of the session interfered with this inquiry. Henry Grunebaum asked about affection, but Jennifer's answer was vague, perhaps compliant, and Larry switched the focus to Jennifer's relationship with her family. I was left with the impression that there were no improvements in this area.

In considering the question of change, one is struck with this couple's pleasure in changes that decidedly do not include a thorough working through of deep conflicts, character change, or even a major shift in roles. They perceive themselves and one another somewhat differently and their typical behavioral sequences have been altered a bit, but the impact and meaning of these modest changes are considerable. Change is, of course, elusive and hard to track. Jennifer *believes* in change; she is committed to it and works hard to describe the extent of personal and relational change as she experiences it. Larry doesn't attach such positive valence to change. He remains skeptical, especially about change within himself. We are dealing with two different value systems regarding psychotherapy and change. We must be careful not to conclude that Jennifer changed and Larry did not.

CONCLUSION

Intimacy is not a unidimensional capacity in each partner or a fixed state in the couple. It is a mutually adaptive, reciprocal, ongoing process. Viable intimacy requires a balance between separateness and mutuality. In a successful couple, each quality enhances the other because an individuated person can risk "giving over [himself] into the keeping of another" (Dicks, 1967, p. 43) and at the same time can mutually affirm and nurture the partner's unique separateness. There are numerous different *workable* styles of intimacy that partly reflect different degrees of individuation and fusion. Viable intimacy requires the capacity to sustain closeness over time throughout the life cycle; to handle inevitable ruptures and variations in the level of closeness; and to learn to come together again after emotional separation, to repair, and to grow.

REFERENCES

Bach, S. (1980). Self-love and object-love: Some problems of self and object constancy, differentiation and integration. In R. F. Lax, S. Bach, & J. A. Burland (Eds.), *Rapprochement* (pp. 171–197). New York: Jason Aronson.

Barnett, J. (1971). Narcissism and dependency in the obsessional-hysteric marriage. *Family Process, 10*(8), 75–83.

Binstock, W. A. (1973). On the two forms of intimacy. *Journal of the American Psychoanalytic Association, 21*, 93–107.

Boszormenyi-Nagy, I., & Ulrich, D. (1980). Contextual family therapy. In A. S. Gurman & D. P. Kniskern (Eds.), *Handbook of family therapy* (pp. 159–186). New York: Brunner/Mazel.

Bowen, M. (1972). Toward the differentiation of a self in one's own family. In J. L. Framo (Ed.), *Family interaction* (pp. 111–173). New York: Springer.

Bowlby, J. (1968). *Attachment and loss: Vol. 1. Attachment.* London: Tavistock.

Dicks, H. V. (1967). *Marital tensions.* New York: Basic Books.

Feldman, L. B. (1979). Marital conflict and marital intimacy: An integrative psychodynamic–behavioral–systemic model. *Family Process, 8*(1), 69–78.

Framo, J. L. (1976). Family of origin as a therapeutic resource for adults in marital and family therapy: You can and should go home again. *Family Process, 15*(1), 193–210.

Greenson, R. (1978). Empathy and its vicissitudes. In R.R. Greenson (Ed.), *Explorations in psychoanalysis* (pp. 147–161). New York: International Universities Press.

Grunebaum, H. (1976). Thoughts on love, sex, and commitment. *Journal of Sex and Marital Therapy, 2*(4), 277–283.

Kaplan, H. S. (1979). *The new sex therapy: Vol. 2: Disorders of sexual desire.* New York: Brunner/Mazel.

Karpel, M. (1976). Individuation: From fusion to dialogue. *Family Process, 15*(1), 65–82.

Klein, G. S. (1976). *Psychoanalytic theory.* New York: International Universities Press.

Kohut, H. (1971). *The analysis of the self.* New York: International Universities Press.

Kohut, H. (1977). *The restoration of the self.* New York: International Universities Press.

Lieberman, E. J. (1976). The prevention of marital problems. In H. Grunebaum & J. Christ (Eds.), *Contemporary marriage* (pp. 315–332). Boston: Little, Brown.

Mahler, M. (1974). Symbiosis and individuation: The psychological birth of the human infant. *The Psychoanalytic Study of the Child, 29*, 89–106.

Meissner, W. W. (1978). The conceptualization of marriage and family dynamics from a psychoanalytic perspective. In T.J. Paolino & B. S. McCrady (Eds.), *Marriage and marital therapy* (pp. 25–88). New York: Brunner/Mazel.

Miller, J. B. (1987, April 24–25). Women's psychological development: Connections, disconnections, and violations. In *Course syllabus, Learning from women: Theory and practice*, The Cambridge Hospital and The Stone Center, Boston.

Paul, N. L. (1976). The role of mourning and empathy in conjoint marital therapy. In G. Zuk & I. Boszormenyi-Nagy (Eds.), *Family therapy and disturbed families* (pp. 186–205). Palo Alto, CA: Science and Behavior Books.

Paul, N. L. (1985). *A marital puzzle* (rev. ed.). New York: Gardner Press.

Sager, C. J. (1976a). *Marriage contracts and couple therapy.* New York: Brunner/Mazel.

Sager, C. J. (1976b). The role of sex therapy in marital therapy. *American Journal of Psychiatry, 133*(5), 555–558.

Weiss, R. (1975). *Marital separation.* New York: Basic Books.

Wexler, J., & Steidl, J. (1978). Marriage and the capacity to be alone. *Psychiatry, 41,* 72–82.

Winnicott, D. W. (1976). Ego distortion in terms of true and false self. In D. W. Winnicott (Ed.), *The maturational processes and the facilitating environment* (pp. 140–152). London: Hogarth Press.

10

From Discourse to Dialogue:
The Power of Fairness in
Therapy with Couples

JUDITH GRUNEBAUM

INTRODUCTION

Few would deny that fairness in relationships and in communities profoundly shapes our lives as humans. Issues of equity between members of a couple, between the generations, and between the peoples and nations of the world have never been more urgently debated than they are in our historic era. Therapists who work with couples are presented perpetually with issues of fairness. The discourse of couples commonly includes such statements as "You're not doing your share of the child care!" and "I don't think I can ever trust you again since your affair." These refrains are familiar, and often the therapist feels struck by their simple and stark reality; they evoke something unique and essential about the human predicament, and at the same time, they often seem refractory to resolution. In helping clients to face inequities and to state claims, grievances, and gratitude, therapists often guide couples away from the ethical realm and focus instead on processes and structures that *appear* to be ethically neutral. It is sadly characteristic of our age that we prefer short-term efficacy to meaning, fixing to healing, and the sanctification of science and technology to the enlargement of the human capacity for relatedness. Attention to human values, it seems, is seen as diminishing the objectivity and therefore the legitimacy of the science of human behavior.

Resisting these tendencies, I choose to work within the framework of contextual therapy, an approach introduced into the family therapy field by Ivan Boszormenyi-Nagy (1972, 1987) and elaborated by him, his co-workers, and others (Bernal, 1982, 1990; Boszormenyi-Nagy & Krasner, l986; Boszormenyi-Nagy & Spark, 1973; Boszormenyi-Nagy & Ulrich, 1981; Cotroneo, 1982; Gelinas, l983, 1986; Grunebaum, J., l987; Karpel, 1986; Karpel & Strauss, l983; Simon, Stierlin, & Wynne, 1985). Contextual therapy emphasizes that trustworthiness and fairness are among the most fundamental ingredients of human bonding, and, I would add, of all cooperative social action. Trust is based on mutually sought standards of fairness. The contextual approach presupposes that the desire for fairness and trustworthiness is basic and universal in human life.

What does a contextual therapist mean by "fairness"? Many philosophers and humanists have recognized the primacy of this desire for fairness, even though they may not agree on the proper criteria for determining what is just, fair, virtuous, or "good." From the perspective of this therapeutic model, fairness is not understood in terms of abstract principles about rights, or universal rules arrived at by rational argument; nor is it even a single notion of the highest "good." Rather, fairness is seen as a *process* of relationships, a process of equitably sharing the burdens and benefits of living over the long term, among members of all generations.[1]

The contextual view of fairness closely resembles women's perception of justice as described by Gilligan (1982) in her classic work on moral development. In both views, life is perceived as an interconnected fabric of relationships, so that if someone is hurt, everyone is affected. Moral decisions are made *in relation to* concrete human situations, and are not predetermined by abstract universal principles. The goal is to minimize injustice and hurt by considering the interests of all those who will be affected.

I am attracted to the contextual approach because I find its emphasis on moral claims and ethical conflicts to be both effective and compatible with the central concerns of families and couples. It is systemic in the broad sense, viewing symptoms and problems as the outcome of a field of relational dynamics. But it is distinctive among systemic therapies in that the dynamics it highlights are the Lifeworld realities of loyalty, gratitude, resentment, owing, and deserving that people in relationships speak of and about which they negotiate. (See footnote 8.)

The contextual therapy model is integrative; it utilizes all sources of knowledge and understanding that may be of benefit to the client.[2] In

---

[1]The essence of the meaning of "history," in fact, can be discovered in the evolving dialogue of trust between the generations (Buber, 1957; Friedman, 1965; Boszormenyi-Nagy & Krasner, 1986; Boszormenyi-Nagy, 1987a).
[2]The frameworks that I find to be particularly compatible with or illuminating of the

reality, the different aspects of relationships which the various treatment models address are inseparable. Therefore, contextual therapists believe that it is crucial to integrate them—without, however, reducing them to one another (Boszormenyi-Nagy, 1987b).

If issues of fairness are so central to couple relationships, why are couples in conflict so often mired in fruitless exchanges of claims of inequity and irresponsibility? From the standpoint of contextual therapy, these couples are not considered improper or immature when speaking of "fairness" in their attempts to address areas of conflict. Unfortunately the scope of their ethical claims is often unilateral and overly present-oriented in their account of who owes what to whom. They are likely to have little appreciation for the profound impact that the justice of their earlier life experiences and other prior relationships has had on the grievances they direct to one another. A couple relationship is but one link in a *multiperson, multigenerational* context. The fact that the struggles of previous generations do not appear in the couple's explicit definition of their problem does not mean that they are inconsequential factors. Nevertheless, each person's experience of the problem in their current relationship is without doubt the place to begin. Ultimately both current and past problems need to be acknowledged and addressed as mutually impinging upon one another. In addition, the particular way in which the future shapes the present, in the form of posterity's claims upon us, is both a distinctive and a crucial therapeutic concern and a therapeutic resource.

The couple relationship is viewed, from the vantage point of contextual therapy, as existing within a *socioethical* framework. Conflicts of interest between members of a couple and within families, as in the larger society, are shaped by vital *human* interests, social practices, and the language we use to both express and shape those goals, values, and practices. The practice of coupling is social and cultural as well as personal. To conceptually strip it of its cultural meanings and social constraints leads to unacceptable distortions in our understanding of

---

contextual approach are the interpersonally oriented "object relations theorists" Balint (1968), Fairbairn (1952), Guntrip (1969), Winnicott (1963, 1971), and Erik Erickson (1964); the philosophers Buber (1965, 1970), Foucault (1979, 1981), Habermas (1971, 1987) and MacIntyre (1984); and certainly the systemic thinkers and clinicians who apply their understanding of pattern in ways that do not violate basic ethical requirements, some of whom are represented in this book. I have been very influenced by Mona Fishbane's (1987) thoughtful article on the dialogic potential in systems-oriented therapies. A number of feminist theorists, clinicians, and colleagues have powerfully shaped my thinking, especially Janna Smith (see Grunebaum & Smith, in preparation). The "bonds" I share with my husband Henry (see H. Grunebaum, Chapter 15, this volume), his father's interest in practical ethics, and my own parents' social and ethical values and contributions have been the most formative influences on my thinking and practice. I am grateful for them, and also for the friendship and colleagueship of Ivan Boszormenyi-Nagy.

couples' relationships. My elaboration and emphasis of the *socioethical* dimension within contextual therapy will suggest the common ground of feminism and contextual therapy, and will highlight the resources each perspective can bring to the other.[3]

Contextual therapists help couples to explore the forces and the facts that have shaped their claims, unmet needs, and negotiations—in the present and in the past—and help them to work toward the openness that will facilitate "dialogue."[4] When dialogue becomes possible, a person's needs, rights, and obligations can be understood and more fairly negotiated.

I will begin my exposition of contextual therapy by contrasting its fundamental goal, the establishment of the conditions for the "unfolding" of *dialogue*, with an inescapable force that often impedes dialogue—namely, *social discourse*. Next, I will discuss some of the key personal, familial, and social dynamics that typically generate and sustain conflicting claims and unmet needs in families. Then I will describe the method of "multidirected partiality," which guides contextual therapists as they attempt to help couples enter into the realm of dialogue. Finally, I will apply the framework of contextual therapy to the case of Larry and Jennifer.

Throughout this chapter, I will present the concepts, methods, and goals of contextual therapy as I understand them and benefit from them. I do not claim to represent all contextual therapists; in addition, I believe that some of the concepts are sometimes used without sufficient explanation of basic assumptions, and therefore I will offer some

---

[3]See Grunebaum, J. (1987). In that article I say that, with its dialectical approach to the "interhuman" issues of fairness, family loyalty, and parental accountability, contextual therapy can transcend the polarization evolving in our field between systems-oriented and feminist family therapy models, while incorporating the important knowledge which those approaches have contributed. I apply the contextual model to *societal* sources of women's "destructive entitlement." See also Leupnitz (1988), who comments on the "great potential for the integration of feminism with contextual therapy" (p. 71). I am in agreement with much of her critique that social and historical injustices related to gender are not adequately addressed in contextual therapy. It is unfortunate, however, that she uses an early text, *Invisible Loyalties* (Boszormenyi-Nagy & Spark, 1973) as the basis of her critique and ignores more recent writings—such as, *Between Give and Take* (Boszormenyi-Nagy & Krasner, 1986) which is a major recasting of the theory. Her critique is partly based on the current radical feminist rejection of "humanism," which I believe is misguided. Why should we not want to preserve what is valuable in the legacy of humanism? We would then be in a position to move beyond its limitations to an understanding of how positive, universal human values and particular social conditions are synergistic or not.

[4]I am using the term "dialogue" to refer to the philosophy of dialogue elaborated by Martin Buber in *I and Thou* (1970) and in a book of essays, which I strongly recommend to the reader, entitled *The Knowledge of Man* (1965), including Maurice Friedman's excellent introductory essay and also his text *The Healing Dialogue in Psychotherapy* (1985).

conceptual ground that I have found helpful in understanding and implementing the contextual approach. Martin Buber's philosophy of dialogue is an inspirational and conceptual source of nourishment for many contextual therapists, and therefore I will make explicit some of his key concepts. My inclusion of the categories of "social practice" and "social discourse"[5] within the contextual framework is an attempt to clarify and elaborate the social and political implications of this important therapeutic model.

THE SOCIAL CONTEXT: DISCOURSE AND DIALOGUE

Relationships of *reciprocity* characterize all social groups. Reciprocity is based on the mutual acknowledgment of vital human interests.[6] Throughout this chapter I will contrast two distinct social phenomena that come about in relation to human interests and needs–the evolving process of social discourse and the ever-present potential for human dialogue.

"Discourse" refers to the ways in which language gives meaning to and shapes a historically specific social reality. Discourse does not merely *reflect* the thinking inherent in our social practices. It also *structures* and *legitimates* new social practices and thought. It shapes the material and social relations of our daily lives, constraining what we can say, do, and (often) think. Discourses attempt to tell us who we are; we are frequently the subjects of language and not the authors of our own experience.

Discourse is organized around those attributes which a culture perceives as significant "differences" (frequently gender, race, or age). Some discourses have more social power and authority than others; many have institutional bases in the family and the workplace. For example, the discourse of intimate relationships in our society has no words like "husband" and "wife" to refer to unmarried couples like Larry and Jennifer or to committed gay partners.[7] The exclusions and inclusions of discourses and practice typically distinguish and promote particular claims to truth, justice, values, and goals (Foucault, 1979;

---

[5]"Discourse" is a term I use to refer to social practices, their language, and their inherent but not static "relations of distribution." The phrase "relations of distribution" denotes those moments of meeting when the potential for fairness is endorsed, ignored, or obliterated.

[6]I am using the term "interest" to refer to a legitimate claim or right that arises in relation to the demands of a particular reality with which a specific group or individual must contend and to which it must respond. This "reality" may be universal *or* a specific social or historic reality (see Ruddick, 1982).

[7]Similarly, there is no word in the discourse of nuclear defense analysts for peace, only "stability," or for human deaths, except "collateral damage" (Cohn, 1987).

Habermas, 1971; MacIntyre, 1984). Acker (1988) sees "relations of distribution" as shaping the quality of relationships by defining and determining the distribution of resources, of rights and responsibilities, and of support and concern. Discourses define power and prestige relations among individuals. They distinguish "legitimate" from "illegitimate" needs, issues, and concerns. The dominant discourse of gender in the 1950s and 1960s, for example, was blind to the limits imposed on many women's lives. Depressed housewives were seen as "dependent," sometimes angry, but not oppressed. In the feminist discourse of the 1970s they were seen as deserving "liberation" from social and economic constraints, while suffering from "learned helplessness." Through the 1980s and into the 1990s, feminist discourses have become more diverse, but most agree that a female consciousness must be articulated that has been previously silent or excluded.

The example of feminism shows us that discourses evolve; they are "contested" and transformed by individuals within relationships whose consciousness is "the site" of many competing discourses. Changes of discourse occur when a gap between human interests and socially defined roles and identities is recognized. Then a space is created for resistance to currently influential discourses, and new discourses and practices may emerge (Foucault, 1979; Weedon, 1987). The recognition of vital human interests, as we shall see, may be facilitated by the human capacity and longing for dialogue.

"Dialogue" reaches beyond "conversation," descriptions of interactions, and social role expectations to the "deep inside" of relationships.[8] It refers to the human capacity to recognize others as unique and to respond to them as independent and existing with their own interests, purposes, and goals; dialogue refers to the encounter that occurs when one person "meets" another in a sphere that Buber called "the between." Reciprocity and mutuality are characteristic of this sphere. In part, because of the ambiguity of spoken language, "mismeetings" also occur. Mismeetings often lead to fruitful dialogue, but the dialogue may also "die in seed."

There is a tendency in recent family therapy formulations to use such terms as "dialogue," "conversation," "language," "consensus," and "discourse" as if they were interchangeable (e.g., Goolishian & Ander-

---

[8]A useful distinction has been made by Habermas (1987) between the systems model of society and his own concept of "Lifeworld." While the systems model of society refers to the differentiated levels and steering mechanisms of society, a description from the "outside," "Lifeworld" refers to the forces of society *as experienced by individuals who live "inside"* it. These forces include the normative "rules" of morality and law, collective consciousness, and forms of mutual understanding. Habermas believes that the systems and Lifeworld paradigms can and should be integrated. The contextual framework suggests a model for such an integration.

son, 1988; Dell, 1986; and others). But I am making distinctions between these terms because I believe, with Buber (1965), that dialogue exists only in a particular kind of relationship and conversation. Further distinction of the meanings of these terms and the exploration of the relations between them can eventually lead to a synthesis of some key but currently polarized ideas within our field.

Dialogue and discourse are in a relation of mutual influence, rather than in simple opposition. The degree to which discourses recognize and meet basic human interests will determine the extent to which they foster or impede truly personal, dialogic relatedness. The longing for fairness and trust, preconditions for dialogue, can lead to transformations of personal relations, evolution of discourse, and social change. For example, in a family with rigid and polarized role definitions, it will be difficult if not impossible for family members to engage in dialogue with each other. To the extent that dialogue is desired and sought, however, it will highlight the discrepancy between personal (or family) interests and needs and *imposed* self-definitions. The search for dialogue may foster change in the prevailing discourse within the family and eventually in the larger social context. Dialogue is both a means and *a desirable goal*. Discourse is a means or perhaps a medium that may permit or prevent social transformation.[9]

Negotiations about rights and responsibilities, and about benefits and burdens, characterize all human social groups and take place at *all* levels of society, even though they may be differently expressed in those different "spheres" (Collier & Yaganisako, 1987).[10] Obligation, indebtedness, entitlement, and exploitation are inevitably "balanced" and "rebalanced" (or not) in human relationships in whatever social domain they occur. In modern life, we tend to relegate ethics and values to the domestic, "private" sphere. Even if the existence or need for dialogue is denied, however—for instance, in the public or political sphere—there is always a "line of demarcation" where the assertion of one group's rights impinges on and provokes an assertion of the rights of others (Buber, 1946/1984). Therefore, politics should be grounded in the "domain of

---

[9]Some social theorists (Foucault, 1979) and therapists believe that power relations *primarily* determine discourses and the relations between them. But clearly people desire power in order to insure that their basic human needs will be met. I believe that all practices and discourse initially arise in relation to human interests (Habermas, 1971).

[10]Feminist anthropologists Collier and Yaganisako assert that feminist theorists have until recently accepted too uncritically such "folk categories" as "public versus private," "domestic versus political," and "nature versus culture," and suggest that these oppositions themselves needs to be understood and challenged. The belief that ethics and values are private matters and that connectedness between people is the province primarily of women, *has* led to the impoverishment of contemporary life. See also Bellah et al. (1985) and MacIntyre (1984).

life," which ultimately requires that people learn to live together, that they consider the interests of others, and "that they compromise and reconcile differences in order to affirm life itself" (Mendes-Flohr, 1984, p. 186). This is as true of couples in their everyday interactions as it is of peoples or nations. Such balances are an aspect of all of life. When imbalances cannot be resolved simply between people, we need courts of law, political negotiations, and *public* debates to decide on values, principles, and priorities.

BUBER'S RELATIONAL THEORY

In developing the contextual approach to family therapy, Boszormenyi-Nagy drew inspiration from and extended Buber's concepts of dialogic relatedness and developed them as they illuminate *family* relationships. However, Buber's "I–Thou" philosophy is an especially important resource for understanding the relationship between members of the adult generation (peers). Buber gives many indications that he views marriage as the quintessential "I–Thou" relationship, because it suggests a commitment and openness to the welfare of another person that transcends transient feelings.

Buber makes a distinction between "social" and "personal" relationships; for him, social membership in no way guarantees the realization of "personal" relationships. Social discourse, as it has been defined here, is the antithesis of the "I–Thou" relationship in the sense that discourse often defines the person *in advance.* Discourse exists in the realm of "I–It" relations, characterized by the *separation* of subject and object; discourse is one way that language may be used—but in this sense, it is the opposite of what Buber meant when he wrote of dialogic "speech-with-meaning." *Personal* relationships are characterized by the potential for "I–Thou" moments. Such moments bring into existence our full humanity and have the properties of contact, presentness, mutuality, authenticity, and spontaneity; they cannot be planned in advance. They involve "turning" to the other as a partner and confirmation of the partner as *other.* They involve allowing the other a full part in the relationship and granting the other a share in one's own existence (Buber, 1965).

"The Between": Buber's Ontology as a Basis for Family Therapy

Distance and relation form Buber's "two-fold principle of human life." They are not primarily experiences or behavior patterns. They are realities of the human condition. "Distance provides the human situation; relation provides man's becoming in that situation" (Buber, 1965, p. 64). Distance is a state of being of which humans are uniquely aware;

"setting at a distance" is the act which acknowledges difference, that is, that others exist independently of us (Buber, 1965). Distance typically points the way back to relation. The rhythmic alternations of distance and relation are the ordinary experience of life, but Buber knew that "the two movements can also contend with one another, each seeing in the other the obstacle to its own realization" (1965, p. 64). He described movingly "the thickening of distance" when such obstacles arise.

Entering into relation involves turning to the other. It expresses both the acknowledgment and the overcoming of the distance that exists most of the time; "imagining the real" other occurs when we enter into the common situation with our partner and are able to imagine his or her unique experience even as we affect him or her—yet remain firmly grounded on our own side of the relationship. "Imaging the real" is contrasted with making the other "an object of contemplation" as in an "I–It" relation.[11]

Existential Responsibility

Buber explicitly applied his philosophy of dialogue to the therapeutic situation. He deplored the failure of the psychotherapy of his day to distinguish between neurotic guilt and "existential guilt"—an "authentic feeling which burns" (1965, p. 127)—and to appreciate the power of realistic, existential guilt as a healing resource in relationships and in psychotherapy. He anticipated the family therapy movement's goal of healing relationships when he encouraged the "doctor of souls" to "cast his glance again and again to where existing person relates to existing person" (1965, p. 122).

Contextual therapy offers a therapeutic method for activating our potential for existential trust and responsibility within families. It calls forth our sense of trust and responsibility for "our personal share" in the world; existential responsibility leads us to repair and heal "an injured order of justice" and to attend to the "actualities of what is happening and has happened between" one person and another (Buber, 1965, p. 122). Buber offers to family therapy a unique and useful epistemology and a radical ontology of "the interhuman." He suggests that the dualism of objective versus subjective ("I–It") knowledge can be overcome by "dialogic" knowing. Reality, according to Buber, is neither simply an objective "given," nor is it primarily constructed by an individual thinking subject. Reality occurs in "meeting" when people enter into relationship.

---

[11]"Imagining the real" refers to the human capacity which enables I–Thou moments to occur. Buber writes "this gift is not a looking at the other, but a bold swinging—demanding the most intensive stirring of one's being—into the life of the other" (1965, p. 81). "Imagining the real" includes but transcends empathy; it implies an "act of the will" and a "seeing through separation" (Stern, Grunebaum, & Friedman, 1989). Buber also calls this relational event "inclusion."

Extension of Dialogue to Family Relationships

The contextual view of relationships is radically dialogic in Buber's sense; contextual therapy heightens our awareness of responsibility to address the particular concrete situations that challenge us and call forth personal and family resources. However, *membership* in particular families or groups *is* viewed as an existentially rooted relationship that often does engender both "existential trust" and "existential guilt." Contextual therapy makes more explicit than did Buber that relationships, especially family relationships, must be *fair* in order to be viable; family relationships afford a unique potential for dialogue and suffer momentously when dialogue seriously fails.

Thus, families, being *social* entities, as well as comprised of relating individuals, are necessarily a complex alchemy of both discourse and dialogue. Both Buber and Boszormenyi-Nagy have given us trenchant critiques of contemporary society and its practices—critiques that are ignored in most therapeutic formulations of family problems.

FAMILY RELATIONSHIPS: RESOURCES FOR TRUST BUILDING AND HEALING

As we have seen, discourse at the societal level powerfully shapes our self-definitions, telling us not only who we are, but also what we deserve and what our obligations are. Discourses about fairness, rights, and responsibilities also exist at the level of the family. These discourses have hidden roots in the dialogue between members of past and present generations. A family's discourse may allow for fruitful negotiation of rights and responsibilities; it may foster a reasonable level of "deserved caring" and allow for the emergence of dialogue. Or it may not. When couples come to therapy, the discourse between them may permit only partial, if any, dialogue about their ethical conflicts. In this section I will describe some ethical dimensions of parent–child relationships and discuss the connection between the consequences of those early relationships and the ethical conflicts that emerge in couples.

"The Parental Imperative" and Filial Loyalty

It is the central axiom of contextual therapy that there are imperatives within families concerning survival interests and basic human needs. When a parent brings a child into existence, an irreversible responsibility toward the child is created. I have called this the "parental imperative"[12] (Grunebaum, 1987). The parental relationship involves an asymmetry of power and competence, and therefore an *asymmetry of giving and responsibility* (Boszormenyi-Nagy & Krasner, l986; Jonas, l984). I will call this the principle of "equitable *asymmetry.*" Parents "owe" more to children than children owe to parents. Children are inherently entitled to unearned care from their parents. This entitlement is due to the universal biological and social conditions of an infant's vulnerability and dependence on his or her parents, even though the pattern of care that is forthcoming is organized by social discourse and practices that vary from culture to culture. The development of a child's capacity to trust requires parental *acceptance* of this asymmetry of obligation. This is an "ethic" intrinsic to family life. It is a premise of contextual therapy that the parental imperative, based as it is in the *universal conditions* rather than specific patterns of parenting, cannot be violated without inducing social, familial, and individual pathology. The quality of care depends on each parent's personal freedom to invest in the child's and the partner's welfare interests. If the parents are not burdened by too much injustice from their own childhood experience or too many societal obstacles, there will be a practical convergence of the parents' existential interests in caring for the child and the child's vital interests in receiving it. "Our understanding of the parental imperative is improved if we make explicit that 'imagining the real' is a key ingredient of 'care.' That is, an essential aspect of parenting is imaginatively recognizing the "Thou" of the child, even though this is more a potential than an actualized reality." (Knudson, personal communication, 1990)

Since family practices originate in the nearly universal *goals* of "preserving the life of the child and fostering its growth" (Ruddick, 1982, p. 79), the equitability of specific cultural patterns of care and actual social practices must be held up to the guideline of the parental imperative. Because the practice of maintaining family life is also subject to social discourse; the parental imperative may be devalued or utilized unfairly to serve other ends, such as simply to reproduce a particular social order (Chodorow, 1978; Ruddick, l982). Furthermore, adults engage in activities other than parenting and participate in discourses and practices pertaining to their own rights and needs for care, meaningful work, and recreation. Coupling is one of the primary ways our society has devised for meeting these adult needs. However, because the parental imperative is nonoptional, it is an intensely

---

[12]Social psychologist David Gutmann (1973) coined this term, but he uses it to mean "the imperative" that women—being the bearers of children—universally are the primary caretakers of children. I am using it in the contextual sense to mean that *parents* have an irreversible, asymmetrical responsibility toward their children.

experienced reality that often conflicts with other adult interests. In contextual therapy, there are no assumptions that family members' interests always converge, or that the interests inherent in the practice of family life do not sometimes conflict. Sorting out both unavoidable and apparent competing interests is frequently the task with which a couple therapist is asked to help. Thus, the ethical implications of both the universal parental imperative and specific social practices may be synergistic *or* in conflict but they are always simultaneously important.

Filial loyalty is another powerful reality of family life. Even when caretaking is inadequate, parents earn merit for having brought a child into existence. The loyalty of the child to his or her parent is based partly on this merit. Adequate caretaking, of course, reinforces and personalizes the child's loyalty. This loyalty is not easily ignored by a child and constitutes a strength and a resource in family relations. In fact, opportunities to express loyalty and spontaneous generosity toward parents are considered to be a child's right (Boszormenyi-Nagy, personal communication). However, it is not and should not be considered to be a static quality of healthy family relations; it must be renegotiated and redefined at each stage of the life cycle as part of an ongoing dialogue with one's family of origin and with one's children and grandchildren.

Parentification and Destructive Entitlement

If excessive support and concern are expected from the child for the parent, the child becomes "parentified." For example, the child may be relied upon by the parent to confirm his or her self-worth at the expense of the child's own need for confirmation. In such a case the child's loyalty to the parent, coupled with the entitlement and needs of the parent, puts the child in a position of having an unpayable debt, because the child is called upon to express filial loyalty in modes that are not possible or fair at his or her age. What the child can give feels inadequate, both to the parent and to the child, and therefore it tends to be dismissed or disqualified. The child then becomes swollen with existential guilt which he or she cannot discharge. This can lead to denial of even realistic guilt and resentment, and later, to a generally distorted sense of guilt and entitlement.

Parentification is one typical and very powerful manner in which an individual can become "destructively entitled." Destructive entitlement is a kind of surplus credit that accrues when one's vital human interests have not been validated, particularly as a child. Destructive entitlement leads people to seek reparation or retribution often in obscure ways, consciously or unconsciously, throughout their lives. The loyalty through which they earned their destructive entitlement and that distorts their new relationships is "invisible," expressed through symptoms, dysfunctional relationships, and other forms of abstract sacrifice.

The sense in which the term "entitlement" is used here is close to the legal meaning; it is not meant pejoratively as indicating an unwarranted claim. Destructive entitlement has its source in *actually* suffered past injuries, especially those sustained in childhood. Because it is based on a valid claim, the person finds it very difficult to transcend and may attempt to seek validation of this debt in new relationships. A person may become desperate in trying to *force* others to become trustworthy; such unjustified actions lead to the continuing accumulation of destructive entitlement in family relationships. Over time, the destructively entitled person becomes more and more depleted because of the dwindling opportunities for mutual give and take.

Marital or other couple relationships are frequently burdened by destructive entitlement. For instance, a man is unable to respond to his wife's request that he go to the doctor with her to discuss her forthcoming operation. He seems unaware and insensitive to her needs for comfort, but also believes that his help will be disregarded. It is discovered in the same interview that when his father died early in his childhood, no one had been available to comfort him, nor was the solace of his company sought by his mother. He was shortly thereafter sent to a boarding school. The comfort that he deserved had not been forthcoming; his need was not met or legitimated. Now he cannot see that his wife needs and deserves his help, nor that he has anything to offer. Moreover, he has defined her problems as "women's problems," problems that he does not understand and does not feel obligated to try to comprehend. This couple's impasse is an example of how interactions may be shaped by social discourse and may be difficult to transcend because of earned "destructive entitlement" and the ensuing failure of dialogue.

Legacy

Parents often feel that their own suffering and the suffering of their parents can be healed or even vindicated if they can provide in a better way for their children. In fact, a crucial aspect of the parental imperative *is* the effort to correct the injustices of the past for the benefit of future generations. This powerful force, called "legacy" (Boszormenyi-Nagy & Krasner, 1986), can be reparative for the parent and of benefit to the child, and it can be evoked in therapeutic work. However, when opposed by too much destructive entitlement, such an imperative can also lead to tragic consequences, such as the parent's envy of the child, or a parent sacrificing a marriage while overgiving to the child. For example, a wife, in her eagerness to have children in order to have a family life better than the one she had, easily dismissed her husband's wish not to have a third child and refused to consider an abortion.

Destructively entitled because of her father's chronic unemployment and eager to "give more" to her own children, she became unwittingly callous to her husband's wishes. Soon thereafter, he took a job in another city and distanced himself from the children, reinvoking the intergenerational pattern of paternal distance and parental irresponsibility.

Clearly, no individual reaches adulthood without having earned some destructive entitlement; therefore partners are, in a sense, always choosing whether to *act* on destructive entitlement or not. The therapist can help them to choose more constructively by helping them to see that demands based on destructive entitlement render them less and less entitled to be "given to" in the present, and that, conversely, generosity in relationships leads to "gains" for the self rather than losses. For example, a couple reported that the husband had been asked by his wife to bring her a cup of coffee, after she had given him a hug. He wondered momentarily if the gesture of affection had been a plot to secure his service to her, but he decided to bring the coffee regardless, along with a flower he had cut from the garden. They were then able to have a difficult conversation that had been postponed for a week. Burdened with some destructive entitlement from his past, he was unable momentarily to give freely to his wife. The social discourse that defines women as "manipulative" and that at times does place women in the position of seeming to exchange affection for economic and other material security provided a particular excuse, a "template," for *acting* on destructive entitlement. Fortunately, in this instance, it was transcended.

The contextual therapist seeks to restore fairness and trustworthiness in relationships, replacing acts of retribution and attempts at compensation with trust—trust that contributions to the welfare of others will be self-reinforcing and self-validating, perhaps not immediately, but over the long term. When trust and fairness are restored to relationships (or perhaps engendered for the first time), both partners gain personal satisfaction, authority, and freedom from cycles of mutually damaging actions.

The Ledger and the Continuity of Contexts

The notion of a "ledger" of the fortunes and misfortunes of a family or group is one of the early concepts in contextual therapy. It is a powerful metaphor for understanding how facts of social existence are given meaning, particularly as they pertain to justice and reciprocity. The ledger is both an account in the sense of a story, and a balance sheet showing what is "owed" and who is obligated. It is the product of the interlocking of discourse and dialogue, interpretation and facts.

Erik Erikson (1964) defines "deeds" as "those actions which make a memorable difference in the shared lives of many" (p. 162); it is a narrative of such deeds and "shared lives" that is recorded in the ledger, especially those deeds through which fairness is expanded or indebtedness is engendered. The ledger contains the narrative meaning of factual, historic events for families and communities. An individual is a link in this chain of events and may be "called to account" for how he or she stands as a person in relation to others. Thus, when a person joins a family through marriage or other committed relationships, the person fatefully places his or her mark on the family ledger for good or ill. How that mark is interpreted and evaluated will be determined to some extent by burdens (indebtedness or destructive entitlement) that the person inherited at birth. For example, a person may be "born guilty"[13] because his or her parents were criminals. The particular mix of inherited guilt and entitlement can be very complex. For instance, if one's parents are survivors of discrimination or genocide, one can be destructively entitled toward the world but within one's family may feel the obligation to compensate one's parents for what they endured. These apparent ethical contradictions are important for the therapist to know about when helping to resolve family conflicts.

SPECIAL ISSUES FOR COUPLES

Ethical Symmetry and Transactional Complementarity

When a couple comes for help, it is assumed that relationships from the past are an active element in their current relationship, although they may or may not be aware of it. The therapist will be particularly interested in the destructive entitlement that may be operating as a consequence of past failures of the parent-child dialogue, and will find ways to make the destructive entitlement explicit. The connections between past and present that the therapist hopes to reveal are not primarily symbolic but rather a matter of the factual consequences of one generation's dialogue with the next.

Thus, a couple therapist must contend with the fact that an individual's several relationships impinge upon one another. A person is a child in one relationship and a partner or parent in another relationship. The therapist must develop the capacity to move back and forth in time in order to address the interlocking of past, present, and future, in both horizontal and vertical relationships.

The most important feature of a couple relationship is that the

---

[13]See *Born Guilty: Children of Nazi Families* by Sichrovsky (1988). He explores how the children of former Nazi war criminals have dealt with the burden of "inherited guilt."

partners are adults, each *equally* capable potentially of the reciprocity required for viable long-term relationships. As contrasted with parent–child relationships, the fundamental requirement for fairness is "equitable *symmetry*." Equitable symmetry does not require identical behavior along the dimension of role behavior; thus, role complementarity is not inherently inequitable. To be equitable, however, role complementarity must be based on choice and negotiation, equality of power and value. Fairness at times may require inequality of give and take. But negotiating such imbalances between adults should not diminish the essential equality of influence and value, which should be intrinsic to adult peer relations. Thus, the therapist must address imbalances of power and coercion and help each partner to understand that he or she can be active and influential, but not unilaterally self-assertive. For a contextual therapist, the goal of "empowerment" implies reciprocity. As J. Grunebaum (1987) wrote, "Within the family, the abuse of power received from the world outside the family is seen as a fundamental statement of despair about the prospects for mutuality and fairness."

The quest to achieve "equitable symmetry" in couple relationships can be quite stressful and complex. The therapist must attend to all relevant contexts, searching for the many potential obstacles to symmetry in the couple's relationship. External factors, such as illness or catastrophic events, drastically alter the balance of give and take between a couple. They will require a new search for balance, which can be healing and growth-promoting or quite disruptive. Each couple keeps a historical "account" of the reciprocity of their relationship. When couples have been together for some time, one of the tasks of the therapist will be to review this narrative accounting. Often, efforts that one person undertook voluntarily to help the other may, in retrospect, seem onerous and self-sacrificial. Here social discourse often plays an important and problematic part. For example, a woman may decide that devotion to her husband as defined by the social discourse of the 1950s no longer serves (and maybe never did serve) her interests. Evolution of discourse and practice can allow couples the social space to redefine their "contract" on a more equitable basis.

The Marriage Commitment and Loyalty to Parents

Adults participate in many loyalty groups that compete for their allegiance. For example, they may have difficulty forming new commitments while continuing a caring dialogue with their parents. Sometimes a therapist has an opportunity to do an extraordinary bit of prevention when two young people who have been intensely parentified request help in deciding to get married or even deciding to "live together." The issue of commitment often leads them to feel disoriented, anxious, guilty, and somewhat depressed. Arguments and power struggles ensue; the relationship feels threatened because they fear their needs are not going to be met. These troubles occur just as they are working hard to establish their right to be an independent couple, and to be less available to their families. When parentified children marry, their relationship is imperiled because it violates the family rule of total availability. One young couple endured cruel punishment: The wife's mother tore up her baby pictures; the husband's father refused to delay his mother's funeral in order to allow him to attend. Couple therapy at this early stage provided the opportunity to interrupt a potentially destructive and perhaps lifelong inability to resolve issues of nurture and entitlement.

Some parentified children find it difficult to make requests but secretly hope that others will read their minds. Some feel entitled to have all their needs met and are outraged when others make demands. Many, like Jennifer, are terrified if they *do* get what they want because their own needs provoke guilt, shame, and disloyalty. Often parentified people fit together in a stable but conflictual union, each harboring resentment. By intervening early, it is possible to prevent their negotiation of needs and rights from becoming a futile activity.

In some instances, conflictual marriages or relationships are formed by young people to avoid facing loyalty conflicts with their parents. For example, a young woman from a fundamentalist family married a nonreligious man without explicitly facing her own searching questions about the teachings of her church. The loyalty conflict then became enacted in the new relationship rather than resolved within the context that engendered it. The new relationship may be conflictual or distant, or end in divorce, but it will continue to serve an important function for new commitments. The first failed or failing marriage serves as a "precious culprit" (Boszormenyi-Nagy, personal communication); it can reduce parental expectations and claims on future commitments and marriages. It can reduce the person's own existential guilt over the disloyalty of individuation.

Split Loyalty

"Split-loyalty" conflicts can also develop when children are caught between divorced parents for whom no collaboration is possible; such offspring are inevitably parentified. In contrast with loyalty conflicts that are developmentally necessary and inevitable, split-loyalty situations erode the child's trust in the parent–child relationship because of the unconditional nature of the bind: He or she cannot be loyal to one parent without seeming to be disloyal to the other. This can happen between parents and grandparents too. Thus, loyalty conflicts and split-loyalty situations of varying degrees of intensity can be interwoven and alternate from one generation to the next. For example, a generation with an unresolved loyalty conflict between parents and spouse may produce a new one, with a child's loyalty "split" between two divorced parents.

Split-loyalty situations also occur in families where there is unresolved marital conflict without divorce. Children are ordinarily aware of this conflict and try to help. While these relational impasses can be described transactionally as "detouring," "triangulation," or the like, clinical experience indicates that such transactional formulations do not adequately describe the consequences for the child of loss of trust in the adult world. The child may be helped not to get involved in an effort to champion one parent or try to heal the rift; however, such functional autonomy may leave the child with an "atrophied personal center" (Buber, 1965), and defensively closed to future healing. With opportunities for spontaneous giving foreclosed, such children may become depressed, suicidal, or delinquent. Thus, when treating couples, a contextual therapist characteristically asks to see the children in order to address and acknowledge their concerns and helping efforts, and to assess their needs for inclusion, direct intervention, or protection from parental neglect or abuse.

Procreation

Intrinsic asymmetries—in particular, women's greater role in biological procreation—also create a necessity for rebalancing between the couple *as parents*. In order to understand this rebalancing, the therapist needs to know how the couple distributes child care *and* breadwinning, and the influence of social discourse and practice on this distribution. The therapist needs to consider, "For whom in the family will the imperatives of child care and of breadwinning be most burdensome?" "How does the social and cultural milieu support or undermine the interests of parents and children?" "What was parenting actually like in the previous generation?" Failure to account for the *social context of parenting* can lead therapists and theorists to idealize the family, especially mothers, and to exaggerate their obligations and capacities to overcome all manner of social hardships, such as poverty, prejudice, or simple indifference to their needs.

The conventional American norm of the heterosexual, married nuclear family with children is supported by a vast cultural establishment. In order to be clinically effective, the therapist must show partiality toward other kinds of families and toward couples who decide not to have children. Deliberations about whether or not to have a child may directly express the presence of unresolved filial loyalty and destructive entitlement. The couple may not feel entitled to have children of their own. They may not feel free to negotiate issues of parental responsibility between themselves or to resist the impersonal dictates of social discourse that define how and when they should become parents. This sense of freedom or lack of it deserves careful exploration, because it often constitutes an entry point for a discussion of both past and current relational impasses. For Larry and Jennifer, the issue of future children is a crucial and almost unspoken topic.

Workaholism

Extraordinary devotion to work or career aspirations may constitute avoidance or sacrifice of personal relationships and parenting responsibilities. It may be the only strategy a person can devise for repaying filial indebtedness. On the other hand, "work" may also represent an important avenue for contributing to one's family and to the future (Ulrich & Dunne, 1986). Men have traditionally been assigned this role. Just as women's work was once invisible, "men's work" is inadequately addressed in family therapy.

How a couple divides responsibility is an important issue in contextual therapy. Conservative discourses have powerfully shaped the division of labor within the family. The division of labor along gender lines of male breadwinning and female child care—the two primary components of the parental imperative—is often accepted as a given. Although feminists have drawn attention to discrepancies of prestige in these two roles, rarely do therapists examine the two roles for their many-faceted advantages and disadvantages. For example, little attention is paid to the sense of imprisonment men may feel even within successful careers, or their desire to be more involved or "empowered" with their children. Clearly, the meaning of work in relation to other opportunities in life varies with the social context.

MULTIDIRECTED PARTIALITY

Therapeutic Goals and Methods with Couples

When faced with clients struggling with conflicting interests, therapists can adopt the individualistic stance characteristic of contemporary Western society and urge individuals to assert their rights and take responsibility mainly for their own happiness. Or, as in contextual therapy, they can urge clients to go beyond these individualistic goals and help clients to seek satisfaction and greater autonomy through engaging with others in a dialogue of reciprocity in which interests are sometimes shared and sometimes competing. They can, as in some family therapies, propose an abstract description of the couple's impasse from a "neutral" position. Or, as in contextual therapy, they can use contextual therapy to reveal and mobilize the relational resources of spontaneity, responsiveness, and responsibility.

"Multidirected partiality" refers to the set of principles that guides the conversation between the contextual therapist and the members of the couple, and ultimately between partners and other family members. It is the term that describes both the *method* and the *goal* of contextual therapy; it is the cornerstone of the approach. As a method, it describes the therapist's stance toward the claims of each partner. The therapist shows "partiality" toward both partners by directing his or her concern to the actual injuries each has experienced and to the sense of injustice that each has expressed. On the other hand, and of equal importance, the therapist also acknowledges contributions that each partner has made to the relationship. Thus, the therapist confirms both the value and the inherent entitlement of each partner as a unique human being and the earned merit of each partner as a participant in his or her significant relationships.

The therapist's acknowledgment of the partners' grievances and contributions makes it more bearable for them to be accountable for their own role in the conflict and helps them to extend acknowledgment, empathy, and appreciation to one another. It mobilizes hidden resources of trust and concern, and encourages people to recognize the *multilateral* nature of relationships—namely, that in any context there are often many valid claims to truth and justice. This recognition of the multilateral nature of relationships is a primary goal of contextual therapy. It is based on the recognition that multiple "goods" exist in the world.

However, the therapist's multidirected partiality does not imply an acceptance of everybody's point of view or claim, nor does it require the therapist to remain outside the system or to maintain "equidistance" from each person. Rather, it involves active openness to each person's respective account. Claims are explored on the basis of their relational "merit." Relational merit is earned by having been interested, concerned, and available for someone when he or she needed and deserved consideration or care. Establishing the relational truth or validity of the claim is an important aspect of the therapeutic process. But it is not the therapist who "decides"; the partners themselves are challenged to establish their own "truths" and engage in a mutual effort to advocate for and negotiate their own standards of fairness. The therapist, however, must be alert to social constraints on definitions of "truth" and seek to broaden the couple's discourse without *imposing* his or her own truths.

Active Elements Leading to Healing

Students often ask, "How does contextual therapy work? Is the therapist a judge, deciding who is fair and who is not?" I will attempt to define in some detail some of the effective elements of this therapeutic method. I will attempt to show how Buber's two-fold principle of "distance and relation" and Winnicott's idea of "potential space" (1971, p. 41) can help us to clarify the active ingredients of this method.

The contextual therapist undertakes an *active search* with clients for differing perspectives, histories, accounts, and the "merit" embedded in each person's story. Together they seek a meaningful account of events relating to reciprocity and fairness. The therapist's openness to the reality of each person's existence creates a space where each person can actually begin to re-engage in living relatedness. I believe that this even is what Buber meant by "imagining the real" and "inclusion."

As we have said, a child's inherent entitlement does not have to be earned. Winnicott indicated that he recognized the ethical dimension of relationships when he wrote of "playing"—a relational mode for which *trust* is a precondition. "Playing implies trust" (1971, p. 51). It is "based on [the] experience" (p. 56) of the parent's or therapist's trustworthiness. Although the child is likely to offer it, trust has to be *justified* by the parent's reliability. "Playing," according to Winnicott, occurs within a "potential space" where a child can begin to trust, to communicate, and to become a spontaneous "true self." This occurs *prior* to the full "acknowledgment of indebtedness" (p. 2). Thus, the parent's reliability is based on his or her ability to make fair demands of children, depending on their age.

This space is what most parents try to create for a child. Yet, when parents have several children, they have to make daily decisions about how to distribute their own resources equitably according to the interests and needs of each unique child and other family members as well. This creates a different kind of space—an interhuman world where fairness, indebtedness, and earned entitlement are realities. Thus, the family becomes the first setting for learning about justice, common "interests," group identity, and loyalty. The contextual therapist's multilateral partiality activates this original group setting and helps to restore its original dynamism.

The therapist's attitude is one of interest in the partners and of humility. He or she does not know in advance what their claims to truth and justice will be nor how they are confirming one another already. The therapist conducts an exploration in order to find out, and credits people who have been contributing in various ways, even in ways that may be obscure. The therapist's inclusive siding with each person helps to actualize the distance that already exists between the partners although they may not be aware of it. The therapist shows that shifts of distance and relation between people are naturally occurring events and that this space *between* the partners may provide the opportunity for *them* to relate differently.

By actively siding with each of them, the therapist recognizes and confirms *distinctness of each person and thus the "distance" between them.* By enabling people to be responsive and accountable, the therapist helps them to complete and to overcome the distance. The therapist's stance of acknowledging uniqueness, inherent entitlement, destructive entitlement, and earned merit and of encouraging people to take "responsible positions" helps to actualize multilaterality, or what Buber calls "the interhuman." *Dialogue emerges in the family as the multilaterality modeled and supported by the therapist is accepted.* Thus, the therapist helps each person both to emerge as an "I" and to express "concern." Each person is enhanced in their potential for meeting the "Thou" of others. In this way, contextual interventions elicit, focus, explore, and catalyze issues of self-delineation, trust, and reciprocity.

Boszormenyi-Nagy, Winnicott, and Buber all emphasize that the essential qualities of this relational space are trustworthiness and spontaneity. Trustfulness is a spontaneous property and cannot be forced. Trustworthiness in one person leads to greater spontaneity and trustfulness in the other. A common reality is created as each person expresses his or her personhood and hears and responds to that of the other. This "common world" (Buber, 1965) may be built with words or constructed in many other ways, such as actions that convey caring and consideration and nonverbal gestures of solidarity and confirmation. The crucial element is mutuality of concern. An aspect of trustworthiness that contextual therapy emphasizes along with Buber and Winnicott, is to show "concern" for the consequences of one's own harmful acts and to engage in reparative actions toward others.

It is expected that dialogue will eventually take place between the partners and other family members as well. This is far more than a conversation; speaking and hearing are the primary modes through which human dialogue can take place. For dialogue to unfold, one must act on the premise that hearing the other person's "story" requires a response. It is mainly through responding that we validate ourselves and each other as human beings. Listening and hearing are not enough. Actions are an important mode through which dialogue can take place. In fact, speaking, hearing, and responding may be viewed as *the relational acts* that most characterize the sphere of the "between." But dialogue cannot be reduced to language or conversation *per se.* Consensus building and cooperative action are essential to all social groups, large and small. But these processes cannot be effective if social discourse imposes a predetermined outcome upon conversation, and thus pre-empts the responsiveness required of dialogue.

Do contextual therapists make judgments? Often, when applying the ethical principles of equitable symmetry or asymmetry, therapists can sense when an old account is being settled unfairly in a new relationship. Sometimes they will know this because their own sense of justice will be activated or offended. They must trust their ethical intuitions and convictions but reflect upon their sources in experiences in their family, community, or culture. Since the therapist's turning to and siding with each family member will to some extent be guided by his or her own standards of fairness, the therapist must be open to feedback from and negotiation with each partner.

Four Dimensions of Relationships

Contextual therapy and its primary method, multidirectional partiality, guide clients through an exploration of the ethical dimensions of their everyday lives as they are illuminated by examining past and future relationships and social forces. It takes the long-term balance of fairness as a crucial determinant of disturbances in relationships and, conversely, of satisfaction. But it does not by any means neglect other aspects of relationships. In fact, it posits four dimensions of relationships that are interwoven but not reducible to one another: (1) the factual context of the relationship, (2) the internal dynamics of each individual, (3) the observable patterns in the relationship, and (4) the dimension of relational ethics. We have seen that contextual therapy is primarily concerned with Dimension 4, but all contextual therapists integrate the other dimensions, depending on the therapist's personal and theoretical convictions and the challenge of the particular situation at hand.

For example, it is important to distinguish the relational processes of Dimension 4 from such intrapsychic mechanisms as displacement, denial, and projective identification; for example, invisible loyalty may be enacted through the psychological mechanism of denial but they are not the same. On the other hand, individual character formation (Dimension 2) can strongly influence relational ethics (Dimension 4)— for instance, when a sense of entitlement from prior abuse is imposed on a new relationship. Similarly, certain mutually reinforcing (circular) patterns of human transactions (Dimension 3) may constitute exploitative forms of "reciprocity" (Dimension 4). Whatever considerations exist in the first three dimensions, contextual therapists believe that it is important to address openly their ethical implications and issues of personal responsibility for the consequences of one's actions. The human longing for trustworthiness constitutes the most potent resource within relational contexts. This longing is activated when interventions are directed to the dimension of relational ethics.

Techniques

Since multidirected partiality is a set of principles and a therapeutic stance based on convictions about the nature of life and relationships, its application cannot be reduced to specific techniques. In fact, many techniques that endorse and generate authenticity and sharing and that foster empathy and reciprocity may be useful. Techniques that deliberately mystify, coerce, assume total responsibility for change, and are disrespectful should not be employed, because I believe that they undermine the goal of expanding trustworthiness and erode the basis of the therapeutic relationship. In practice, the method of multidirected partiality structures the turning to and the siding with each partner, and therefore no special techniques are necessary. I will address specific techniques that I find compatible with this approach in the next section.

CLINICAL APPLICATION

In this section of this volume, each author applies a particular therapeutic approach to the case of Larry and Jennifer as it was described by their couple therapist and by the four presenters who participated in the demonstration interviews. It is important to note that the clinical data we are given are unavoidably the product of substantial editing by each of these therapists. Their editing, of course, reflects their theoretical frameworks, just as my theoretical framework has led me to select different information and exchanges as more relevant. Nevertheless, I found the case report and the reports of the four demonstration interviews to be sufficiently detailed to allow me to identify some initial *points of entry* into the ethical realm of the couple's relationship, or what I often refer to as their "domain of deserved caring." A point of entry is indicated by whatever ongoing discussions the partners are having about giving and receiving and about rights and responsibilities, whether those discussions are characterized more by accusations or by fruitful dialogue. Blaming and complaints are valuable indications that hope for relatedness about these issues is still alive. Feelings of anger, guilt, and disappointment are important indicators of such hope; by contrast, some issues seem lifeless, and the couple's relationship when discussing them is disengaged and ethically "stagnant." These issues may not be ripe for entry and should be reserved for later exploration.

I, and the other workshop leaders, had the advantage of imagining rather than performing a clinical intervention. We were located outside the therapeutic field and thus not subject to its full force nor burdened by the direct and weighty responsibility for protecting the central protagonists in this drama from exposure and exploitation. Thus it is relatively easy for me to assert what "I would do" based on the model of my choice. However, I will do so without undue apology, using the case to illustrate how this contextual therapist thinks and works.

I will present my hypothetical intervention in five sequential phases. This model is not intended as a rigid program, but as one example of how the therapeutic process might develop.

Step 1. Establishing a New Discourse: "Healing Resources"

A distinctive perspective of contextual therapy is its resource orientation. When establishing a therapeutic relationship with clients, I present myself as interested in helping them to discover and activate the resources in their own relationship. Thus, I attempt to establish a relationship of collaboration between myself and them, just as I present their task as a couple as one involving active collaboration. At the same time, I am careful not to let the necessity for collaboration in a therapeutic relationship obscure the asymmetries of power and responsibility that necessarily exist between us.

While I typically address issues of unequal power and responsibility in the therapist–client relationship at some point in the process, in the case of Larry and Jennifer I would have thought it urgent to address the ethical context of the teaching conference itself early in the session, because the ethical implications of the therapeutic relationship would be magnified by the unusual nature of these interventions. The facts that (1) Larry and Jennifer were paid for their participation and (2) no therapist was expected to develop a lasting relationship with them or their families exacerbated the asymmetry of the relationship and left many openings for harm. The fact that the couple was paid not only put them in a position of owing cooperation; it also raised the possibility that the "business contract" would obscure the clients' vulnerability, and thus the therapists' responsibility.

If I had interviewed the couple as part of a large public conference, I would have explicitly addressed issues of power and responsibility at the beginning of my contact, especially when Larry suggested that he and Jennifer suspend "judgment" because they were "in the experiment." I would have expressed my gratitude for their participation and acknowledged their courage and vulnerability. To my knowledge, the only therapist to have done this was Sluzki, and his acknowledgment was made only in passing: "in addition to your contribution to our endeavor, what brought you . . ." without giving them a chance to respond. Also, I would have taken it upon myself to protect the couple from undue exposure and other potential ill effects of their and their families' participation. For example, I would have made explicit my availability for follow-up services for the couple and their families after the interviews. At the conference, I would have asked that the audience refrain from laughing during the taped presentations.

The therapists in their demonstration interviews did not fail the couple; in fact, they deserve much credit for the degree to which they shaped and conducted their interventions according to the ethical requirements of the situation. That the interviews evolved as they did indicates to me how powerfully the "trust context" must and often does shape the therapy itself. But the absence of direct discussion of the ethical context of the conference itself missed an important *therapeutic* opportunity to show caring in the face of vulnerability, and thus to partially redress the imbalance through acknowledgment. However, Norman Paul did show sensitivity to and concern for Larry's parents as persons in their own right when he took up the issue of Larry's mother's weight and suggested that Larry's father support her in carrying forward her weight reduction project.[14] Demonstrating explicit concern about health issues is a characteristic contextual intervention.

I typically begin a consultation by asking the couple how I can help them to create the kind of relationship they want now. Thus, I frame my relationship to them as meaningful and personal, but give critical importance to their own collaboration and goals—to *their* dialogue. I also encourage the couple to value the resources they bring to their relationship and to take a constructive and future-oriented approach to addressing areas of conflict (see also Chasin & Roth, Chapter 7, this volume). For example, I might say, "I know that the two of you must have pain and grievances in your relationship, but I believe from what I know of your history that there are also reasons for being hopeful. There seem to be many resources and strengths in your relationship, such as the fact that you have been available to each other through hard times and the fact that your relationship is moving in the direction of more commitment. While we will undoubtedly need to go over past history, both your own and your families', the purpose of reviewing the past will be to find the hidden resources there and to expand them." If I had known what had happened in the Framos' interview (see Chapter 4) at the time of my hypothetical interview with the couple, for example, I would have acknowledged the intense loyalty that Jennifer felt toward her parents, as expressed in her protectiveness of them. I might have said, for example, "It's good, Jennifer, that you want to protect yourself and your parents from being hurt today. That's a plus for you and your family. But you are being very careful at the expense of any improvement in your relationship. Maybe we can find another way to be protective without keeping things at a standstill in your present relationship."

---

[14]Editors' note: This occurred in a portion of the interview not transcribed in Paul's chapter.

I might then make a statement to the couple communicating hope for the future—for example, "If there isn't enough trust in your relationship now, we will try to find ways to generate it." Then I would underscore my interest in the future by asking for a brief statement from each of them about how they would like things to be better, and how perhaps each would like to "do" better. Note that these opening statements serve to propose a new discourse, one that uses the language of trust, acknowledgment, responsibility, negotiation, and collaboration. This resource framework will be the basis of treatment from the first moments of meeting to the last moments of contact.

Step 2. Exploring and Identifying Opportunities for Dialogue

In the second part of the interview or therapy, I would begin to convey a multilateral perspective—one that validates differing perspectives and claims. A contextual therapist would be particularly interested in the couple's own discourse of caring, reliability, or teamwork and in statements about being "let down" or about "selfishness." He or she would notice whether the conversation was characterized by accusations or by openness to the response of the other.

In the case of Larry and Jennifer, I would begin to activate a multilateral process by acknowledging their willingness to engage in couple therapy. Despite the differences in their degree of enthusiasm, both Larry and Jennifer came. I would indicate that Jennifer deserves credit for taking the lead, but that Larry also deserves credit for cooperating. This stance might be compared with Sluzki's approach, which reframes Jennifer's leadership as a "plot to change Larry." My offer of "partiality" based on the unique contributions of each partner would establish an atmosphere in which differences between the partners could safely emerge. This stance would convey to the couple that I expect to have different relationships with each of them and that I am prepared for shifts of "distance and relation" with me and with the difficult process of the therapy itself.

I expect to feel closer or more sympathetic to one or another partner at various times (see Lamb & Hare-Mustin, Chapter 13, this volume), and often I say that my siding with one *or* the other, and especially *with both simultaneously*, is a transient but important part of the process and that I will do my best to be "fair," as I hope they will.

Step 3. Entering the Domain of Deserved Caring

As each partner presented his or her account of these issues, I would listen and consider these questions: "Who is speaking?" "Who is being addressed?" "Does the conversation feel authentic?" "Is each partner addressing each other as a *person*, or are they appealing to social stereotypes or mythic images in framing and justifying their claims against one another?"

I would attempt to locate the couple socially and historically. For example, in the case of Larry and Jennifer, I would note that they are members of a cohort known for its rejection of established ways of doing things. In a positive sense, they are social innovators. Had they been born 10 or 20 years earlier, they may well have married early or ended their relationship in order to pursue marriage with another partner. They would not have lived together unmarried for several years to "try out" their commitment.

Why they chose this course for their relationship is, of course, not a simple question. Many factors influence such choices, including the outcome of the interplay between individual and family history and shifting modes of relationship within a changing cultural context. But I believe that many people in their cohort chose this course because the prevailing discourse of marriage and family did not legitimate equity and "deserved caring" in intimate relationships sufficiently to foster the emergence of dialogue. In addition, Larry's and Jennifer's personal and family histories did not engender enough trust to allow them the confidence they needed to overcome such constraints. Thus, personal histories and their place in the larger social and historical context seem to have converged and provided an opportunity to participate in a new social practice and to develop their relationship at their own pace without premature commitment or separation. In therapy, they would examine the ways in which their daily interactions either foster or obstruct the achievement of goals they define for their relationship.

In this phase, I would expect them to raise issues related to their relationship "accounts." I have reason to believe from the case report and the four interviews that they would. For example, we learn from the case report that Larry's struggles with Jennifer's unfaithfulness and with his cancer led him to claim the right to a redistribution of support; they made him want to become more "self-centered" and make fewer sacrifices for Jennifer. At the same time, we see that Jennifer wants more from Larry. She presents a strong desire for her feelings to be validated by Larry and has a history of feeling unloved and unwanted by her parents. Both partners want something more from the other. Jennifer wants understanding and attentiveness; Larry wants more trustworthiness from Jennifer. Both want more confirmation and acceptance. Yet neither is comfortable with the vulnerability they associate with receiving and being cared for. We know from the therapist's report that Jennifer sometimes feels "empty" when Larry fulfills one of her needs; though she wishes to receive, she is more comfortable with the role of giver. When Larry feels vulnerable, he prefers withdrawal to support. Issues of giving and receiving are confused with concerns about loss of self, efficacy, power, and control—a not uncommon consequence of childhood trauma and injustice.

Larry's and Jennifer's statements would provide the opportunity to offer partiality to each person. I would hear validity in each person's complaints, encourage both partners to hear the merit in each other's statements, and invite them to give a caring, crediting response. For example, "Jennifer, can you imagine what it felt like to Larry when you let him down early in your relationship?" "What did it mean to you that Larry was 'always there'?" Or, "Larry, in what ways did Jennifer show how much she cared for you when you were sick, or even now, how does she show she cares? Could you tell her?"

As a next step in identifying the couple's resources for achieving "equitable symmetry," I would enlarge the field of inquiry to include their own past history as a couple. I would note that Larry's illness seemed to have provided an opportunity for rebalancing in the couple's relationship. The "needy" and "undependable" Jennifer became a source of strength, support, and protection for Larry. Larry, the "pursuer" and "protector", became vulnerable. It is vital to remember, however, that the decision to live together—a shift toward commitment—was made *before* the cancer was diagnosed.

It is most surprising that these important changes in the couple's relationship were not addressed in the material presented by the interviewers. Perhaps the interviewers felt it would be difficult to address the cancer in the conference setting and therefore avoided focus on that period in the couple's relationship. I would ask the couple to discuss both their decision to live together and the cancer. I would ask them how they had come to the decision and how they had resolved the imbalances in their previous relationship. I would specifically acknowledge the unfairness of Larry's cancer and would explore how the illness had concretely overburdened each of them, especially in light of their new commitment.

Throughout, I would present issues of trust and mistrust as central and would encourage both partners to consider how each habitually responds to the experience of the other and how reliable and trustworthy each had been in terms of "being there" for the other. (Compare with Sluzki, Chapter 6, this volume, when he tells Larry that he is not interested in such "sophisticated" issues as "trust.") I might ask, for example, "How have each of you contributed to the relationship? How have you been hurt or disappointed or betrayed?" In this discussion, the therapist usually begins to hear clues about sources of destructive entitlement in the childhood events of each partner. For instance, Larry's unilateral overgiving to Jennifer and Jennifer's intense need to be needed by other men would be seen as clues to old hurts and imbalances. Focus on the couple's relationship might recede temporarily as the therapist deepened the conversation to include their experiences of childhood injustice.

Step 4. Recognizing and Exploring Sources of Destructive Entitlement

In the previous phases of the interview, my multidirected partiality will have helped Jennifer and Larry to express both their subjectively felt and objectively demonstrable grievances. At this point, I would further explore clues regarding destructive entitlement, guided not only by clinical experience and theory, but also by my own personal convictions regarding the centrality of fairness in relationships. In this phase of the therapeutic process, all dimensions of relationships converge: the historic facts and their culturally specific meanings, as well as the psychological, transactional, and ethical dynamics. In my search to identify ways in which each partner might be seeking compensation for actual injuries suffered in the past, or might be unavailable for new commitments, all of these dimensions would be relevant. But the ethical dimension would be regarded as the most inclusive and the most penetrating.

The mix-up of contexts and generations is partially addressed in this phase. Insight and learning are important steps, but the main goal is to reassess relational balances with families of origin through actual re-engagement, facing conflicts, and the discovery of ways to renew dialogue.

Larry and Jennifer came to their relationship burdened by different degrees and patterns of parentification and destructive entitlement. Jennifer's parentification is clearly more onerous. She was delegated to take care of her frail father who was presented to her as on the verge of death. She slept with him and sometimes lay awake, fearful that he might stop breathing if she didn't watch the rise and fall of his chest. She was terrified and overwhelmed by this confusing responsibility. Moreover, from her perspective, her inherent entitlement to exist seems to have been called into question. She told Jim Framo that she never felt "valued, needed, useful, appreciated, or wanted."

By contrast, Larry's basic right to be alive, to be loved, and to make requests of others was not compromised. Yet he too experienced parentification, although less severe and more subtle than Jennifer's. His parentification seems to have occurred in relation to his cousins. Asked to conceal his academic success to preserve his mother's sisterly loyalty and solidarity, he constrained his own imagination and ambitions and confined his aspirations to winning in sports. We can only speculate about his role in his parents' relationship, but the interviews revealed that Larry's mother is rather lonely in her marriage. Perhaps Larry used distancing behavior to prevent himself from becoming her confidant, thus attempting to contend with a covert "split-loyalty" situation.

I would explore these historic events first with the couple alone, with one partner listening as witness and potential resource (Boszormenyi-Nagy & Krasner, 1986). If family of origin meetings are planned, it is often best to conduct them, at first, as Paul and the Framos did, without the person's spouse present. The goal would be to help the spouse to withdraw from playing an active part between the partner and his or her parents, and later, perhaps, to be available as a supportive resource. I would explore the sources of destructive entitlement from the standpoint of that individual's experience and also from his or her parents' standpoint. Inclusion of the parents' vantage point is possible even if the parents are dead.

Paul and the Framos called forth multiple perspectives in their family of origin interviews; however, their interviews differed in key respects from a contextual family of origin meeting. Both interviews were directed primarily to the psychological and interpersonal dimensions. Though they reviewed experiences of suffering and injustice of individuals, the interviewers did not invite the family members to acknowledge and respond to each member's recollection of *actual* injustice. Rather, they assumed that immaturity, inadequate information, and "misunderstandings" led Larry and Jennifer to develop inaccurate images of other family members. These childhood images (even if partly accurate) were seen by Paul and the Framos largely as anachronisms that did not fit the current personalities or intentions of other family members—anachronisms that impeded the achievement of the major goal of creating new, up-to-date relationships.

In my opinion, the Framos may have been induced to rush toward that goal because of the pressures and pitfalls of a demonstration interview. Thus, that approach bypassed the essential processes necessary for dialogue. From the contextual viewpoint, one unfortunate result was an expectation of premature, inauthentic forgiveness. Jennifer understandably reacted strongly to this. A contextual therapist would have been guided by the premise of "equitable asymmetry" in the parent–child relationship and would have made an attempt to elicit from the parents an *effort* to hear, to recollect, to understand, and to validate the actuality of the injuries suffered. When parents are struggling with the therapist's challenge is just the moment to offer partiality to them for their own difficult or unjust life experiences. But the children's destructive entitlement has priority in terms of the temporal sequencing of the therapist's partiality. Challenging the parents to acknowledge their children's suffering offers *the parents* themselves the opportunity to earn entitlement and self-validation (Boszormenyi-Nagy & Krasner, 1986). This dialectic of ethical challenge and fair crediting is the key to *partiality*. Often parents respond over time with an increased sense of worth and self-esteem. Then it may be possible for children to consider possible misunderstandings and for family members to engage in a less ethically stagnant form of relating. But it would be necessary to guide the family through this process beyond one all-or-nothing interview. Therefore, in a demonstration interview, it is preferable to delineate these issues as topics for work with the couple's therapist.

Had the Framos been less pressured, presumably, they would have examined carefully Jennifer's grievances but would have given equivalent attention to Beth's parentification. Her mother's abandonment and her father's premature departure from his home and homeland would have been placed on the agenda as well. Nonetheless, the Framos' interview did exemplify many values and goals important to a contextual therapist; for example, Jim Framo kept his promise to Jennifer that he not ask her mother about her past, and the Framos did enable Jennifer to hear from her mother that she *was* wanted. Mary Framo was extremely helpful in introducing acknowledging comments and in slowing down the process.

Paul's interview seemed more "multilateral" because it emphasized not just outdated images but the *actual consequences* for the child of the parents' behavior, such as the impact on Larry of his parents' failure to mourn their own parents' deaths. A three-generation context was outlined for further exploration. As in the Framos' interview, some genuinely healing moments occurred, as when Larry learned of his father's great affection and concern for him in the brief discussion of his illness. Yet one wonders: Had the source of destructive entitlement been other than denial of the *emotions* associated with illness and loss (e.g., his father's abuse by his stepfather), would Paul have recognized and developed these issues? Often, it is precisely the *unfairness* of a loss that leads to its denial, rationalized by cultural or religious beliefs. Prohibitions against recognizing and discussing injustice should be addressed both as loyalty imperatives and as concrete social constraints.

If I were to conduct a family of origin meeting with Larry's or Jennifer's family, I would search not only for familial sources of destructive entitlement but also for societal sources. I might wonder, for example: Would Jennifer have been designated as caretaker for her father if she had been a boy? What were the migration and immigrant experiences of these families, and what impact did they have on them and their parenting practices? We would expect each parent's invisible loyalties and destructive entitlement to be linked to these historical, cultural, and social factors which they experienced not only as children, but also *as parents*.

Step 5. Interlocking Ledgers: The Partner as Resource

At this point I would use what has come before in the therapeutic process to help Jennifer and Larry face and renegotiate the imbalances in their relationship as a couple. I believe it is essential for the therapist to guide the couple in freeing their relationship from the family "ledgers" that are woven into the fabric of their own accounts. The explorations of each partner's family of origin will have helped both partners to understand that neither lives in circumstances entirely of his or her own making. Each has been shaped by earlier relationships. Each brings into the current relationship burdens inherited from the past. It is often a relief for couples to gain insight into the prior sources of their partner's needs and claims. But insight is not enough. The ultimate goals for the contextual therapist are to elicit acknowledgment from each partner of the basic human merit of the other, to restore trust, and to renew efforts toward a caring and mutually responsible dialogue with the previous generation. Active efforts toward these goals will free the couple to establish their commitment as a new priority and to be available as a resource to the other.

We would now turn to an examination of the complementarity and relational balances of their early relationship. In their first five years as a couple, Larry and Jennifer played distinct roles with each other. Larry seemed to do all the giving, Jennifer the receiving. He could be "relied on." She was "mixed up" and "in need of care." Through affairs with other men, Jennifer gave to others at the expense of trustworthiness and fairness in her relationship with Larry. A systemic therapist might argue that this complementarity constituted a "contract" to which they had both implicitly "agreed," and thus might view their problems as due to a pattern of rigid role polarization. A contextual therapist, however, will examine such a "contract" from the perspective of fairness and will hypothesize that destructive entitlement may be fueling inequities. The contextual therapist will see such a complementary relationship as ethically nonreciprocal and locked in an impasse that blocks the couple from engaging in fair negotiations about their claims, needs, fears, and desires.

For example, I might hypothesize that Larry was acting on an invisible intergenerational loyalty to his mother when he found a woman who badly needed his support. He may have wanted to be more supportive to his mate than his father was to his mother, but through loyalty to his father would have chosen someone who could not accept his support. He may also have been seeking a way to be more spontaneously giving as an adult than he felt he could be as a child and young adult.[15] Thus, compelled to be an unrequited "giver," Larry was still bound by a split-loyalty predicament. Invisibly loyal to his parents, he may have chosen a woman who at that time could protect them both from *reciprocal* closeness.

Jennifer, at the time, was unavailable for commitment. She was still invisibly loyal and destructively entitled as a consequence of the stressful and overwhelming responsibility she suffered as keeper of her father's life. The lack of acknowledgment that she received as a child left her loyally believing that she did not deserve Larry's unqualified care and support. As Erik Erikson points out, "Too much mistrust leads to an inhibition of the wish to take." (1964, p. 184) Thus, she sought to be giving in relationships with less trustworthy men who could provide her with safety from the terrors of a committed relationship. As I see it, the problems that Larry and Jennifer experienced in their relationship were not due primarily to competition or role polarization around intimacy and distance, but to their deeper confusion of adult receptivity and interdependence with past experiences of overwhelming powerlessness, vulnerability, and loss of autonomy. The dichotomy of vulnerability versus autonomy that our cultural discourses promote and which foster this confusion is an untenable one for closely relating partners.

As mentioned earlier, we never learn how Larry and Jennifer were grappling with the imbalances in this early period of their relationship when they decided to live together, because Larry's illness provided an unexpected and traumatic opportunity for Jennifer to reciprocate the consistent devotion that Larry had provided her for so many years. Because of the frightening nature of the illness, however, Larry returned to a *nonreceptive* position, avoiding dependency and striving for self-sufficiency—precluding direct validation of Jennifer's support. At this time in his life, Larry was entering adulthood and a professional life; he had been well trained in the male gender discourse of mastery, control, and independence. Thus, a serious illness was for Larry, as it would have been for most men, a relational and cultural as well as a medical challenge. For Jennifer, Larry's illness created a familiar if recently avoided role: that of being a caretaker in a frightening situation. As in her earlier parentifying situation with her father, Jennifer was once again watching over the man she loved, told that he might die, wanting and needing to be helpful, but unable to assess or significantly enhance

---

[15]Chodorow (1978), Dinnerstein (1976), and others have made the point that the structure of the contemporary nuclear family, which makes the mother central and the father peripheral as parents, leads to later difficulties in the capacity of men and women to form stable, intimate relationships. On the other hand, this kind of family structure also tends to reproduce itself, by virtue of a "(sadly) efficient feedback system" (Ortner, 1974, p. 87).

his chances of survival. Yet what is *most* significant is that both Jennifer and Larry gained much self-validation and entitlement during this period for their courage and teamwork in facing the extreme challenge of Larry's illness. Each earned the right to receive.

As we would shift our focus back and forth between the past and present and discover the threads of old family ledgers in the ledger of the couple's relationship, a circular, self-reinforcing pattern would become apparent. Each partner would now see how he or she had inadvertently contributed to the anxiety and mistrust early in their relationship. Fuller understanding of their contributions would emerge in the safe context of multidirected partiality, where they would be encouraged to acknowledge and respond to each other's perspectives and claims. The discourse of accusations and labels (e.g., "He's trustworthy and she's undependable") would fade as openness, spontaneity, and risktaking began to emerge.

Encouraged by my openness to the wholeness and uniqueness of their relationship, and by my entering into our "common situation" of couple therapy, I would hope that Larry and Jennifer would come to appreciate their own resources and to recognize in their pain and grievances a basic human longing for dialogue.

COMPATIBLE TECHNIQUES

Many of the techniques described in this book are helpful to me in fostering the emergence of dialogue between family members. Papp's (Chapter 3, this volume) wonderfully evocative structured fantasy elicited many images and themes of longing for connection and trustworthiness, as well as conflicts of obligation, which indicate both the goals of the couple and their difficulties in achieving them. Chasin and Roth's (Chapter 7, this volume) dramatic enactments of the ideal future and disappointing past are uniquely helpful in evoking the partners' destructive entitlement and often liberate the couple's own resources for negotiating a new "present-oriented," more "just" relationship and for a courageous renewal of dialogue with the previous generation. "Future questions" (Penn, 1985) are useful for generating hope and, by "imagining the real," for enabling people to think about the future consequences of their current behavior. Such techniques are fruitfully employed within the ethical and methodological framework of multidirected partiality.

CONCLUSION

Contextual therapy is a discourse that identifies long-standing injustice in relationships as a major source of dysfunction. It is a model based on the conviction that trust and reciprocity are not arbitrary distinctions, but intrinsic to human nature and to all group and family relationships. I believe that the contextual model offers a unique and "generative" discourse. Nonetheless, the *application* of any model will unavoidably be shaped by the person of the therapist in particular relationships with couples. A theory can never be judged by its discourse alone; the power of a model can be discovered only in the struggle to comprehend its implications and to assess honestly its human value through interpretation and application in "the between" created by therapists and couples together.

Thank you, Larry and Jennifer, for sharing your lives with us.

Acknowledgments

I would like to thank Roger Knudson for his close reading and valuable comments – and Richard Chasin and Margaret Herzig for their inspiring editorial assistance. They have helped me to "imagine the real" of this chapter..

REFERENCES

Acker, J. (1988). Class, gender, and the relations of distribution. *Signs, 13*(3), 473–497.

Balint, M. (1968). *The basic fault: Therapeutic aspects of regression.* London: Tavistock.

Bellah, R., Madsen, R., Sullivan, W., Sundler, A. & Tipton, S. (1985). *Habits of the heart: Individualism and commitment in American life.* Berkeley: University of California Press.

Bernal, G. (1982). Parentification and deparentification in family therapy. In A. S. Gurman (Ed.), *Questions and answers in family therapy* (Vol. 2). New York: Brunner/Mazel.

Bernal, G. et al. (1990). Development of a contextual family therapy: Therapist action index. *Journal of Family Psychology.* 3(3).

Boszormenyi-Nagy, I. (1972). Loyalty implications of the transference model in psychotherapy. *Archives of General Psychiatry, 27,* 374–380.

Boszormenyi-Nagy, I. (1987a). Transgenerational solidarity: The expanding context of therapy and prevention. In I. Boszormenyi-Nagy (Ed.), *Foundations of contextual therapy: Collected papers.* New York: Brunner/Mazel.

Boszormenyi-Nagy, I. (1987b). Contextual therapy and the unity of therapies. In I. Boszormenyi-Nagy (Ed.), *Foundations of contextual therapy: Collected papers.* New York: Brunner/Mazel.

Boszormenyi-Nagy, I., & Krasner, B. (1986). *Between give and take: A clinical guide to contextual therapy.* New York: Brunner/Mazel.

Boszormenyi-Nagy, I., & Spark, G. (1973). *Invisible loyalties: Reciprocity in intergenerational family therapy.* New York: Harper & Row.

Boszormenyi-Nagy, I., & Ulrich, D. (1981). Contextual family therapy. In A. S.

Gurman & D. Kniskern (Eds.), *Handbook of family therapy*. New York: Brunner/Mazel.

Buber, M. (1957). Religion and modern thinking. In *Eclipse of God; Studies in the relation between religion and philosophy* (M. Friedman, Trans.). New York: Harper & Row.

Buber, M. (1965). *The knowledge of man: A philosophy of the interhuman*. New York: Harper & Row.

Buber, M. (1970). *I and thou*. New York: Scribner.

Buber, M. (1984). A tragic conflict? In P. Mendes-Flohr (Ed.), *A land of two peoples: Martin Buber on Arabs and Jews*. Oxford: Oxford University Press. (Original work published in 1946.)

Chodorow, N. (1978). *The reproduction of mothering: Psychoanalysis and the sociology of gender*. Berkeley: University of California Press.

Cohn, C. (1987). Sex and death in the rational world of defense intellectuals. *Signs, 12*(4), pp. 687–718.

Collier, J., & Yaganisako, S. (Eds.). (1987). *Gender and kinship: Essays towards a unified analysis*. Stanford, CA: Stanford University Press.

Cotroneo, M. (1982). The role of forgiveness in family therapy. In A.S. Gurman (Ed.), *Questions and answers in family therapy* (Vol. 2). New York: Brunner/ Mazel.

Dell, P. F. (1986). Why do we still call them "paradoxes"? *Family Process, 25,* 223–234.

Dinnerstein, D. (1976). *The mermaid and the minotaur: Sexual arrangements and human malaise*. New York: Harper & Row.

Erikson, E. (1964). *Insight and responsibility: Lectures on the ethical implications of psychoanalytic insight*. New York: Norton.

Fairbairn, W. R. D. (1952). *An object-relatedness theory of personality*. New York: Basic Books.

Fishbane, M. D. (1987). Buber and couple therapy: An integrative systemic approach. Presented at conference *Martin Buber and his influence on psychotherapy.*Washington, DC. (S. Kepnes & H. Abromovich, organizers).

Foucault, M. (1979). *Discipline and punish*. Harmondsworth, England: Penguin Books.

Foucault, M. (1981). *The history of sexuality: Vol. 1. An introduction*. Harmondsworth, England: Pelican Books.

Friedman, M. (1965) Introductory essay. In M. Buber, *The knowledge of man: A philosophy of the interhuman*. New York: Harper & Row.

Friedman, M. (1985). *The healing dialogue in psychotherapy*. New York: Jason Aronson.

Gelinas, D. (1983). The persisting negative effects of incest. *Psychiatry, 46,* 312–332.

Gelinas, D. (1986). Unexpected resources in treating incest families. In M. Karpel (Ed.), *Family resources*. New York: Guilford Press.

Gilligan, C. (1982). *In a different voice: Psychological theory and women's development*. Cambridge, MA: Harvard University Press.

Goolishian, H., & Anderson, H. (1988). Human systems as linguistic systems: Preliminary and evolving ideas about the implications of clinical theory. *Family Process, 27*(4), pp. 371–393.

Grunebaum, J. (1987). Multidirected partiality and the "parental imperative":

An answer to the feminist critique of systems theory. *Psychotherapy,* 24(35), pp. 646–656.

Grunebaum, J., & Smith, J. (in preparation). Beyond roles: Family and friends as the paradigms of group treatment. In B. A. DeChant (Ed.), *Women, gender, and group psychotherapy.* (Originally presented at a workshop, "The Ideal Mother and the Actual Mother: Their Encounter in the Consulting Room." Conference on *Women.* Harvard Continuing Education, 1988, Cambridge.) New York: Guilford Press.

Guntrip, H. (1969). *Schizoid phenomena, object relations and the self.* New York: International Universities Press.

Gutmann, D. (1973). Men, women and the parental imperative. *Commentary, 56,* 59–64.

Habermas, J. (1971). *Knowledge and human interests.* Boston: Beacon Press.

Habermas, J. (1987). *The theory of communicative action: Volume 2. Lifeworld and system: A critique of functionalist reason* (T. McCarthy, Trans.). Boston: Beacon Press.

Jonas, H. (1984). *The imperative of responsibility: In search of an ethics for the technological age.* Chicago: University of Chicago Press.

Karpel, M. (Ed.). (1986). *Family resources.* New York: Guilford Press.

Karpel, M., & Strauss, E. (1983). *Family evaluation.* New York: Gardner Press.

Leupnitz, D. A. (1988). *The family interpreted: Feminist theory in clinical practice.* New York: Basic Books.

MacIntyre, A. (1984). *After virtue: A study in moral theory* (2nd ed.). South Bend, IN: University of Notre Dame Press.

Mendes-Flohr, P. (1984). Prefatory note. In P. Mendes-Flohr (Ed.), *A land of two peoples: Martin Buber on Jews and Arabs.* Oxford: Oxford University Press.

Ortner, S. B. (1974). Is female to male as nature is to culture? In M. Z. Rosaldo & L. Lamphere (Eds.), *Woman, culture and society.* Stanford, CA: Stanford University Press.

Penn, P. (1985). Feed-forward: Future questions, future maps. *Family Process,* 24,(3), pp. 299–310.

Ruddick, S. (1982). Maternal thinking. In B. Thorne & M. Yalom (Eds.), *Rethinking the family: Some feminist questions.* New York: Longman.

Sichrovsky, P. (1988). *Born guilty: Children of Nazi families.* New York: Basic Books.

Simon, F. B., Stierlin, H., & Wynne, L. C. (1985). *The language of family therapy: A systemic vocabulary and sourcebook.* New York: Family Process Press.

Stern, A., Grunebaum, J., & Friedman, M. (1989). *The philosophy of Martin Buber and overcoming stigma.* Workshop presented at the meeting of the American Psychiatric Association, San Francisco.

Stierlin, H. (1975). Book review of *Invisible loyalties. Psychiatry, 38,* 96–98.

Ulrich, D., & Dunne, H. P., Jr. (1986). *To love and work: The effects of families on performance.* New York: Brunner/Mazel.

Weedon, C. (1987). *Feminist practice and post-structuralist theory.* Oxford: Basil Blackwell.

Winnicott, D. W. (1963). *Maturational processes and the facilitating environment: Studies in the theory of emotional development.* New York: International Universities Press.

Winnicott, D.W. (1971). *Playing and reality.* New York: Basic Books.

11

Treating Communication Problems from a Behavioral Perspective

VICTORIA M. FOLLETTE and NEIL S. JACOBSON

A great deal of research has been conducted over the past 15 years on the efficacy of behavioral marital therapy (BMT) (Jacobson, 1984a). Based upon that research, we can draw two broad conclusions. First, we know that BMT leads to relationship improvement for many couples (Jacobson, 1984b). Indeed, many married couples can truly be described as happily married after completing a standard behavioral treatment program (Jacobson & Follette, 1985). Second, marital discord is a pernicious clinical problem and there are more treatment failures and relapses than we would like (Jacobson, Follette, Follette, Holtzworth-Munroe, Katt, & Schmaling, 1985; Jacobson, Follette, Revenstorf, Baucom, Hahlweg, & Margolin, 1984). While the "good news" reinforces us for our hard work and perseverance, the "bad news" reminds us that we still have our work cut out for us.

The two main components of BMT, as implemented in our program, are behavior exchange (BE) and communication/problem-solving training (Jacobson & Margolin, 1979). However, we do not now consider either or both of these components sufficient by themselves for satisfactory marital therapy. We generally offer these elements with additional components (Jacobson & Holtzworth-Munroe, 1986; Wood & Jacobson, 1985). When conducting BMT in a clinical setting, clinicians can pick and choose from various approaches to design a treatment plan that seems most relevant for any particular couple, and thus one less likely to allow for relapse.

In this chapter, we will present a treatment plan that incorporates the basic components of BMT as it is currently practiced within our group, and emphasizes areas that are especially significant for Jennifer and Larry. Since we did not have an opportunity to interview the couple, our recommendations for therapy must be based on the evidence obtained by other therapists. We mention this because our own assessment instruments would have focused on areas other than those emphasized by the therapists who interviewed this couple (Jacobson, Elwood, & Dallas, 1981). Our typical evaluation procedures involve two or three interviews devoted exclusively to questions of assessment. Although this is an unusually lengthy assessment procedure, it is necessary for two reasons. First, without it we cannot obtain an adequate baseline against which to subsequently assess the effects of our intervention. Second, it takes us two or three weeks to collect the information we need to develop a treatment plan tailored to the needs of a particular couple.

Our assessment procedures are of three types: self-report measures, direct observation of interaction, and clinical interviews. Quite often, the self-report questionnaires are collected from couples prior to the first clinical interview to afford the therapist an opportunity to plan the initial interview with the information derived from them. Moreover, the questionnaire data help the therapist pinpoint potential obstacles to "treatability" as early as possible, so that plans can be made for further evaluation without needlessly delaying the onset of treatment. For example, if the possibility of organic brain syndrome is indicated, the therapist can include a neurological evaluation early enough so that the evaluation and treatment processes can proceed expeditiously.

Assessment interviews are conducted with the couple first, followed by one session with each spouse. The initial interview with the couple focuses on current precipitants of marital difficulties and includes a review of the developmental history of the relationship. To the surprise of many couples, they spend about half the interview reminiscing about their early courtship. This is a pleasant occurrence because they frequently enter the initial interview expecting to recite a litany of complaints about each other. While information exchange about conflicts needs to occur at some point during the evaluation, we believe that the initial interview with the couple is not the optimal time for it. In part, this is because such information can be obtained with greater candor through the use of self-report questionnaires. Perhaps more importantly, however, if the initial interview focuses on each person's complaints, it is likely to leave the couple feeling demoralized (see also Chasin & Roth, Chapter 7, this volume). In contrast, if the therapist can direct the couple to contemplate and discuss happier times, clients can derive some immediate benefits from marital therapy, and leave the session feeling better than they felt when they came in. When they experience some relief during this initial contact, it is usually because they are reminded that the relationship has some positive aspects, or at least it once did.

The separate sessions with each spouse provide the therapist an opportunity to explore individual concerns that the couple might be hesitant to broach during conjoint sessions. It is important for the therapist to know about these concerns when devising a treatment plan. It is only in these individual sessions that virtually no attempt is made by the therapist to control any intense negativity that may be expressed by a spouse.

This routine use of individual sessions represents a change from the prescriptions discussed by Jacobson and Margolin (1979). At that time it was believed that individual sessions detract fundamentally from the dyadic focus of the treatment. Although some still advocate the exclusive use of dyadic sessions (e.g., Stuart, 1980), we have changed our position. It seems to us that the benefits derived from new information more than compensate for the minor costs to the relationship focus.

After the assessment phase has been completed, the therapist meets with the couple for a round-table discussion. The major purposes of this discussion are to present a treatment plan and to convey to the couple what they can expect from the therapy and the level of commitment that will be required of them. The therapist begins with a formulation of the present problem that refers to both the strengths and the weaknesses of the relationship. Then a treatment plan is presented, proposing intervention strategies designed to address the couple's problems. Although the session has didactic elements, it evolves into a dialogue between therapist and couple, in which the therapist's formulations are qualified and modified by the responses of the couple. Toward the end of the discussion, a decision must be made by the couple regarding their commitment to therapy. They are encouraged not to make this commitment without recognizing that therapy will require some major adjustments in their lifestyle; they will be expected to work hard, both during and between sessions, to improve their relationship. It has been our experience that successful marital therapy is rare unless the couple maintains a collaborative set and complies with homework assignments. If couples understand the nature of the commitment required and actively make this commitment, the probability of success is greatly enhanced.

BEHAVIOR EXCHANGE (BE) PROCEDURES

Although BE has been an integral part of BMT from its inception (Baucom, 1982; Jacobson & Margolin, 1979), it has undergone a great deal of revision over the years (Jacobson, 1984a). Early BE interventions taught couples to exchange positive behaviors in a contingent manner. These interventions, which were based on a *quid pro quo* or reciprocity-based model of a good relationship, seem to have been misguided (Gottman, 1979; Jacobson, Follette, & McDonald, 1982). Recent research indicates that only distressed couples are so sensitive to immediate contingencies and so highly reciprocal that they require daily exchanges of positive behavior. Interventions that focus on immediate contingencies may be self-defeating if the goal is to promote a happy long-term relationship. As a result of this research, our version of BE now promotes exchanges that are parallel but not contingency-based, exchanges that more closely approximate the types of interactions that characterize happily married couples.

BE interventions consist of directives from the therapist designed to increase the frequency of positive behavior exchanges in the couple's natural environment. When employed at the beginning of therapy, as they typically are, BE directives serve several functions: They offer relatively "low-cost" ways to increase marital satisfaction on a day-to-day basis; they help to consolidate the collaborative set; and they demonstrate to demoralized couples that they can indeed enhance the quality of their relationship. This last purpose is particularly important. Couples often enter therapy complaining that they are powerless to change their interaction patterns. If we can show them that change is possible through systematic attention to day-to-day exchanges, the impact can be, and often is, quite dramatic.

The first BE directive often promotes the acquisition of "pinpointing" skills. Each spouse is asked to identify or "pinpoint" behaviors already in his or her repertoire that, when enacted, have a reinforcing impact on the partner. Thus, from the beginning, spouses focus on themselves and what they can do to enhance the quality of the relationship for the partner. This runs counter to the typical practice of having each spouse ask for what he or she *wants* from the partner. This departure from traditional procedures has a number of favorable consequences. First, it is a directive that is almost always new for the couple, and thereby minimizes the likelihood that the therapist will simply be asking for "more of the same." Second, it allows spouses to begin the change process without exposing either partner to the vulnerability involved in asking the other for something. Finally, it enhances the likelihood that any change that does occur will be favorably received, since positive behaviors are increased at the initiative of the giver rather than at the request of the recipient.

Various strategies can be used to teach the skill of pinpointing. At times we begin by generating lists in the sessions; at other times couples are taught to collect data at home on a day-to-day basis. Whatever the specifics of the task, the goal for each partner is to generate a large menu of behaviors that he or she believes to be pleasing to the other spouse. The next step is to increase the frequency of these behaviors. The directive for this task is usually general rather than specific, and leaves as much of the initiative as possible in the hands of the giver. Generally, the request involves enacting some of the items on the menu at an increased rate, and observing the impact of these positive behaviors on the partner.

We encourage couples not to commit themselves during the session to increasing particular behaviors, but to decide during the course of the week which ones to enact. Additionally, they are urged not to increase behaviors that would lead to resentment on their part. The point of the task is to have each giver decide what to give and how to give it rather than leaving the decision up to either the therapist or the recipient. The range of behaviors that couples are willing to enact varies widely, running the gamut from making the partner a cup of coffee to initiating sexual intercourse.

Subsequent BE sessions expand on the groundwork laid down through the use of these early directives. The material generated during the course of doing the homework provides the grist for later sessions. The debriefing of previous homework assignments and the generation of subsequent ones are major foci of therapy sessions following such assignments. Routinely, the therapist wants to know how and to what extent each assignment was completed. If both spouses complied with the task, and each was in fact successful in improving the partner's subjective sense of satisfaction, then the therapist is free to move on to more challenging assignments. However, often something goes wrong the first time the assignment is attempted. In some cases, one spouse attempts to generate numerous positive behaviors but none successfully increases the recipient's marital happiness. When this happens, the therapist must discern which of two possible causes accounts for the lack of success. It may be that the particular behaviors chosen were the wrong behaviors and that additional pinpointing is required, or it may be that the recipient is indeed benefitting from these positive behaviors but for one reason or another is withholding credit or praise. Since we generally have no way of determining which of these two possible explanations accounts for the lack of increase in marital happiness, we assume, until proven otherwise, that the giver has simply chosen the wrong behaviors.

Couples vary in terms of their need for BE. For some couples, it occupies center stage for a number of sessions. For other couples, for whom day-to-day satisfaction is not a problem and the ultimate success of the relationship hinges upon resolving particular major problems, BE might play a minimal role. In the case of Jennifer and Larry, it does not appear that BE would constitute a central part of the treatment. It is difficult to know for sure, however, since the quality of the day-to-day relationship was not systematically assessed by the therapists who interviewed Jennifer and Larry. We can be more confident, however, in our speculation about what would come next for Jennifer and Larry. Judging from the information we have, their treatment would focus on communication and problem-solving training.

COMMUNICATION/PROBLEM-SOLVING TRAINING

There is much evidence, both clinical and experimental, that communication training is the *sine qua non* of effective marital therapy (Jacobson, 1978). We practice many different types of communication training with attention to both process and content. Thus, we are concerned not only with the efficiency and clarity of information transfer, but also with couples' learning to use the process of effective communication to make concrete changes in the areas of their relationship that cause discord.

The material on Larry and Jennifer provides much evidence for communication difficulties in their relationship. Moreover, the case report written by their therapist (see Chapter 2) indicates that they came to therapy stating as their goal "to improve communication with each other and to identify and resolve their problems." We are told that Jennifer has said to Larry, "I miss you most when we are together." This is a classic message that we hear from couples entering BMT. Jennifer and Larry, both bright and articulate individuals, do not seem to be able to use communication to enhance closeness and intimacy. This particular function of communication would receive a great deal of emphasis in our work with them. They also report that they lack a satisfactory method for discussing problems. Although the ability to communicate in a way that fosters closeness and intimacy will help them when they begin to discuss conflict areas, we would also spend some time focusing specifically on this rather highly specialized set of communication skills. But we would start by attending to receptive and expressive communication skills, without special reference to conflict resolution, because such skills are both easier to teach and less demanding.

We are struck by the lack of attention paid to communication and problem-solving by the other four therapists who interviewed Larry and Jennifer. Sluzki asked them what brought them to the consultation:

JENNIFER: Well, we were having problems in our relationship, and the nature of the problems revolved around a sort of lack of communication, an inability to interact with one another. I felt the need for more interaction, and I was hoping that we would learn how to interact better. I felt that we had been living sort of parallel lifestyles, in the sense that we weren't really interacting and communicating with one another. I felt like we had become just roommates, rather than partners or friends or comrades, or, you know, people that we could share our emotions with, that could actually exchange ideas and feelings with one another.

SLUZKI: Uh huh.

JENNIFER: I would say that that's probably the nuts and bolts of the real problem. We were hoping to see whether we could improve that.

SLUZKI: Uh huh. (*To Larry*) And what brought you?

LARRY: Well, I agreed that there was something that could be improved in our relationship and one of the things was why the interaction between us wasn't what Jennifer thought it should be, and what I thought it should be, and also how our long history together affected the interaction now, and to try and get a grip on how we can improve our relationship, possibly by understanding what went on in the past and what's happening in the present, with some objective help.

SLUZKI: (*To Jennifer*) You were mentioning communication. What does it mean? What were you talking about?

JENNIFER: Well, when I say "communication," I mean an exchange of feelings and ideas and thoughts, you know, a sharing of these things. I mean exposing one's vulnerabilities and feeling that it's safe to do so. And my feeling is that if you can do that with somebody, you establish a closer relationship with that person.

SLUZKI: That makes sense.

At this point, Sluzki chose to concern himself with achieving equidistance between himself and each member of the couple. Toward that end, he joked about Jennifer's desire to bring Larry into the world of therapy, to the "mode or language" that she had developed in individual therapy. He then recast Jennifer's need for communication as a style complementary to Larry's less communicative style. While Sluzki's interview attended more to communication patterns than the other three interviews, he failed to respond directly to the couple's clear request for help in dealing with communication deficits. Sluzki's intervention may have been useful, but it was not as likely to have long-term benefit, in our view, because it did not give Larry and Jennifer enough specific guidance on how to change their entrenched style of communication. A basic tenet of our treatment has always been to address a couple's request for change in a straightforward manner, assuming that they are indeed experts in knowing what will be helpful to them in their relationship.

Communication Training

The early focus on listening or receptive communication skills has two functions: to help each partner become a better listener, and to teach both how to communicate to the other partner that they are, in fact, listening, and that they understand what they are being told. Many of the skills taught during this phase are quite similar to those taught to beginning therapists. Modeling is frequently used during the session, with the therapist demonstrating both poor attention skills and optimal ways of showing that one has attended to what the partner is saying. By demonstrating extremely inattentive behavior (interrupting, looking away, etc.), the therapist can inject humor into the session. Despite the exaggerated nature of the therapist's demonstrations, couples are usually able to see the relevance to their own more subtle manifestations of nonattending. Whenever the therapist models particular "listening skills," there is always some discussion or "debriefing" afterwards to insure that the rationale for the skills is apparent. Moreover, when the therapist models particular skills while role-playing with one spouse, it is important to obtain feedback from the other spouse about how it feels to be listened to and understood.

One of the primary listening skills taught to the couples is paraphrasing. Paraphrasing involves not only listening to what the partner is saying, but also restating it to make sure that it was correct. Paraphrasing is not mind reading; in fact, mind reading is avoided in the early stages of marital therapy, since distressed couples usually use mind reading as a weapon. Paraphrasing involves simply summarizing what the other person has said, and avoiding reading into the statement any motivation, intent, or underlying personality trait. When paraphrasing, partners simply report what they observe.

The subject matter for the listening and paraphrasing exercises should be restricted to relatively benign or neutral topics, such as how each partner spent his or her day apart from the other. Each individual has the opportunity to both provide and receive information; the therapist provides feedback and opportunity for further practice. Couples are asked to practice paraphrasing and other listening skills at home between sessions as well as during the sessions.

The second phase of communication training involves the development of more sophisticated expressive skills. Critical to this phase of treatment is the understanding on the part of both spouses that most observations have "relative and multiple viewpoints" (Wood & Jacobson, 1985; see also J. Grunebaum, Chapter 10, this volume). Many arguments revolve around futile attempts by spouses to reach agreement on the objective reality of the particular situation. Not only is it impossible to grasp an objective reality, but the search for "truth" is often self-defeating for couples in distress. As an alternative, we encourage couples to be as clear as possible in expressing their qualified, subjective experience in a neutral manner. Gottman and his colleagues (Gottman, Markman, Notarius, & Gonso, 1976) list a variety of expressive behaviors to be avoided in such discussions, such as accusations, "kitchen-sinking" (presenting a potpourri of issues), and character assassination. The therapist encourages both spouses to use "I statements" to link feelings and behaviors. For instance, Jennifer might say to Larry, "When you watch TV in the evening when I would like to talk, I feel lonely and a little angry." Larry would be asked to paraphrase what Jennifer said, essentially validating her experience. This is often a very difficult task even for verbally sophisticated couples. They feel that by validating what their partner has said that they have lost the argument and have agreed to change. Thus, it is important for the therapist to point out that this is not the case. Validating simply means that one partner understands the other person's position and can understand why he or she is taking it, given his or her premises (see also Chasin & Roth, Chapter 7, this volume).

When spouses are unwilling to validate what the other has said, discussions become stuck and ultimately produce one of two negative outcomes: escalation or withdrawal. Escalation refers to the process whereby both partners continue to restate their positions in an attempt to get the other to "hear" what is being said. The negative affect escalates, whereas the verbal interchange may be repetitive and ritualized. Withdrawal usually occurs with a great deal of negative affect, quite often amounting to feelings of hopelessness that the other person will never really understand.

The therapist would coach Jennifer and Larry in these new communication skills and continue to give them feedback on their progress. At this point, we frequently have couples practice their skills by spending time talking together about what they did while apart during the day. This gives the couple a chance to communicate without the stress of discussing an affectively charged topic. However, it has an additional benefit that may be even more important for Larry and Jennifer. Sharing experiences and expressing feelings on safe subjects make it easy for the partner to show understanding and caring; thus, the sense of intimacy may increase between them and some of the positive aspects of earlier times in the relationship can be revived. It would be particularly important to monitor their reactions to this phase of therapy. How are they reacting to the homework? Do they feel that these communication skills are producing benefits for them? When maximum benefit has been reaped from these techniques, the focus then shifts to the more demanding task known as problem-solving training.

Problem-Solving Training

Problem-solving training is a structured communication format for reaching specific agreements regarding relationship problems. (Specific guidelines are described in Jacobson & Margolin, 1979.) Communication skills training always precedes problem-solving training because communication skills facilitate the acquisition of problem-solving skills. In addition, when the early therapy sessions are devoted to BE (assuming that the emphasis on increasing positive behaviors has met with some success), couples are more likely to work collaboratively on the demanding tasks associated with conflict resolution. Problem-solving training itself is useful not only in helping couples to solve long-standing relationship problems, but also in teaching a process that can be used to deal with unforeseen conflicts that occur after therapy ceases. Thus, not only is the "content" of the issue important, but also the process by which issues are discussed becomes very significant.

At first, when couples are taught conflict resolution skills, they practice them only in the therapy sessions. This restriction affords them the opportunity to learn the process with maximum feedback from the therapist, and at the same time minimizes the frustration resulting from unsuccessful attempts at home. A mastery experience is much more likely if the therapist is providing continuous feedback.

Prior to the initial problem-solving training session, couples are given copies of our training manual (Jacobson & Margolin, 1979) to read. They are encouraged to underline parts that seem particularly important, make notes in the margins, and write down any specific questions that they have about the procedure. It is not uncommon for couples to express initial reservations about the format. The most common reservation is that the procedure appears to be excessively encumbered by rules, thus rendering the communication process too mechanical. It is very important that these reservations are adequately dealt with by the therapist before the training process begins, in order to avoid covert resistance. Therapists are taught to acknowledge that problem-solving communication *is* mechanical when one first learns it. It is explained that in order to overcome long-standing habits and substitute new communication patterns, the process must be mechanical at first; however, once the skills are learned, the approach is tailored to fit the communication styles of each particular couple. If this idiographic tailoring process is underemphasized, generalization and continued use of these skills after therapy are unlikely.

We begin problem-solving training by setting some guidelines for the couple. Larry and Jennifer, for example, would be encouraged not to attempt to solve problems at the "scene of the crime," but rather to set up a specific time to discuss the problem. This is in part an attempt to insure that problem solving occurs during times other than those of peak emotional intensity concerning the issues at hand. Although productive work can be done during such periods, they tend to be inopportune times to attempt conflict resolution, and couples are much more likely to work collaboratively in a conflict area if they have some emotional distance from it.

The problem-solving process involves two distinct components: problem definition and problem solution. The failure to maintain this distinction is responsible for many failed attempts at conflict resolution. At the beginning, the focus is exclusively on problem definition. More often than not, each individual has his or her unique conception of what the problem is. When couples launch into a discussion of possible solutions to the problem prematurely, often the result is that neither feels "heard" by the partner. Moreover, inadequately formulated and articulated problem definitions result in each spouse discussing a different problem without either knowing it; in other words, each partner attempts to solve a problem while assuming a common definition, when in fact each is trying to solve a different problem. Taking time to clearly define the problem allows each partner to develop his or her position fully.

As couples are taught to pinpoint the specifics of a conflict area, they are encouraged to emphasize the behavioral, affective, and cognitive aspects of the problem. They are taught to place particular emphasis on the affective consequences of upsetting behaviors. Jennifer and Larry, for example, seem to have some difficulty sharing areas of vulnerability with one another, a common difficulty in distressed relationships. The therapist can gently encourage some affective disclosures in the relatively safe environment of the therapy session. For instance, Larry may complain that Jennifer does not call when she is going to be late coming home from work. To Jennifer, it may seem that Larry is unreasonably demanding and is focusing on something that is relatively trivial. However, when Jennifer is late, it may remind Larry of times in the relationship when Jennifer was dating another man. A seemingly innocuous behavior can become extremely salient because of the meaning it has for the complaining spouse. Unless one's cognitive and affective context is known, the partner has no way of understanding the significance of the issue.

When one partner offers a definition of a problem, we ask the listener not to interrupt, but simply to respond by paraphrasing what the other has said. Paraphrasing during the problem definition phase can have a number of benefits. First, the person expressing concern about some area in the relationship has the experience of being fully listened to by his or her partner. This experience of being listened to is often quite unusual for distressed couples, where interruptions and cross-complaining are typical patterns in problem discussion. Second, communication is much clearer, since distortions are immediately nipped in the bud. Moreover, when paraphrasing is done properly (with or without coaching), it is nonjudgmental and thus decreases the temptation to interrupt and cross-complain. A smooth problem definition process, in and of itself, can constitute a major change in the relationship. Often the information that is provided about thoughts and feelings, which has been withheld in the past, generates compassion instead of defensiveness in the partner. Resistance to behavior change is thus diminished; in some cases the conflict simply loses its intensity and desperation.

During the second phase of a problem-solving discussion, the focus shifts to the search for resolution. Here, the collaborative set faces its sternest test. The first step during the resolution phase involves brainstorming, a method designed to generate a large number of possible options, including ones that involve some behavioral and/or cognitive changes. The sheer number of possibilities provides some relief for the couple, as many apparently irreconcilable differences have resulted from a battle over one particular solution. When a variety of alternatives are considered without initial concern about their quality, it is easier for each partner to be flexible and avoid the pitfalls of an "all or nothing" stand. Additionally, the creative brainstorming process can often generate novel solutions that would not have surfaced under normal circumstances. For example, Jennifer and Larry might identify the division of household chores as a problem in the relationship. Some of the proposals made during the brainstorming session might include the following:

1. Making a list of all the chores and dividing them by drawing lots.
2. Each taking full responsibility for the house on alternate weeks.
3. Hiring a team of servants.
4. Having the therapist come to the house to help with chores.
5. Having someone come in to do the heavy housework and dividing the smaller tasks between them.
6. Having Larry do all the indoor work and having Jennifer take responsibility for all the outdoor chores.

After a discussion of the pros and cons of each suggested option, the problem-solving session concludes with a written change agreement specifying the resolution. A good change agreement will generally require some modification in behavior by both spouses and will be specific enough so that each spouse can judge whether or not it is being carried out. Furthermore, the agreement is typically structured to insure that what is agreed upon will be implemented. Finally, all agreements are temporary when they are first negotiated; they are designated as trials for a limited period of time. Provisions are made for re-evaluating, and if necessary renegotiating, once the trial period is past. Modifications are often necessary, as unforeseen developments occur.

TREATING SEXUAL PROBLEMS WITHIN THE CONTEXT OF MARITAL THERAPY

The majority of couples who present themselves for marital therapy experience some dissatisfaction with their sexual relationship (Melman & Jacobson, 1983). Although in some cases the sexual dissatisfaction involves a classic dysfunction, more commonly it involves boredom and/or decreased desire. Jennifer and Larry seem to fall into this latter category, reporting that although sex was once "terrific," it is now "tepid and mechanical." It is incumbent on the marital therapist to address sexual issues directly as part of the marital therapy process. We can state most categorically from our own research that sexual enhancement does not occur routinely as an indirect consequence of relationship improvement in other areas (Melman & Jacobson, 1983); in other words, no matter how successful marital therapy is in resolving other presenting problems, unless sexual issues are addressed directly, they continue to pose problems. It is unfortunate that the treatment of sexual problems is a neglected area in the literature on marital therapy, since sexual satisfaction plays an important role in overall marital satisfaction and fosters emotional intimacy for many couples. We know that a lack of emotional intimacy is a major concern for Jennifer and Larry, especially for Jennifer.

Assuming that the assessment phase of therapy has not revealed a sexual dysfunction, the therapist might follow the problem-solving phase of therapy with efforts to enhance sexual intimacy. Usually, affection is the initial focus of this phase. We use a number of guided fantasy exercises based on techniques described by Barbach (1983). The goal is for each spouse to generate ideas regarding his or her ideals for the expression of affection in the relationship. In the case of Jennifer and Larry, affectionate interactions might be increased when they are engaged in parallel activities such as watching television. It is important for the therapist to facilitate more effective ways of exchanging information about affection and sexual expression. Using the skills developed during the communication phases of therapy, it is often useful to have each spouse define how he or she would like to talk about sex. Couples are then given homework assignments in which they are asked to try some of the behaviors of affection mentioned by their partner, and to begin keeping a sexual journal.

Much of this sexual enhancement phase involves more communication training about issues related to sex. One important area involves communication about sexual initiations, and partners' responses to such initiations. Another involves the issue of giving positive and negative feedback about particular kinds of sexual stimulation. Sensate focus exercises are used as a vehicle for discussion.

Fantasy exercises are also used to facilitate the quality of sexual interaction *per se*. One of the purposes of these fantasy exercises is to generate new ideas about what would be pleasurable from the perspective of each spouse. Such exercises are often perceived as less threatening if a therapist frames them as "information," than if there is an implied demand for change in accordance with each spouse's fantasies. Subsequent homework assignments involve attempts to introduce some of this information into the communication and/or sexual interaction during the course of the subsequent week. The lists of desired sexual behaviors are expanded further in subsequent sessions, and in some cases, change agreements are formed to focus on conditions that would be likely to improve the quality of the couple's sex life.

GENERALIZATION AND MAINTENANCE

One of the tasks of a marital therapist is to help couples retain continuity from one session to the next. Otherwise, couples may leave a session and not think about it again until the next contact. Specifically, the therapist must remind the couple of what has happened up until now, and in what direction therapy is moving. At the beginning of a session, the therapist might refresh the couple's memories about the content of the previous session, and at the end of a session might summarize the important issues discussed. Such efforts to maintain continuity contribute to the overall treatment progress by allowing gains to accumulate and to be consolidated from one session to another.

As termination approaches, couples are encouraged to assume increasing amounts of responsibility for providing this kind of information. They begin to describe the important points of a previous session, or summarize the most salient aspects of a just completed session. The major emphasis becomes "How can the material discussed during the session be used at home?"

Toward the end of therapy, therapist and clients look in detail at the gains made and the extent to which therapy has accomplished the clearly specified treatment goals established after the initial assessment. Problem areas that have not changed as a result of therapy, along with new problems that have developed subsequent to the onset of therapy, can be tackled with the couple acting as their own therapist. Couples are encouraged to have "state-of-the-relationship" sessions on their own at home in between therapy sessions. Gradually, these sessions substitute for therapy sessions. The important point is that couples begin to take time to discuss the quality of the relationship, and to re-engage the skills learned in therapy at points where they are clearly needed. When a couple can successfully conduct their own state-of-the-relationship sessions, termination is indicated. These final meetings are generally less structured than therapy sessions, but they include a discussion of past change agreements and any problem-solving that still needs to be done. We imagine that for Jennifer and Larry these sessions would focus on communication and problem-solving skills. The relationship meetings could serve as gentle reminders for both of them to continue to engage in behaviors that foster a sense of intimacy between them. Or if they feel their overall marital satisfaction has deteriorated, they might use this time to determine what action might ameliorate the problem.

Recently, we have been experimenting with the use of booster sessions following the termination of treatment. During these sessions, the skills learned in therapy can be reviewed, crisis intervention can occur, or new problems that had not been foreseen during the period of treatment can be considered. Although some therapists and clients view a return to therapy as a failure (there was a time when we did as well), we now see booster sessions as a resource that can enhance the long-term effects of therapy. If neither therapist nor clients view a return to therapy as a negative outcome, couples are more likely to return and less likely to have the gains of therapy slip away.

CONCLUSION

The treatment interventions described in this chapter are typical of those used in a BMT approach, and central to it. However, by no means do they exhaust the realm of BMT. Had we conducted an evaluation with Larry and Jennifer, we might have discovered aspects of their individual and relational lives that would steer us in different directions than those highlighted here. We are confident, however, that the overall approach described, in one particular manifestation or another, could have helped Larry and Jennifer to clarify the nature of their conflicts over intimacy and to make concrete progress toward resolving them. Our confidence that a wide range of types of couples can be helped with our approach has deepened considerably in recent years, as what began as a relatively standardized treatment model (particularly in research settings) has been enriched with options and variations. The current state of the field would be barely recognizable to its pioneers. We expect this evolutionary process to continue.

REFERENCES

Barbach, L. (1983). *For each other.* New York: New American Library.

Baucom, D. H. (1982). A comparison of behavioral contracting and problem-solving/communications training in behavioral marital therapy. *Behavior Therapy, 13,* 162-174.

Gottman, J. M. (1979). *Marital interaction: Experimental investigations.* New York: Academic Press.

Gottman, J. M., Markman, H., Notarius, C., & Gonso, J. (1976). *A couple's guide to communication.* Champaign, IL: Research Press.

Jacobson, N. S. (1978). Specific and nonspecific factors the effectiveness of a behavioral approach to the treatment of marital discord. *Journal of Consulting and Clinical Psychology, 46,* 442–452.

Jacobson, N. S. (1984a). A component analysis of behavioral marital therapy: The relative effectiveness of behavior exchange and problem solving training. *Journal of Consulting and Clinical Psychology, 52,* 295–305.

Jacobson, N. S. (1984b). The modification of cognitive process in behavioral marital therapy: Integration of cognitive and behavioral intervention strategies. In K. Hahlweg & N. S. Jacobson (Eds.), *Marital interaction: Analysis and modification.* New York: Guilford Press.

Jacobson, N. S., Elwood, R., & Dallas, M. (1981). Assessment of marital dysfunction. In D. H. Barlow (Ed.), *Behavioral assessment of adult disorders.* New York: Guilford Press.

Jacobson, N. S., Follette, V. M., Follette, W. C., Holtzworth-Munroe, A., Katt, J. L., & Schmaling, K. B. (1985). A component analysis of behavioural marital therapy: One-year follow-up. *Behaviour Research and Therapy, 23,* 549–555.

Jacobson, N. S., & Follette, W. C. (1985). Clinical significance of improvement resulting from two behavioral marital therapy components. *Behavior Therapy, 16,* 249–262.

Jacobson, N. S., Follette, W. C., & McDonald, D. W. (1982). Reactivity to positive and negative behavior in distressed and nondistressed married couples. *Journal of Consulting and Clinical Psychology, 50,* 706–714.

Jacobson, N. S., Follette, W. C., Revenstorf, D., Baucom, D. H., Hahlweg, K., & Margolin, G. (1984). Variability in outcome and clinical significance of behavioral marital therapy: A reanalysis of outcome data. *Journal of Consulting and Clinical Psychology, 52,* 497–504.

Jacobson, N. S., & Holtzworth-Munroe, A. (1986). Marital therapy: A social learning/cognitive perspective. In N. S. Jacobson & A. S. Gurman (Eds.), *Clinical handbook of marital therapy.* New York: Guilford Press.

Jacobson, N. S., & Margolin, G. (1979). *Marital therapy: Strategies based on social learning and behavior exchange principles.* New York: Brunner/Mazel.

Melman, K. N., & Jacobson, N. S. (1983). The integration of behavioral marital therapy and sex therapy. In M. L. Aronson & L. R. Wolberg (Eds.), *Group and family therapy*. New York: Brunner/Mazel.

Stuart, R. B. (1980). *Helping couples change: A social learning approach to marital therapy*. New York: Guilford Press.

Wood, L. F., & Jacobson, N. S. (1985). Clinical applications of behavioral marital therapy. In D. H. Barlow (Ed.), *Behavioral treatment of adult disorders*. New York: Guilford Press.

PART IV

ISSUES IN COUPLE THERAPY

12

Women in Couples:
How Their Experience of
Relationships Differs from Men's

NATALIE S. LOW

Women and men bring to a couple relationship different experiences, different notions of how it is supposed to be, and different expectations of what each will get from the other. Because these differences shape the interaction of the couple and the structure of the relationship, they have to be understood by the couple therapist. Some differences are best understood as gender-based.

Psychological differences between men and women have been discussed and conceptualized in a variety of ways. Until recent years, they were seen simply as "natural" differences, so much a part of the human condition that they invited no examination (Hare-Mustin, 1987). Even in the current family therapy literature, it has often been assumed that couple relationships can be described in terms of symmetry between the behavior of men and women (Haley, 1976; Minuchin & Fishman, 1981; Willi, 1982). As Virginia Goldner (1985, p. 33) writes, "the category of gender remains essentially invisible in the conceptualizations of family therapists." Further confounding the family therapist's understanding of the couple relationship is the grounding of descriptions of a couple's behavior in the male's experience of the relationship. Drawing attention to gender differences, therefore, will not only invite exploration of male–female differences, but will also help us to introduce the woman's experience into our descriptions of the interaction.

As a consequence of dramatic changes wrought by the women's movement, preconceptions about women are now open to inquiry. In the last two decades we have witnessed an outpouring of work leading to new observations about women's experience in history, literature, political science, and, of course, psychology (Heilbrun, 1979; Keller,

1985). This work has led to a more complex understanding of gender differences as a phenomenon varying historically and across cultures, but always as an important part of the social system. In this chapter I will examine the clinical implications of our enhanced understanding of gender differences, particularly as they apply to the practice of couple therapy. I will focus on two gender differences that are particularly powerful in shaping the functioning of the couple system: differences in power (and perception of power) and differences in the ways in which men and women characteristically experience relationships. Typically, in a couple relationship, both partners tend to act on the assumption that the man has more power. The woman usually concerns herself more with the quality of the relationship and attends to maintaining communication and closeness. The man, on the other hand, often tries to shape the relationship to preserve his independence and continued autonomy. These differences can create difficulties, particularly when the man's greater power (and the woman's acceptance of it) results in both members assuming that his way of experiencing the relationship is the more valid one.

THE POWER DIMENSION

Historically, the distribution of power between men and women has been unequal in economic, political, and religious institutions, as well as in family life. These inequalities have persisted for a variety of complex reasons that clearly go beyond biological destiny. The growing evidence of the extent of male physical abuse of women and children and sexual abuse of both male and female children (Herman, 1986) is startling testimony to the corruptibility of physical and psychological power. While these abuses, particularly sexual abuse, are considered aberrant by most of society, they do reflect the power of the man to keep his family hostage to the satisfaction of his needs, even when such satisfaction is manifestly destructive. In trying to understand the male use of power in apparently better-functioning couples, we have to look for its more subtle and socially accepted expressions.

One of the primary sources of the man's greater power in the nuclear family has been his provision of the income on which the family unit depends. Women, especially middle-class women, are taught by their mothers, their fathers, and various institutions of society that their husbands will provide for and protect them and their children. In exchange for this, wives agree to be feminine—that is, loving, caring, dependent, and less powerful (Stiver, 1984). Underlying women's response to the demand for "femininity" is their need for safety. It is not safe for a woman to act in her own self-interest. To seek equal power with a man, to be independent, breaks an unwritten and unspoken rule, provoking anxiety and raising the spectre of possible abandonment. These cultural "rules" lead both men and women to participate in a deeply ingrained differentiation of roles based on gender. The derivatives and ramifications of these rules are likely to inform both the conscious and unconscious layers of a women's concept of herself.

Jean Baker Miller (1976) was one of the first mental health professionals to discuss this gender-based inequality in power positions and its effects both on women's sense of themselves as individuals, and on the structure of male–female relationships. As Miller says, "the woman is not encouraged to take her own needs seriously, to explore them, to try to act on them as a separate individual. . . . Instead the woman is encouraged to concentrate on the needs and development of the man." (p. 18).

In typical couples, even through the 1980s and into the 1990s, the man and the woman share the assumption that the man has more power. If a woman should find herself exercising power in the relationship, she will likely experience herself as selfish and destructive. All of the psychological mechanisms that support the development and maintenance of the self in relation to others are involved in order for women (and men) to maintain this particular power structure. While we recognize that society declares men to be more powerful, we would do well to study how this prescription is integrated into the psyches of individual women and men and how it is psychologically maintained by the couple.

Although we say that the man has more power, we recognize that his power would be diminished if the woman did not respond with a receptive complementarity. In order to understand how male power is maintained in the couple relationship, let us look at a couple interaction. A successful lawyer tells his wife, a college professor who is overweight but far from obese, "You do have a problem with being fat that we have talked about over and over again, and because you are fat, I'm not attracted to you sexually, and that is why I'm having affairs." The wife responds by confessing that by not losing weight she is treating her husband as she had treated her father, who had also complained of her being fat when she was a child. She says, "I know that that was my way of defying my father, and now it is how I defy you." Only a woman who felt clearly subordinate could accept the cruelty and self-righteous justification of the husband's remark and respond with a confession of culpability. Only someone who assumed the more powerful, controlling side of a relationship could have struck out at his wife with so little awareness of his punitive attitude. There is no doubt that the roles in this example could be reversed. However, if one were to study the frequency with which this pattern of male-female exchange takes place, there is no question that it most typically involves the sex roles illustrated above.

In seeking to understand this type of interaction we could also refer to the man's narcissism and sadism and the woman's masochism, but if we did not include in our analysis of the interaction the couple's assumption of the man's power over the woman, we would neglect the context that provides a structure for his narcissism and her masochism. As Virginia Goldner says so well, "Male privilege and female masochism are structured into the psyche and into the arrangements of everyday life. A challenge to these structures requires no less than a momentous social upheaval, and that is now in progress" (1985, p. 44).

In order to keep the balance of power in favor of the man, the woman has to cooperate by maintaining certain psychological positions, which in some couples may become exaggerated, as in the example above. The woman has to consciously and unconsciously defer to her husband because he is the man, even though at times such deference may do violence to her own self-image. She may also have to idealize him, to exaggerate his talents and abilities, in order to justify her less powerful position. By marrying a man who is typically older, taller, smarter, and more educated, a woman places herself in a position in which it seems natural to be less powerful. The converse is also true: Most men marry younger, smaller, less intelligent, and less educated women, which helps them to maintain their more powerful position.

Neither the man nor the woman need consciously recognize that their choices are shaped by power considerations. The man's socialization to power and responsibility can preclude an awareness that he uses power and the woman assists him in maintaining that role. Where a woman might attribute volition to the man in his exercise of power, a man may experience himself as merely carrying out his "natural" function or role. He might even, in some cases, relinquish a particular responsibility or explicit power if asked. But the woman does not dare to ask, because it would threaten the balance of power as she understands it has to be maintained.

How does the fact that more women are earning their own money and having fewer children affect the traditional marital relationship? Among other changes, the divorce rate has risen to 50%, more women are remaining unmarried, and middle- and upper-middle-class women are purposely having children without husbands or legal fathers of the children. These changes of demography and family structure, however, particularly in the middle and upper middle class, have not clearly changed the power arrangements between men and women, at least as seen every day in the consulting room. It may be that there is a time lag in the psychological adjustments we make to social change. Changes in "external" social institutions can sometimes be effected rapidly, but the ways in which we retain meaning in our lives are so deeply rooted in our upbringing that changes in that realm may have to proceed more slowly. Women now in their 20s, 30s, and 40s were born into families in the 1940s, 1950s, and 1960s, where they learned from their mothers and fathers how to be responsive to the needs of men. The contradiction between women's newly emerging opportunities for experiencing power in the workplace and their learned patterns of accommodating to their husbands' power is seen in the following case.

A highly successful academic woman lawyer in her 30s is married to a man equally well educated, but struggling with a faltering career and periodic unemployment. At the end of a demanding and long day, the wife comes home to her bored and restless husband, who has been at home all day while their child was in day care. She cooks him a fine dinner and then feels obliged to cater to his need to go out in the evening. With her eyes half-closed with fatigue and her child in her arms, she joins him in his quest for social stimulation. Despite this couple's role reversal in the realm of economic and worldly success, the wife still places her husband's needs above her own and acts the part of the caring, dependent wife. The husband assumes, according to male tradition, that he is the head of the household and that he has the right to make these demands on his wife. It would be a mistake to see this example as a special instance of a woman's individual masochism or a male's self-indulgence. Rather, it is a case of failure to adapt to the changed realities of the husband's and wife's daily life, which serves to highlight the cultural tradition of the man's greater power over the woman in the life of the couple. It should be noted that this is the reverse of the typical story of the bored housewife demanding attention from the busy husband. In that case, he probably would not have acceded to her complaining request for diversion, and she would have been made to feel frivolous and guilty.

WOMEN'S RESPONSIVENESS TO RELATIONSHIPS

There is another readily observable and acknowledged difference between men and women, and that is the difference in their sensitivity and responsiveness to emotional and interpersonal issues. While the talent of women for tuning in to emotions and relationships has been acknowledged, it has not been highly valued. It has been treated as a second-class capability that is not especially worthy of study since it does not contribute much to making the world go round, although it may make the household go round. Recently, largely because of the women's movement and a growing interest in studying female development, women's behavior has begun to be investigated in a context that values women's experience. Researchers have been able to determine, for example, that women's orientation to emotions and relationships is systematic, moral, purposeful, and worthwhile.

Carol Gilligan (1982), a developmental psychologist, has been a ground breaker in differentiating the female from the male experience. Her work legitimizes the observation that men and women develop in different ways. Prior to Gilligan's work there had been very little independent observation of women's behavior and its underlying meaning. It had been assumed that women were supposed to be like men; to the extent that they were not like men, they were assumed to be inferior. Not until the last decade did it occur to psychologists that women have an independent and different psychology from men that can be studied, understood, and valued on its own terms.

Gilligan, as well as many others (Jordan, 1986; Miller, 1983; Surrey, 1985), characterizes male development as moving along a trajectory that has as its goal separation from others and autonomy. This is in sharp contrast to women, whom she sees as living their lives so as to center themselves in a context of relationships. The major concern of women is to be responsible in caring for others. Their main ethical and emotional injunction is not to cause hurt to another person. The main ethical injunction for men, according to her analysis, is to guarantee and protect the rights of the individual.

According to Nancy Chodorow (1978), the female child is taught sensitivity to the feelings and needs of others early in life, usually by her mother. Chodorow also states that it is the mother who teaches her male child to leave her, to loosen the attachment, and to be clear in his definition of his ego boundaries. The message given to girls is to be kind, loving, empathic, and responsive to the needs of others. This message tends to make ego boundaries less firm. Women experience themselves in a network of relationships where connection with others, rather than autonomy, enhances self-esteem. Women feel that they have failed when something has interfered with their capacity to be effectively involved in loving and caring for others.

Men typically seek independence. They become anxious and feel that they have failed when their autonomy is threatened (Weiss, 1985). The language of relationships is more foreign to them than to women. Indeed, some men will see a psychotherapist only in the context of couple therapy. Since the process of therapy operates in a framework that resonates better with women's experiences than with men's, many men choose to avoid it. The man often comes to couple therapy only because he feels blackmailed by the woman's threat to end the relationship if he doesn't, and even then he sees it as being "for her sake—to help her."

The experience of the couple relationship for women includes a need for intimacy that depends in part on sharing with her partner an ongoing dialogue she has with herself about how she affects and is affected by others. That internal dialogue, which reflects her experience of self-in-relationship, provides the database that women depend upon in order to maintain their relationships and guard against hurting others. A woman can be very disappointed if her husband has difficulty in relating to that part of her experience. Further, a woman is likely to believe that when her man does not share his personal, internal dialogue with her, he is being withholding and rejecting. This can lead to frustration and anger. What she does not realize is that the man's way of experiencing is different from hers and that his failure to share may be due to his own way of experiencing himself and the events in his life. In short, he may not have an internal dialogue quite like hers to share, or a desire to connect with her through self-disclosure.

A man's internal dialogue seems more often to be goal-directed, concerned as he is with the struggle for achievement, with the struggle to be successful as a man (Pleck, 1977). Given a problem, he is more likely to reach for a solution than to share the feelings that the problem stirs up. For example, a couple was suddenly presented with the news that their closest friends' newborn infant was in danger of dying. The husband wanted to leave immediately for the hospital. The wife wanted to be held and to hold her husband. He looked for comfort in doing something; she looked for comfort in sharing the pain. She felt abandoned by his lack of responsiveness to her need. He was hurt and confused by her disappointment in him.

In couple relationships the man typically offers himself as someone to be relied upon for providing material things and safety, but not as someone who wants to share his internal, emotional experiences or hear about those of others. It is not that he necessarily regards these emotional exchanges as bad or good; he simply is not as attentive to the experience of relationships in himself or in others. It is not that connection is not needed by men, but rather that it is repressed. A man typically assumes that his wife will provide the connection and that it will be there as a necessary background against which he can realize his other goals.

If the man is not centered on connecting with his wife, but more centered on his work and preserving his separateness, and if the woman is seeking to make a connection with him, there is inherent conflict in their relationship. The woman is threatened by the failure of connection, and the man withdraws from her overt attempts to connect, seeking to preserve his autonomy. This conflict between men and women is so basic that only a rare couple does not deal with it at some level. Even when other conflicts are more central, it is safe to assume that in most instances this gender difference will intensify other difficulties.

In *The Heart of the Matter*, Graham Greene (1948) creates a vivid portrait of a man listening to his wife talk. The account is so familiar that it is almost a stereotype. In the context of this chapter, it will be useful to penetrate the stereotype in order to better understand both the man's and the woman's experience.

> . . . Scobie made the right reply. He never listened while his wife talked. He worked steadily to the even current of sound; but if a note of distress were struck he was aware of it at once. . . . He could even work better while she talked than when she was silent, for so long as his ear drum registered those tranquil sounds—the gossip of the Club, comments on the sermons preached by Father Rank—he knew that all was well. It was silence that stopped his working—silence in which he might look up and see tears waiting in the eyes for his attention. (p. 27)

This excerpt from Greene's novel is likely to be read by both men and women as a presentation of a prattling woman and a serious man engaged in important work, particularly if both devalue the woman's need for connection and value the man's right to be supported in his quest for autonomy. The characters can also be interpreted as a man who is withdrawn and unavailable and a woman who is unseen, unheard, and therefore hurt. However, since the novel is written from a man's perspective, we do not actually hear the woman's voice and are at a disadvantage if we try to empathize with her. When a "man's perspective" is taken by a woman—when she accepts a silencing of her own voice—she may experience internal turmoil or seemingly unjustified depression. Her dissatisfaction is grounded not only in the gender differences themselves, but in the fact that she joins her husband in devaluing her way of experiencing life events.

Gender differences in power positions thus interact with other differences in the way that men and women experience themselves in their relationship. If the man in the couple is assumed to have more power, then both he and his wife will assume that when there are differences, his view of events is the one to be more highly valued. For example, a statement by a husband that his wife shouldn't be so involved with her mother can be heard by the wife as a sound judgment about her behavior, rather than simply another point of view. Unless one understands that women attribute power to men, one cannot understand an important source of the difficulty that women have in valuing their own experiences and judgments. The greater power of the man suggests to the woman that he knows more about how she should be than she herself does.

Difficulties can arise in couples when they attribute different meanings to the same signals. For example, a woman may intend her anger as a signal that there is trouble in the relationship and that the couple should jointly examine their problems in an effort to improve their connection. The woman's anger may be intensified by her fear that her concern will not be considered important by her husband. This sequence may occur in part because she has difficulty in valuing her own observations, especially if they are different from his. In devaluing her own experience, she is thrust into conflict about her own needs and may end up not listening to her own inner voice. Her frustration may finally explode into anger, causing her to fight to protect herself. But even in the fighting, her intention is to join with her husband in trying to solve the difficulty. A man, on the other hand, may expect his anger to be taken as a signal that her troublesome behavior must stop. His anger is an assertion that some boundary has been crossed, that some right has been violated. It is not, therefore, an invitation to increase the connection, but rather an assertion that the couple should at least temporarily increase their separateness.

To the extent that the man in the couple is less expert and less concerned with maintaining the emotional climate of the couple's life together, he depends on the woman to make the necessary adjustments to keep them comfortable. She can, therefore, exert power over the man in that arena, where she is both expert and responsible.

A man can be made to feel very inadequate and guilty if his wife accuses him of emotional insensitivity. Paradoxically, if he is feeling guilty, he is likely to withdraw, since separating himself when anxious may be his way of restoring his equilibrium and re-establishing his autonomy. If he does withdraw, his wife will feel even more alone, left with a power that has not served her well. This male gender-linked tendency to withdraw is particularly hard on women, since it is so antithetical to their need to stay connected.

Another paradoxical turn of events can occur when a woman demands that her husband express his feelings: If he complies, she may become frightened by evidence of his vulnerability. His vulnerability makes him seem less powerful and, therefore, less dependable and protective. Sometimes this will cause the woman to turn away from her husband's expression of feelings, thereby discouraging him from expressing them again. Only if a woman feels strong enough herself can she accept her husband's vulnerability.

A couple with a conflicted marriage of 20 years described in a session one of the husband's many affairs, this time with a colleague. When the focus was shifted to his business, it became clear that he had a long history of failed enterprises. However, he had managed to produce enough income to obscure his chronic difficulties. The high income was important, since the couple's life was heavily concentrated on having the right possessions. While the husband seemed willing to talk about his business concerns, his wife resisted and kept returning to his extramarital affair. It became clear that she was actually more anxious about her husband's business difficulties than about his affairs. Indeed, she had had a number of affairs herself. However, her fear of his not being able to earn enough could not be neutralized, and was intensified by her own conviction that she was incapable of earning any money. In order to manage her own anxiety about not being able to work gainfully, she had to deny his vulnerability in that area. They colluded about identifying the affairs as the source of their trouble. This couple was eventually helped by the wife's recognizing her own strength so that she could accept her husband's weakness, and by the husband's acknowledgment and solution of some of his problems at work, which allowed him to become less defensive, distant, withdrawn, and authoritarian at home.

Another reason a woman might turn away from her husband's expression of his needs, even though a part of her really desires it, is the belief that if she learns what he wants she will have to comply with his wishes. A couple in therapy was instructed to talk to each other about a long-standing conflict about where they would live. The wife was surprisingly inept in her efforts to learn what her husband wanted. When questioned about this, she realized that she was afraid that if she were to clearly perceive what her husband wanted, she would automatically feel his wish to be her command. She did not consider the possibility that the desires of both might be met in a fresh solution to their conflict. Sometimes women who know themselves to be overly solicitous of their husbands' needs will stubbornly resist understanding and attending to particular needs in a confused effort to maintain some sense of autonomy.

Not all couples present gender differences in a typical pattern. Some husbands have a greater desire than their wives for connection and relatedness and some wives have a greater desire for power and autonomy than their husbands. Some women are distancers and some men are pursuers. But even in couples that are atypical, the expected gender differences remain powerful determinants in shaping their behavior. For example, in the case of a husband and wife who were both doctors, the wife was considerably more ambitious and more successful than her husband. She was not only outstanding in her profession but also an expert in a specialized field of art, which led to considerable financial reward. Despite her talents, the wife experienced and presented herself as a helpless woman who had long been deprived by her husband's lack of love and as suffering, along with her children, from his rages. In the consulting room, it was easy to recognize the husband's attempts to hide his poignant need for her love and approval, which when denied to him, would cause him to become demanding and angry. The wife, although claiming to be helpless, was actually very powerful and controlling. For example, when she decided to divorce him she deftly arranged to insure that her husband had no part of the fortune she had accumulated from her art collection. Although the divorce was clearly her idea, she disclaimed it and acted as if he had rejected and victimized her. She was unaware of how she used power, and of how powerful she could be. She saw herself in the more feminine role of being loving, caring, and only defensively self-protective. She was unaware of and dissociated from her own power. The husband felt uncared for, unloved, manipulated, and mystified by his wife's uses and denial of power. His frustration bred the kind of aggression typical of adolescents. He fought back by having affairs, which made his wife intensely jealous, and by going off on long trips, leaving her with the responsibility of the children and household. Both struggled with denying the parts of themselves that were atypical of their gender. She needed to disown that part of herself that could be autonomous and powerful; he needed to disown that part of himself that sought love and affection. In trying to appear as a typical couple (i.e., a strong, demanding man and a loving, helpless woman), they were presenting a very inaccurate picture of who they really were.

The psychological differences between men and women make it very difficult for them to live in the semi-isolated lifestyle that is the norm for many couples in modern American society. The lack of an extended family intensifies the demands that men and women place on each other for the understanding, support, protection, and approval that is needed for each to maintain a sense of well-being. Gender differences in couples can be tolerated more readily in the absence of an extended family if the couple has managed to establish a supportive network of friends, where each can find someone else more like himself or herself. The women's movement has encouraged women to find support with each other. Men's support groups are still rare.

A couple's isolation tends to accentuate gender differences, particularly when there is stress in the life of the couple. Each will use characteristically male or female defenses. "When in doubt, connect," might be a woman's motto. "When in doubt, withdraw," might be a man's. When the ready possibility of divorce is added to the isolation of everyday life, it serves to intensify the awareness and intolerance of these differences. Dissatisfaction with the relationship is exacerbated when gender differences are perceived not as culturally prescribed patterns of thought or behavior, but as ways in which the other is willfully disappointing. The couple therapist can provide a place where gender differences can be explored safely.

A couple in their late 30s came to therapy when the wife was in the early months of her first pregnancy. The fact that they were in the same profession, doing exactly the same kind of work, served to obscure characteristic gender differences. The wife angrily told her husband, who was being trained to assist her in childbirth, that he could not possibly offer her the comfort she would need when she was in labor. Her husband was deeply hurt by her remark but he accepted her criticism as valid, even though he couldn't understand the nature of his failure, since he knew that it did not reflect his intentions. Clearly, he had given her the power to be the expert about their emotional life. He protected himself from her criticism by withdrawing. His wife's anger was then fueled by her belief that he had the ability to help her, but was withholding his help.

The wife in this case had meant her provocative, angry statement to serve as an opening for sharing her fear of labor with her husband. She wished her anger to be understood by him as an invitation to come closer, but he took her anger as a signal for him to disconnect. He was unwilling to express his anger because he was afraid that this would conflict with his need to be protective of his pregnant wife. He avoided an exchange of anger and any further discussion of the subject. His withdrawal left his wife feeling abandoned. At the same time, she was ashamed of her angry and insulting remarks. Her husband felt hurt and a little in awe of the mystery surrounding the coming birth, as if he had already failed in his responsibility to his wife and future child.

It was important for the couple therapist to move beyond the couple system and explore the wife's fear of labor. She lived far from her family and did not have women friends with whom she could share experiences of childbirth. Her fear of labor had its origins in her own mother's several stillbirths and miscarriages during her adolescence. When the wife began to understand the origin of her fears, she was freed from focusing on her husband as the source of her difficulty. She spontaneously arranged to fly home to visit her mother. Her talk about the miscarriages increased her feeling of connection with her mother, which reduced her excessive dependence on her husband, thereby decreasing the tension in the couple relationship. With the tension decreased, the husband could be more supportive of his wife in a manner consistent with his personality style.

This couple's attempts to deal all alone with a major life event served to highlight and exaggerate their male–female differences. While husbands and wives can be expected to be major supports for each other, there are limits to the kind and amount of support they can provide. One of the limitations is based on their gender differences, which are highlighted and can become polarized at stress-laden times. Therefore, it is helpful for both to have others of the same gender involved in their lives when they are in a crisis. This decreases the possibility of polarization and makes what each has to offer to the other more satisfying. In this case, once the woman had connected with her mother and the tension in the couple was reduced, they were able to continue without further therapy concerning their gender differences.

PROJECTIVE IDENTIFICATION AND THE MAINTENANCE OF GENDER DIFFERENCES

Having described and illustrated some gender differences, I would like to focus now on projective identification as a mechanism through which these differences are maintained in couples. In projective identification, the subject projects the undesirable, unwanted, or unused and unintegrated parts of himself or herself onto the object and then perceives the object as if it contained these qualities. In addition, the subject provokes behavior in the object that conforms to the subject's projection and selectively does not attend to any behavior that contradicts the projection. The object, or other person, accepts the projection because of the pressure to do so, and also because it is consistent with some of his or her needs. The object then acts in accordance with the projection. The originator of the projection vicariously experiences those parts of himself or herself as they appear in the other person and identifies with the other through recognition of the projected parts of his or her personality (Shapiro, 1978; Ogden, 1979).

The normal developmental process of gender differentiation begins early in the life of the child (Haviland & Malatesta, 1981). This process is not yet well understood, but we can assume that it involves a very complex mixture of biological programming and social learning. Ultimately, the gender-appropriate behavior is woven into the core identity and into the daily experience of the self. Taking independence and dependence as examples of a gender difference, let us see how these differences are maintained by individuals in their life as a couple.

Traditionally, the female child is socialized into dependence and the male child into independence (Chodorow, 1978). When the male and female are joined as a couple, they can, to the degree that they find it necessary, project onto the partner the part of themselves that has not been developed. The wife who has learned to deny expression of independent impulses may project those feelings onto her husband, thus reinforcing his behavior in the gender-appropriate direction. Her identification with him in his independent stance vicariously gratifies her, and she is encouraged to further support his independent behavior. The same thing happens, of course, in the opposite direction. The husband, because he cannot easily express his dependency needs, projects them onto his wife and then identifies with her expression of them. An internal struggle to deal with lost or repressed aspects of identity is played out and mutually stabilized in the couple's relationship through this process of projective identification. On the outside, however, we see only a couple playing "natural" sex roles. As clinicians, we need to appreciate that this "natural" picture can be adaptive and comfortable, but can also become distorted and maintained by extreme and inflexible projections that preclude psychological authenticity in one or both members of the couple. For example, if the couple's mutual projections result in a helpless woman who has lost the capacity to exercise her own judgment and cannot make realistic observations regarding her husband's behavior, and an autocratic man who acts as if his wishes, without question, should be the basis for his wife's behavior, then we have a situation where the mutual projections have gone out of control. (See also H. Grunebaum, Chapter 15, this volume.)

The view of mutual projective identification that is most helpful in understanding its role in the maintenance of gender differences is one that recognizes projective identification as a defense mechanism operating along a continuum from the normal to the pathological (Zinner & Shapiro, 1972). In its more normal uses, it is one of the ways in which societal prescriptions for gender behavior are woven into the psychological fabric of the couple relationship.

GENDER DIFFERENCES IN THE CASE OF JENNIFER AND LARRY

The case of Jennifer and Larry illustrates clearly several of the points discussed above. Jennifer brings Larry to couple therapy with the classical woman's complaint that they do not communicate well enough. She says that he is riveted to the TV set and does not make room for her. She asks for greater connection, and he appears to press for distance.

The way in which couples manifest typical gender roles may vary according to other factors in their lives. In the earlier years of their relationship, Larry pursued Jennifer. Later, their roles were reversed and Jennifer became the pursuer. In the interview with Peggy Papp, Larry explained that this shift in his behavior occurred as a result of his taking on a more committed professional identity. In other words, as Larry grew older he adopted the more traditional masculine role expected of him in the workplace, which affected his relationship with Jennifer.

LARRY: In the beginning years, she was always of primary importance. My career and school were always secondary. I'd cut classes to go visit her. . . . she might take it that I care less about her, but I don't think it's true. I've just grown as an individual, and I just felt that in order to interact, to be happy with her, you have to be happy with yourself first. And although my career is still secondary, it is not as far away.

The trauma of Larry's foot amputation for cancer also threatened him with the possibility of dependency, to which he responded with a powerful thrust toward autonomy. In his interview with Norman Paul, he spoke about the time of the amputation:

LARRY: . . . how I handle something like this is, you have to do it for yourself first. I mean, she wasn't around every minute of the day, and my parents weren't around. I was the one who had to get up on the crutches and take one step, and then with the prosthesis— painful as it was—take the other step. No one is going to take my foot and move it for me.

Both the push toward achievement and the trauma of the cancer propelled Larry into a more autonomous posture than he had taken earlier. It is possible that without the threat of cancer and the resulting amputation, Larry might have become less guarded against dependency. Instead, he developed into a man more like his emotionally closed father, and less like his more emotionally open mother. He says in his interview with Norman Paul, "I'm more like my mother in nonpersonal interactions . . . My interactions with Jennifer probably put me closer to my father."

Larry's strong push toward independence during this period left Jennifer confused. When he would not allow her to share his difficulties she felt excluded, unwanted, and unneeded. Jennifer may have her own difficulties with intimacy, but she assumed that in a couple relationship with a man she was supposed to care for him and share feelings with him. When he excluded her, she was disoriented. She says to Norman Paul in a comment at the conference, but not in his chapter.

JENNIFER: Many times I felt that he's feeling all these things, but he's not telling me what his feelings are and I'm supposed to read his mind and it makes me feel very uneasy . . . I mean it's better to hear, for instance, that he's upset with me or that he's angry or that he's frustrated, rather than not hearing anything at all.

The fantasies that Jennifer and Larry developed in their interview with Peggy Papp also illustrate gender differences inherent in their views of themselves in relation to others. Jennifer's fantasy is one of caring for and nurturing a hurt and lonely child who will then be her friend and end her loneliness. Larry's fantasy is one of experiencing himself in the pleasures of competition with his male friends. He wants Jennifer as a witness and admirer of his activity. His attraction to her and her demands on him place him in conflict with his ambitions. Jennifer hopes to satisfy her need for closeness with a man by giving to and nurturing him. He will then be dependent on her and stay with her. Larry, on the other hand, desires and expects the closeness of someone who stands off and admires him. In his fantasy he wants to hold her at a distance and share with her a focus on his achievement.

There are two sources of frustration for Jennifer in her attempts to befriend the boy of her fantasy. The first is his hesitation in responding to her. The second is her fear that if he does join her in the play then he is likely to take it over and shape the experience for both of them. The following statement by Jennifer in her interview with Papp illustrates how she tries to protect her own experience as the valid one for her, while at the same time she believes that Larry's way of experiencing may be closer to the truth.

JENNIFER: When I feel like he's telling me what to do . . . and I guess how I should feel, is the thing that really gets me upset. He tells me how I should feel. That is even beyond controlling the games, that's controlling the feelings. I'll be very upset one day coming home . . . and he'll say, "Oh, that's not a big deal, you shouldn't feel upset.". . . Well, then I start feeling, well, maybe he's right . . . and I start doubting how I should feel about a certain situation and it gets me very confused.

Larry tries to teach Jennifer to be more like him, less emotional. Jennifer attributes power to Larry assuming that he knows best. Jennifer attempts to follow Larry's construction of experience, only to find that in so doing she denies her own experience. She avoids this conflict by withdrawing. The couple disconnects, leaving both partners unhappy.

Of the therapists who interviewed Larry and Jennifer, only Carlos Sluzki directly addressed the gender issues as a source of conflict. Although, the Framos, Paul, and Papp did not deal directly with gender, their work reflected gender issues. The Framos' work addressed Jennifer's isolation from her family members. Jennifer's isolation as an adult reproduces her isolation in her family of origin and is reflected in involvement in her work, which absorbs her from early morning until late evening. The Framos, by meeting with Jennifer and her mother, father, and sister, helped her reconnect with her family, thereby reducing her dependence on Larry as a sole source of emotional support. A generation ago, Jennifer and Larry, who at the time of the interview were 29 years old, would have had children, which would have reduced the intensity of their need for full satisfaction from each other.

Norman Paul's interview with Larry's family of origin revealed that Larry's parents' relationship followed the gender-prescribed patterns of an emotionally expressive mother and an emotionally constricted father. Larry reproduced their marital pattern. However, Larry's mother, unlike

Jennifer, found a rich source of direct emotional support in her own family of origin, which made it much easier for her to accept emotional distance in her marriage than it is for Jennifer to accept such distance in her relationship with Larry.

The fantasy that Peggy Papp elicited from Larry and Jennifer revealed not only their adoption of typical gender roles, as discussed above, but also their own less well-expressed and integrated desires to experience satisfaction in the domain of the opposite gender. Jennifer's fantasies showed very ambitious, autonomous goals, as well as goals of being nurturing. Larry's fantasies included satisfying his dependent needs as well as his needs for autonomy. The gender-based expression of the self, while important and usually the most evident, does not preclude other desires and potentials for self-expression that characteristically belong to the other gender. Papp was able to demonstrate that both Jennifer and Larry had aspects of themselves that were not consistent with gender assignment of roles. One can assume that Larry and Jennifer used mutual projective identification as a way for Jennifer to deal with her needs for autonomy and for Larry to deal with his dependency needs, thereby intensifying their differences and complicating their present conflicts over closeness.

In his work with Jennifer and Larry, Carlos Sluzki responded immediately to the gender differences that their conflict revealed. He saw Jennifer as presenting herself as the expert on emotional life and, therefore, at the moment of the interview, the more powerful member of the couple. He attempted to equalize the power between Jennifer and Larry by devaluing Jennifer's ability to express her feelings in therapy; at the same time, he was respectful of Larry's stereotypical male behavior.

In reframing the differences in their modes of experiencing themselves in relation to each other as complementary rather than antagonistic, Sluzki described Jennifer as a "balloon" and Larry as a "rock." It is important to consider the meaning of this metaphor. While it was helpful to the couple to have their differences seen as complementary rather than antagonistic, it is questionable whether a woman's self-esteem is enhanced by her being likened to a balloon. A balloon is, at best, cheerful; but it is also a childish and lightweight object. The implication was that Jennifer's desire to increase the connection between herself and Larry, to find a way to share their emotional life, was flighty and not solidly anchored in reality. She needed a man, a rock, to ground her, to keep her from taking off in emotional flights into outer space.

In this metaphor one can find a strongly biased male view of the couple and their problems. It implies that Jennifer's desire for greater closeness reflects a flightiness and emotionality. Sluzki's metaphor might quiet the couple's difficulties for a while; the implicit message was that Jennifer should stop being so demanding of Larry's emotional responsiveness, and Jennifer, like many women, might indeed accept instruction from an authority who placed the burden of protecting the relationship largely on her. But Sluzki clearly created a solution that would maintain the status quo: The woman is asked to be sensitive to the man's needs, while the man remains safely in his autonomous and more powerful position.

While I am sure that Sluzki meant to keep himself equidistant from the two, he did not altogether succeed. This provides us with an example of how even the most talented among couple therapists can bring biases of gender to their work.

In spite of Sluzki's recommendation that Larry resist dampening Jennifer's emotions, the interview ends with a beautiful example of the couple acting out their usual roles: Jennifer expresses a feeling and Larry dampens it. Jennifer then tries to comply with Larry's judgment and Sluzki laughs in seeming approval. (Note that the end of this excerpt was presented at the conference but is not in Sluzki's chapter.)

JENNIFER: You are also the first therapist who brought out something positive in our relationship, which is very nice, very interesting. I mean, most people say, "OK, what's the problem?" and "Let's tear apart the problem," instead of looking at what's there.

LARRY: But our couples therapist has brought out positive . . .

JENNIFER: Sure, sure. But I'm just talking about the people who've interviewed us so far. And they're looking for snags.

LARRY: Jennifer, we're in the experiment. We can't judge . . .

JENNIFER: I know. All right . . .

SLUZKI: (Laughs.)

RECOGNIZING GENDER-BASED DIFFERENCES IN COUPLE THERAPY

Gender differences are part of the structure of the couple relationship. As discussed above, mutual projective identification functions to maintain and exaggerate these differences. Jennifer projects that part of herself that wants autonomy and distance onto Larry, and in doing so encourages him to exaggerate his own impulses in that direction. In accepting her projections, he is discouraged from tuning in to that part of himself that is more emotionally available and dependent. Larry, in his turn, projects his dependency needs onto Jennifer, and in receiving his projections, she exaggerates her dependency needs and denies her needs for autonomy and emotional distance. As in all projective identification, the result is that Jennifer vicariously identifies with Larry's autonomy and ambition and Larry vicariously identifies with Jennifer's expression of needs for greater closeness, and neither of them can adequately deal with what they have projected. With most couples who are in conflict over stuck and impacted gender differences, the goal should be for each of the partners to reinternalize the projected parts of themselves. This would not necessarily alter the direction of the gender differences, but it would allow for more flexibility regarding these issues.

Part of the work of the couple therapist is to be someone who listens to, understands, and values both the man and woman without taking sides. This serves to create a safe environment in which gender-based as well as other differences can be tolerated. It helps the couple to feel a little less stuck and less dependent upon projective identification, which only serves to polarize them and make their differences less workable.

The couple therapist cannot expect to improve matters by encouraging the man to be more like a woman or the woman to be more like a man, or the man to be more manly or the woman more womanly, but rather by helping them to better understand and negotiate their differences. The couple therapist must be aware of gender differences, so as not to consciously or unconsciously take sides. The most obvious pitfall is for the male or female therapist to more readily identify with the same-sex patient and to disapprove of and attempt to change the behavior of the other. Another pitfall is for the therapist of the same sex to try to teach the patient to be more like the typical male or female is supposed to be, so that the woman might be expected to be more accommodating and the man more authoritative. As therapists become more aware of the different characteristic frames of reference of men and women, as well as more aware of their own assumptions, they will be in a better position to understand the interactions of each particular couple and their conflicts.

Today, men are being encouraged to pay more attention to the tender, nurturant parts of themselves, especially as they are asked to share in the care of the children. Women are being encouraged to pay more attention to their autonomous sides as they enter the world of work. A new ideal is springing up in the mental health profession that encourages men and women to be both more autonomous and more tender, more like each other. The profession reflects, of course, changes in the culture, and is not an independent source of wisdom. What the nature of heterosexual intimacy will be like when there is greater equality and less difference between men and women is not as yet clear. As couple therapists, we should be aware that these are going to be important issues in our work and in our own lives.

REFERENCES

Chodorow, N. (1978). *The reproduction of mothering.* Berkeley: University of California Press.

Gilligan, C. (1982). *In a different voice: Psychological theory and women's development.* Cambridge, MA: Harvard University Press.

Goldner, V. (1985). Feminism and family therapy. *Family Process*, 24(1), 31–45.

Greene, G. (1948). *The heart of the matter.* New York: Viking Penguin.

Haley, J. (1976). *Problem solving therapy.* San Francisco: Jossey-Bass.

Hare-Mustin, R. (1987). The problems of gender in family therapy theory. *Family Process*, 26(1), 15–27.

Haviland, J., & Malatesta, C. (1981). The development of sex differences as nonverbal signals. In C. Mago & N. Healey, (Eds.), *Gender and nonverbal behavior* (pp. 183–208). New York: Springer.

Heilbrun, C. G. (1979). *Reinventing womanhood.* New York: Norton.

Herman, J. (1986). Histories of violence in an outpatient population. *American Journal of Orthopsychiatry*, 56(1), 137–141.

Jordan, J. V. (1986). The meaning of mutuality. *Works in Progress*, No. 23. Stone Center, Wellesley College, Wellesley, MA.

Keller, E. F. (1985). *Reflections on gender and science.* New Haven, CT: Yale University Press.

Miller, J. B. (1976). *Toward a new psychology of women.* Boston: Beacon Press.

Miller, J. B. (1983). The construction of anger in women and men. *Works in Progress*, No. 4. Stone Center, Wellesley College, Wellesley, MA.

Minuchin, S., & Fishman, H. C. (1981). *Family therapy techniques.* Cambridge, MA: Harvard University Press.

Ogden, T. H. (1979). On projective identification. *International Journal of Psycho-Analysis*, 60, 357–373.

Pleck, J. (1977). The work-family role system. *Social Problems*, 24, 417–427.

Shapiro, E. R. (1978). The psychodynamics and developmental psychology of the borderline patient: A review of the literature. *American Journal of Psychiatry*, 135(11), 305–315.

Stiver, I. (1984). The meanings of "dependency" in male–female relationships. *Works in Progress*, No. 11. Stone Center, Wellesley College, Wellesley, MA.

Surrey, J. L. (1985). Self in relation: A theory of women's development. *Works in Progress*, No. 13. Stone Center, Wellesley College, Wellesley, MA.

Weiss, R. S. (1985). Men and the family. *Family Process*, 24, 49–58.

Willi, J. (1982). *Couples in collusion.* New York: Jason Aronson.

Zinner, J. & Shapiro, R. L. (1972). Projective identification as a mode of perception and behavior in families of adolescents. *International Journal of Psycho-analysis*, 5(3), 523–530.

13

Therapists' Fantasies in Working with Couples:
The Unstable Triad

SHARON LAMB and RACHEL T. HARE-MUSTIN

Therapists bring to their work with couples explicit theories about couples—theories about what holds couples together, what tears them apart, what games they play with each other, and how they each view themselves and the other partner. Therapists also bring their personal experiences, cultural biases, needs of the moment, anxieties, and values. These factors serve as implicit theories about the way people are and the way they ought to be. Such implicit theories typically stand apart from the explicit theories we espouse. For example, therapists may be implicitly influenced by high divorce rates and underestimate the strength of a couple's connection, forgetting that couples usually have a special unidentifiable linkage to each other beyond our comprehension. We know very little about what keeps couples together.

In the four interviews with Larry and Jennifer, we see examples of four explicit theories, each with some recognized validity. What is less apparent is that each of the therapists who conducted the interviews has implicit needs, biases, stories, and fantasies that by their very nature are relatively unscrutinized. Furthermore, these implicit factors can unwittingly affect therapeutic interventions, sometimes to the detriment of the effectiveness of the therapy. For example, the therapist influenced by that small glow of pleasure that arises when achieving an alliance with at least one of the couple may succumb to the tug of the inherently unstable three-person system and become overinvolved with one member of the pair and disengaged from the other.

When faced with the confusion of a new encounter with a couple, as therapists we need to be aware of our fantasies, recalled stories, myths, and personal daydreams. Such fantasies and stories select and crystallize universal human experience and our personal experience in a comprehensible drama. It is through examination of such fantasies that we can begin to look at one of the most common problems therapists have in remaining effective in their work with couples: suction. In this chapter we will describe a number of fantasies that a therapist might have about Larry and Jennifer, drawing from the work of the therapists who interviewed the couple as well as the therapists who attended our workshop. We will discuss how such fantasies might have informed the therapist of areas of vulnerability, particularly the vulnerability to forming an alliance with one member of the couple over the other.

A FANTASY OF TREASURE ISLAND

Imagine a therapist who has been meeting with Jennifer and Larry, the couple in this case, who have lived together for five years after an on-and-off relationship for the previous five years. Three times the couple decided to marry, but these engagements ended when Jennifer changed her mind. They have rarely talked about the foot amputation Larry had five years earlier to stop the spread of cancer. Their story reveals that formerly he had seen himself as her protector, but now he is more self-centered. She finds him lively with friends but withdrawn and unresponsive to her, a perpetual television viewer.

Suddenly there may flash through the therapist's mind the image of Long John Silver, the pirate with the peg leg, and Jim Hawkins, the young cabin boy in Robert Louis Stevenson's *Treasure Island*. It is a tale of adventure, of a relationship, of a tragedy. Long John Silver admires the plucky and honest lad, and Jim responds to this admiration despite his fear about the relationship. Although they are opponents in complex ways, Jim and Long John are shipmates, partners, and pals; each comes through in need and saves the other's life.

What does the fantasy mean? There Jennifer sits with her fair skin and silky black hair, yet there is an asexual, sturdy, boyish quality about her in her Frye boots. Like Jim, she has the innocent appearance of one on an adventure, or, if you will, a quest. She is willing, she tries hard, cooperating with the therapy and what is asked of her. She has the agility to climb the rigging. But what of the crotchety pirate, Larry, roistering with his crew, but not dependable for Jennifer? Appearing aged and scarred, Larry, like Long John, will not climb the rigging again, but he seems unbowed, sage, wily, a little shrunken, his eyes shifting from one speaker to another. He has endured. The bond between the two is one of loyalty; they have exchanged the magic handshake. Or is there love? Long John sees the boy as he himself once might have been, and Jim responds to this vision.

What can the fantasy reveal about the therapist and her response to these patients? Does the therapist find Jennifer's goodness admirable or is it merely tiresome? Does the therapist envy her youth? Why is the image of the pair not more sexual? Is it her boyish eagerness or Larry's disability? Is the therapist denying the couple's sexuality in order to remain the most sexual of the three? Or is the image asexual because that feels comfortable for the therapist? Does the amputation engender respect and compassion for suffering, or is the therapist repelled? How can such a pair have a future?

The therapist having the Treasure Island fantasy might be pulled into an alliance with either member of the couple. There could be a competitive relationship with Larry to win Jim/Jennifer's loyalty and engage her interest. It would be easy to go with her openness, cooperativeness, and determined quest for the answer in therapy. On the other hand, the therapist might find her goodness offensive and tiresome and want to put her in her place with the common crew, to make sure she realizes she is no one special. Toward Larry, the therapist might feel challenged to be part of what Jennifer cannot join, the male roistering. Or there might be a nurturant or protective stance because of Larry's injury. On the other hand, the savageness represented by the pirate, the grimness that is necessary if one is to be a survivor of the seven seas, might make some therapists fearful of getting close to Long John/Larry.

THE THREE-PERSON SYSTEM

In family therapy, Minuchin (1974) has used the term "suction" to describe the way the therapist can be unwittingly drawn into the family's characteristic mode of interaction. When the family pulls the therapist toward certain coalitions and ways of relating that are contraindicated for change, the therapist can resist the power of the system by aligning with other, less empowered members of the family to unbalance the usual disabling patterns. Although a useful technique with families, this does not work with couples. To join with either member of the couple rebalances the system at the cost of excluding one member. Because the pull for such an alliance in the three-person system is strong, the therapist may not always be aware of how the choice was made.

Many family therapy theorists have pointed out that couples tend to bring in a third party when a marriage is in trouble. Minuchin, Haley, Madanes, and Palazzoli all speak of the symptomatic child who serves to bring distancing parents together, with a common goal centered on parental responsibilities rather than on their own relationship. In like manner, an extramarital affair shifts a couple to a three-person system and creates distance in a couple having difficulties with intimacy. A parent from the older generation can become a third party to a troubled couple, and take over some of the functions and responsibilities usually assumed by one of the pair. It is easy to see how the act of going to a therapist also fulfills this pressure to bring in a third party to provide a distance regulator, tension alleviator, and fresh focus.

The therapist as the third party is in danger of being drawn into the role of "the other woman" or "the other man" with individuals and couples. Avoiding this role is particularly difficult, since therapists typically, and quite naturally, like one member of the couple better than the other. When we see individuals, the fact that we find one patient more likeable than another does not create major difficulties. However, when we see couples, preferences may become apparent, and favoritism may be interpreted as or evolve into flirtatious or seductive behavior. It has been said that seductive patients are those who can't resist us and hostile patients are those who don't admire us. Sympathizing, aligning, or flirting with one member of a couple, whether by intent or lack of awareness, isolates the other in a way that can maintain the difficulty between them rather than unbalance the system to bring them together.

A couple may also use a therapist as they do a symptom-bearing child, to take the focus off their own difficulties. The therapist can be drawn into this kind of system by becoming the problematic one, as evidenced, for example, by forgetting appointments, not finding convenient meeting times, or putting the couple "on the spot" with overly aggressive questioning, like the child who demands to know "why?" Forgetting appointments raises the question of commitment in the therapist for a couple having difficulties with commitment. Such a wayward therapist will unite the couple with respect to their handling of the therapist, but will address neither their crucial issues nor the therapist's.

Since members of a couple usually enter therapy feeling somewhat unconnected to each other, the strongest pull for attachment is between one of them and the therapist. Couples often are well aware of this. Thus, it becomes essential for us as therapists also to be aware of the pulls and pushes drawing us into these dramas.

ANOTHER WAY OF VIEWING SUCTION

The therapist's feelings toward the patient were referred to by Freud as "countertransference," and were seen at first as a weakness of the therapist. Freud believed that the existence of such feelings should not be widely acknowledged lest patients and the public become disillusioned with psychoanalysis. Given this negative view of such feelings, therapists who were supposed to remain uninvolved sometimes became angry when they discovered in themselves an emotional bond with a patient. This reflected the original view of countertransference as a hindrance, a sign of unfinished analysis in the therapist. Those who have undergone the rigors of psychoanalytic training aimed at isolating this very phenomenon may be particularly sensitive about it. On the other hand, theorists like Racker, Winnicott, and Langs have pointed to the usefulness of countertransference as a source of information, not only about the patient, but also about the therapist and the process of therapy itself (Epstein & Feiner, 1979). Nevertheless, there is a powerful tradition that tempts us as therapists to deny our involvement and believe that we must and can take an impartial therapeutic stance.

Perhaps more than any other theorist, Robert Langs has contributed to the communicative view of countertransference which considers the material produced by the patient to be a response to the therapist's inner life (Silverstein, 1984). Patients can be exquisitely sensitive to the therapist's needs, and so they seek to adapt to them. We see how Jennifer and Larry behave differently with each therapist they see at the conference. Langs's solution to the therapist's tendency to give out covert messages is for the therapist to maintain firm boundaries and ground rules. Among the covert messages, it has been suggested, are those that serve the unconscious need of therapists to defend their professional image (Gottsegen & Gottsegen, 1979).

Although therapists are more inclined to investigate their clients' difficulties than their own, a few warnings appear in the literature about couple therapy concerning suction or the pull on the therapist when working with couples. Walker and White (1975) describe three kinds of competition that can evolve within the therapeutic triangle, each of which leads to vulnerabilities with regard to suction. The first is "political competition," by which they mean the vying of each of the partners for the therapist's support. Second, "sexual competition" occurs when one partner is attracted to the therapist and the other tries hard to win back the partner's affections. Finally, they identify "sibling rivalry" where the competition is possibly more internal to the couple. In the case of political competition, the pull will be for the therapist to cast his or her vote for one of the pair more than the other. In the case of sexual competition, the therapist, perhaps flattered by the attention of one of the pair, or attracted to that person, will be tempted to return this attention or express the attraction. This is often justified by therapists on the grounds that it will lead the neglected member to become more active. In the case of sibling rivalry, the therapist will be drawn into parental behavior, such as scolding the couple for not doing an assigned task or mistakenly viewing their relationship as asexual.

Noting that the triangular situation evokes powerful feelings and

memories of early experiences, Herta Guttman (1982) discusses parental, child, symmetrical, and asymmetrical countertransference reactions.
Writing from a psychoanalytic perspective rather than a systemic one,
she too notes that a common pattern is for a therapist to respond
asymmetrically to the pull of one member of the couple, as may happen
in a seductive alliance. What follows is that the uninvolved partner in
the couple, the outside party, feels excluded, unheard, and unhelped.

We propose that the use of the therapist's fantasy can be the most
fundamental guide for discovering one's own heart in the therapy
session. Fantasies are clues, clues to patterns of response. Fantasy is a
naturally occurring phenomenon that calls us to further investigation.
Following some observations about the nature of fantasy, we will
discuss various fantasies therapists had about Jennifer and Larry.

FANTASY AND REALITY

Fantasy and mythmaking can be understood as the means we use to fill
in gaps in knowledge. Actually, we never reach the point of explaining
any event in purely literal terms. A literal statement has been defined as
merely one whose metaphorical character has been forgotten (Boas,
1961). Out of a need to create order and familiar patterns in our
environment, we draw from the past, from our culture's symbols, and
from familiar narratives. Indeed, our recollections of our families are
fictionalized tales of family life, which often provide an illusion of the
past that hides a secret (Grolnick, 1983).

Fantasy also is characterized by an energy and playfulness that, as a
response to ambiguity or complexity, is a form of what has been called
"regression in the service of the ego." However, once a particular
fantasy emerges, we may find it as difficult to shift to another metaphor
or fantasy as it is to reframe the behavior before us in the session. When
a fantasy emerges, it organizes the field and its images guide our
thoughts and impulses.

Traditional myths and fairy tales as well as our own fantasies reflect
society's stereotyped roles for young and old, male and female, rich and
poor. As therapists, we may maneuver patients into those stereotyped
roles that best fit our needs and make us as therapists less anxious. For
example, many therapists are uncomfortable with patients who violate
sex-role stereotypes. Thus, if the female in a couple seems strong and
the male weak, this is often defined as a problem. Male therapists have
been found to be bothered more by deviations from stereotypes, while
female therapists seem more troubled by excesses in stereotyped behaviors, such as the macho male or the superfeminine female (Kahn, 1980).
We would expect therapists' fantasies to reflect common stereotypes.

Such fantasies provide a convenient clue to the presence of bias against patients who deviate from traditional norms.

A theme in many traditional myths that we as therapists may share is the just-world hypothesis: that justice will be done, that equality will prevail, that wrongs will be righted. But we need to be aware in working with couples that each person in a relationship may view morality differently. Zuk (1972) has pointed out that the powerful tend to advocate the virtue of rules and rationality while the weak espouse justice and compassion.

Jackson's (1965) idea of a natural *quid pro quo* speaks to the elusive myth of equity in claiming that there is an implicit marriage contract in which each party gets something in exchange. However, it has recently been suggested that belief in the *quid pro quo* may lead therapists working with couples to sanction inequities to which they may not be sufficiently sensitive (Margolin, Talovic, Fernandez, & Onorato, 1983). Often the therapist will assign the husband some family work usually done by the wife in exchange for the wife's doing a task designed for the husband's personal pleasure. The assumed reciprocity unwittingly accentuates the inequality in status and resources traditionally available to men and women (Hare-Mustin, 1987). Also, women's goals of affection, appreciation, and understanding may be less easily achieved than the behavioral goals men may desire. In general, therapists' assumptions of equality can be at variance with couples' perceptions, and so a couple may view the therapist's idea of a *quid pro quo* as off the mark.

The theme of overcoming hardships is a frequent motif in fantasies and myths. In traditional myths, the relief of suffering typically comes about in one of the two ways described in *The Golden Bough* (Frazer, 1890/1980): either directly by ritual or indirectly by scapegoating (Kahn, 1980). Guided by his or her own fantasy, the therapist tries to relieve suffering by prescribing a ritual or selecting a scapegoat, often a different scapegoat from the one presented to the therapist. A most tempting scapegoat in our society is the mother of either member of the couple. Or perhaps the scapegoat will be the excluded member of the couple.

Because the family is the ancestral land of heart's desire, families and couples exert a powerful pull upon our own memories and call up images from our early experiences in childhood (Thompson, 1971). Yet, as therapists we are not always aware that our fantasies can be paths toward understanding not only our clients, but also those roles we play as therapists that emerge from our own childhood fantasies. The question may occur whether the therapist should impose his or her fantasy on the couple. Since we cannot help but be influenced by our fantasies, the answer is that we need not impose them on the couple but we must be aware of them ourselves. In any case, the therapeutic task with a couple is not to be merely an interpreter of reality but to be a disrupter of reality. Some typical fantasies of both therapists and patients about the role of therapists include: the omnipotent rescuer; the avenger; King Solomon; the perfect lover, husband, wife, mother, father, or friend; the sage; the truth speaker; the oracle; the disinterested bystander; the free spirit; the scientist; the detective; the policeman. In the case of Larry and Jennifer, varied fantasies reveal the different ways this couple is seen by different therapists.

THE PURSUER AND THE PURSUED

When a fantasy is widely held, it comes to serve as a theory. Such a fantasy about couples is that one member is the pursuer, the other the pursued. As one member seeks to come closer, the other increases the distance. This approaching and retreating can sometimes oscillate so that like children on the playground, first the girls chase the boys and then the boys turn and scatter the fleeing girls. Larry reveals this fantasy when he tells Peggy Papp in his play enactment that the boys really want the girls to chase them.

When working as part of a three-person system of the therapist and the couple, therapists often picture a pursuer and a pursued in regard to themselves. One of the couple wants an alliance with the therapist, whereas the other wants to keep a distance. Carlos Sluzki describes the pull from each of the couple; his fantasy is that each is pursuing him for an alliance, each one seeking the therapist's sympathy.

We note how Jim Framo pursues Jennifer; he wants her to say certain things. His fantasy is that he can provide a transcendent transforming event if he can get Jennifer to tell her family the secret of how she feels. He believes that crying together brings change. In trying to realize this fantasy, Jim Framo and his cotherapist, Mary Framo, become parents, and urge Jennifer to say what would evoke the affective experience they believe is necessary.

On the other hand, Norman Paul allies with Jennifer in pursuing Larry to express his feelings. Paul keeps asking Larry, "Did that touch you?" Paul is indeed the pursuer of feelings: His theory–fantasy seems to be that the problem with Larry's family is that they do not express emotions. Some other therapists have the fantasy that chasing feelings is like chasing a rainbow; as one approaches, the rainbow strangely recedes. Jennifer seems to be viewed as the pursuer by Sluzki, Paul and Jim Framo—a demanding woman who is overwhelming Larry (and perhaps the therapist) by wanting too much.

THE FANTASY OF THE COTHERAPIST

Given the fantasies of power that tempt us as therapists, we often are a little disparaging of the patient whom we see as seeking the role of the therapist's assistant. Often that person is rejected or put through an ordeal like the Sorcerer's Apprentice for presuming to share our powers. The fact that we conceive of one of the pair as cotherapist does not necessarily indicate a preference for that member or dislike for the outsider; rather it simply points to an engagement, friendly or threatening, competitive or helpful. As therapists, we may feel competitive with the partner in the couple who has traditionally played a therapist role in the relationship. A game of one-upmanship can rapidly ensue in which the "outsider" feels powerless because the "two therapists" are both focusing on helping that person. But the "cotherapist" may also feel useless since the official therapist has taken over the role of expert and helper.

Although the "cotherapist" may feel relief at not being part of the problem, he or she must also feel abandoned, because he or she also came for help and is in some sort of psychological pain. Jennifer and Larry nicely illustrate this situation in that Jennifer, who has been in her own therapy, thinks "psychologically" and joins by using psychological terminology, which may be interpreted as wanting to help the therapist "cure" Larry. Some therapists might welcome such support which allows them to lapse into individual therapy with one of the couple rather than face the problems of the three-person system. On the other hand, it might irritate a therapist, as it seems to annoy Sluzki, who rejects Jennifer's approaches to align herself with him and chooses to align himself instead with Larry. Sluzki, in rejecting Jennifer as cotherapist, leans toward Larry and ironically whispers, "Secretly, this couples therapy is for you."

If we imagine that Jennifer's attempt to be cotherapist is one of Sluzki's fantasies, in part evoked by her actions and language, and that another therapist might have had a different fantasy, we can further investigate what such a fantasy reveals. Jennifer is not blind to Sluzki's alliance with Larry. She asks Sluzki if he has a degree in engineering because he sounds just like Larry. Sluzki subsequently acknowledged in his lecture at the conference that he prefers Larry's engineering language to Jennifer's psychological language; he prefers terms like "amplifying" and "dampening." In becoming aware of one's preferences in expression, a therapist might recognize the sex-role stereotypes underlying the male rational talk that Sluzki prefers and the female talk about feelings and intentions that the couple's previous female therapist may have responded to more positively, and in fact encouraged, in Jennifer. Sluzki's maneuver has the effect of modeling and encouraging traditional sex roles.

Sluzki reacts to Jennifer's encroachment on his territory and her attempts to align with him by doing the opposite: He forms an alliance with Larry. His aligning himself with Larry seems to raise Larry's level of confidence, for Larry becomes more involved and open. But it seems to deflate Jennifer, who becomes more guarded and confused, now the seemingly powerless outsider in a male-dominated system. Watzlawick, Weakland, and Fisch (1974) have pointed out that attempting to solve a problem by switching to the opposite solution can result in "more of the same" problem. Thus, to build up Larry and ignore Jennifer makes Jennifer try even harder for an alliance with Sluzki. However, this may have been a price Sluzki decided to pay for Larry's greater engagement during the relatively brief consultation.

CHILDREN AT PLAY

In considering Peggy Papp's use of fantasy, we will focus on the couple's imaginings rather than the therapist's, since Papp's fantasies are so much less accessible than those of the couple which are richly elaborated. Papp uses fantasy to lead a couple into play. She asks Jennifer and Larry to recall when they were children, when their imaginations were freer and more vivid, in order to help get them into the mood of fantasy, play, and pretend.

PAPP: It's like a game that children play. . . . But if you remember, as a child, you had a very vivid imagination. . . . You may remember that as a child, when you saw people in these fantasies and dreams, they often took different forms. . . . if your father was authoritarian [he may have been] a policeman. If your mother was cross with you, you may have seen her as a witch . . .

The fantasy imagery each partner reveals is provoked by the nature of their relationship as well as by Papp's introduction and warm yet directive style. As she becomes motherly or like a fairy godmother, they become even more childlike; in fact, each member of the couple imagines a scene in which both of them are children. While Jennifer imagines she is a little girl attempting to make a shy, orphaned boy her friend and playmate, Larry's fantasy is that she and her girlfriends are teasing him and interfering with his basketball game with the boys. The presence of the therapist as director and the conference as audience undoubtedly also influences their images of themselves as children participating in a performance or play, since being asked to perform and being studied are somewhat infantilizing.

Can a preference for one member of the couple be discerned? Larry states that in his fantasy "the girls" are bothering him, and he wants to ignore the girls. In fact, he threatens to "beat their heads in" if they interfere with his game. In this fantasy "the girls" may mean Papp and Jennifer, whom he may view as colluding to ruin his game. It is possible that Larry is perceiving some subtle alliance between them, and if so, this perpetuates his position as the consistent outsider.

How the therapist may have stimulated Jennifer's fantasy is less apparent. Is the therapist the family who abandoned the little boy? Is she the horse brought in to entice the boy into joining in? Or is Papp the one who will help Jennifer "bring out" this quiet and frightened orphan? If the latter is true, Papp must exercise care not to "abandon" Larry throughout the play, since it might intensify Jennifer's tendency to focus on his needs rather than her own.

The idyllic childlike fantasies, the dreamy innocent quality Papp encourages as the couple pick flowers and catch butterflies, are as romantic as their subsequent powerful fantasies of success. The latter fantasies have themes of death, but while Larry's is of Thomas Jefferson writing the Declaration of Independence while his wife is dying, Jennifer's is of Mozart whose creativity was cut short by his own death. In the follow-up interview (see Chapter 18), both Larry and Jennifer acknowledge that Papp's technique brings out how competitive they are, which seems to have been an unacknowledged aspect of their relationship.

THE BALLOON AND THE ROCK

Sluzki openly shares his own fantasy imagery of the couple with them. One fantasy is that Jennifer is like a balloon "shooting into space" if it were not for a weight, Larry, holding her down. He informs them that their complementarity is useful for balance in the relationship, since one would not want two balloons drifting in the wind or two rocks at the bottom of the lake. This is a delightful fantasy, and one the couple found useful months later. It reveals nothing about his alliance with either member of the pair, but his preference becomes apparent when Sluzki shares another fantasy. Speaking to Jennifer, he says, "It sounds like you are one of those fanatics that jump onto any bandwagon with all her soul, and you [Larry] say, 'Hey, wait a minute, reality testing, one, two, three.'" The phrase "with all her soul" may indicate some affection for Jennifer, but the word "fanatic" is clearly pejorative. In his fantasy, Sluzki describes Larry as using the phrase "reality testing," which may suggest Sluzki's preference for the implied rationality and solidity of Larry as well as a feeling of comradeship with him. If Sluzki were unaware of communicating a preference for Larry, a danger would be that he might unwittingly exclude Jennifer and render her powerless while he takes over the role of Larry's partner which she is striving to achieve. In fact, Sluzki has allied himself more strongly with Larry for therapeutic purposes. According to the couple in a later interview, Sluzki's intervention with the balloon and rock image seemed the most useful.

THE PRINCE AND THE PRINCESS

Couple therapists are, in general, romantics about relationships, and so it is not surprising that one conference participant's fantasy was a fairy tale with a happy ending. This participant imagined that Larry was like the fairy tale prince who overcomes numerous hurdles to win the princess. In this unelaborated fantasy, both characters are presumably likeable. However, the prince has the added virtues of being persistent, determined, and brave, while the princess is a passive ideal. Would the holder of such a fantasy conceive of the therapy session as one more hurdle and thus try to make the experience easier for Larry? Does this therapist begin with the assumption that the pair will and should stay together? By joining Larry and treating Jennifer as a much-sought-after object to be won, the therapist would unwittingly focus on the needs and activity of the questing individual—Larry. The therapist could instead use the fantasy to understand his or her own preferences and inclinations. Perhaps the therapist's fantasy has picked up on a theme in the couple of proving one's love—a theme that might be made explicit and examined in terms of each partner's need for ritual proof of such love, as in the overcoming of obstacles to achieve a romantic union.

FRANKENSTEIN'S MONSTER AND THE GIRL

Another fantasy the interviews with Jennifer and Larry evoked in one of our workshop participants was that of Frankenstein's monster and the little girl he encounters. One might safely assume that a therapist with this fantasy feels more comfortable with the small girl and probably likes the girl more than the monster. The notion of a monster has the unpleasant connotation of overwhelming power, even if the monster is ultimately calmed by the childish innocence of the little girl. Also present is the threat of imminent danger which the girl does not recognize, so the therapist might be drawn into protecting her from what may be seen as hidden rage in Larry. This fantasy of a monster also suggests that the therapist may be uncomfortable with Larry's amputation. It may further reveal the perhaps misplaced image of Jennifer as a naive child who is powerless and has little anger herself. Since angry people often seem threatening to us as therapists, we may be drawn into covertly rewarding those who express pleasantness. In examining such a fantasy, a therapist might gain some clues to look more broadly for the hidden "monster" in Jennifer, and also become more aware of his or her own anxiety about the silent, awkward Larry.

THE PRISONER AND THE KEEPER

In another fantasy offered about Jennifer and Larry's relationship, one participant saw Jennifer as a prisoner and Larry as her keeper. It would appear that a therapist's natural sympathies might be with the prisoner. Would a therapist having this particular fantasy be motivated to help the prisoner escape? Is the prisoner actually using therapy to exit from the relationship? The suggestion of restraint, confinement, and possible violence might move the therapist to be protective of Jennifer. Moreover, imagining Larry as the prison keeper seems to imply that the therapist may not believe that Jennifer finds Larry attractive or could love him without coercion. The question also arises as to why she needs to be confined and punished. Is she too dangerous when she is free?

The therapist who remains unaware of the implications of this fantasy might be drawn into alliance with Jennifer—an alliance that would most likely confirm not only her power, but her need for a therapist to save her by freeing her from Larry and the confining relationship. Larry would become the outsider, and although the power of his position as keeper is self-evident, his being left out might leave him with feelings of low self-esteem. Further examination of this fantasy might lead a therapist to see his or her own difficulties with holding a couple as a "captive" audience within the therapeutic situation. The therapist would also need to question his negative feelings toward Larry, as well as the prisoner. Reframing the prisoner–keeper fantasy as one in which each partner is prisoner to the other—for a prison keeper is in turn dependent on a prisoner—would help the therapist to overcome what might be an asymmetrical preference for one of this pair. The therapist might attempt to free them both by clarifying the choices they have made in order to remain locked together in their present situation.

THE LION AND THE LIONESS

The fantasy suggested by one therapist of a lion and a lioness presents both Larry and Jennifer as powerful, but in different ways. The animal pair also suggests a sexual metaphor, for this is a bestiary male–female pair. But in nature, the behaviors shown by the lion and lioness are very different. The lion in folklore is the king of the jungle with his mane and mighty roar, but actually, in the wild, the lion is a lazy beast who lies about dozing in the sun. The lioness is the hunter, the one who, with the other females, patiently stalks, outruns, and brings down the kill. The lioness is the fierce and active one, training and protecting her cubs, seeking food, and stalking her prey.

In this fantasy, Larry is the powerful king of the beasts, but it is Jennifer who is the more active one who provides for the pair. Does the therapist hold the view that women as well as men can be strong? Is the therapist annoyed by the empty posing of the male? Or does the therapist view the relaxed male as part of the natural order in allowing the female to do the ordinary tasks of daily life? Would the therapist with this fantasy see this as the natural way for a couple to be, not unlike the accepted roles in the human family? Or does the fantasy reveal an impulse to provoke and stir up the dozing lion, perhaps to rage, or relieve the lioness of responsibility for the kill? Does this fantasy also reflect Larry's injury, as in the legend of Androcles and the Lion? The therapist who examines such a fantasy might become aware of feelings of admiration for the raw but noble savagery in the lion and lioness, and perhaps for the primitive bond between Larry and Jennifer. The powerful nature of this pair may also incite fear, making the therapist timid and hesitant to intervene.

REPRISE

Fantasies often draw on myths and fairy tales, which reflect unproven collective beliefs about human relationships. They reveal to us the conventional and stereotypical ways we have of looking at the world and our limited ability to step outside that shared framework. Thus, when we think of a typical couple, we find it hard to free ourselves of the images that remain from childhood stories. After all, the prototypical couple of the Western world is Peter Pan and Wendy, not Adam and Eve. Peter is the adventurer, out with the lost boys, their acknowledged and daring leader. Wendy, making a cozy nest for him to return to, sits at home sewing on buttons. Tinker Bell, the fairy, is the third party in the unstable three-person system, as is the serpent in the Garden of Eden. In today's world, Peter Pan and Wendy truly live in Never-Never Land, but this magic place still exists in our fantasies.

And so does the tale of *Treasure Island*. Returning to that fantasy, perhaps we see a therapist enthralled by the adventure of working with Larry and Jennifer—attracted by the risks, cautioned by the dangers; seeking to understand the nature of the therapist bond with each one of the pair, as well as their loyalty and allegiance to each other. Fantasy is an elegant simplification of reality that helps us make sense of our experience. Like play, it offers images and roles that can extend our understanding of the world.

Fantasy can reveal the limits of our choices and our human tendency to project images onto patients and then seek to satisfy those images. We have been trained to focus on patients' fantasies for understanding the complexities of patient–therapist interactions. However, following our own fantasies may lead us to recognize how our alliances and preferences influence us in working with couples.

REFERENCES

Boas, G. (1961). *The limits of reason.* New York: Harper.

Epstein, L., & Feiner, A. H. (1979). Countertransference: The therapist's contribution to treatment. *Contemporary Psychoanalysis, 15,* 489–513.

Frazer, J.G. (1980). *The golden bough: A study in magic and religion.* London: Macmillan. (Original work published 1890)

Gottsegen, G. B., & Gottsegen, M. G. (1979). Countertransference: The professional identify defense. *Psychotherapy: Theory, Research and Practice, 16,* 57–60.

Grolnick, L. (1983). Ibsen's truth, family secrets, and family therapy. *Family Process, 22,* 275–280.

Guttman, H. A. (1982). Transference and countertransference in conjoint couple therapy: Therapeutic and theoretical implications. *Canadian Journal of Psychiatry, 27,* 92–97.

Hare-Mustin, R. T. (1987). The problem of gender in family therapy theory. *Family Process, 26,* 15–27.

Jackson, D. D. (1965) Family rules: Marital quid pro quo. *Archives of General Psychiatry, 12,* 589–594.

Kahn, L. S. (1980). The dynamics of scapegoating: The expulsion of evil. *Psychotherapy: Theory, Research, and Practice, 17,* 79–84.

Margolin, G., Talovic, S., Fernandez, V., & Onorato, R. (1983). Sex role considerations and behavioral marital therapy: Equal does not mean identical. *Journal of Marital and Family Therapy, 9,* 131–145.

Minuchin, S. (1974). *Families and family therapy.* Cambridge, MA: Harvard University Press.

Silverstein, E. A. (1984) Langsian theory and countertransference. In J. Raney (Ed.), *Listening and interpreting* (pp. 99–126). New York: Jason Aronson.

Thompson, W. I. (1971). *At the edge of history.* New York: Harper & Row.

Walker, J. L., & White, N. F. (1975). The varities of therapeutic experience: Conjoint therapy in a homosexual marriage. *Canada's Mental Health, 23,* 3–5.

Watzlawick, P., Weakland, J. H., & Fisch, R. (1974). *Change: Principles of problem formation and problem resolution.* New York: Norton.

Zuk, G. R. (1972). Family therapy: Clinical hodgepodge or clinical science. *Journal of Marriage and Family Counseling, 2,* 229–304.

14

Navigating Among the Theories:
An Eclectic Approach to Couple Therapy

WALTER ABRAMS and NICHOLSON BROWNING

This book presents a number of coherent and compelling theories about couple therapy. Among its readers there are undoubtedly many couple therapists and students of couple therapy who are left wondering: Which theories and techniques should I employ in my own work? Can I integrate aspects of them all into one eclectic plan for the conduct of therapy without feeling confused and adrift?

In this chapter we explore some of the strengths and challenges of eclectic approaches to couple therapy with the aim of addressing this concern about drifting. We begin our exploration by presenting and commenting on the case of Larry and Jennifer as we imagine it might have been handled by a fictional eclectic therapist. Next we discuss the use of theory and identify some of the factors that shape—consciously or unconsciously—the eclectic therapist's repertoire. Then we highlight three aspects of clinical work that require of the therapist particularly well-reasoned and skillful choices: diagnosis, tailoring the therapeutic work to the couple's learning style, and utilizing feedback. Finally, we discuss paradigms for systematic eclecticism and make recommendations for training. It is our hope that this exploration will lend to the practice of eclectic therapy a sense of value and coherence not always apparent even to its practitioners, while at the same time identifying challenges for more skillful and effective eclectic practice.

All therapists have a common goal when a couple enters the office: to help the couple resolve their pain and conflict. Like other service professionals, from surgeons to auto mechanics, we try to restore or enhance function. Unlike most service professionals, however, we find ourselves in a field that enjoys little consensus about how to approach and resolve the dilemmas our clients present to us. Ten out of 10 auto mechanics are likely to tell you that your broken fan belt is making your engine overheat; 10 couple therapists may give 10 different reasons why a couple is overheating. What is more confusing is that all may be "right" and all may have something of value to offer the couple.

Many therapists (ourselves included) appreciate the value of multiple perspectives on a case and routinely make use of a variety of approaches and methods. We like to think of ourselves as eclectic, open, and pragmatic, able to adopt whatever methods might be helpful to the client. Yet our eclecticism at times seems random and incoherent. One day the psychoanalyst within us makes an illuminating interpretation that gives a couple a new and useful understanding of their relationship. In the next session we suggest a structural change in the couple system and, without any new insights, the couple seems freed from some previously intractable constraints (MacKinnon & Slive, 1984). As we move from one theoretical orientation to the next, we can easily lose our sense of direction and begin to drift aimlessly. Even when we arrive safely on shore, metaphorically speaking, we wonder what winds, currents, and features of our ship shaped our meandering course, and if a more direct route might have been apparent to us had we understood these influences more clearly.

THE ECLECTIC THERAPIST: A HYPOTHETICAL CASE

To begin our exploration of the factors that shape a therapeutic course, we will present the case of Larry and Jennifer as it is handled over the course of several sessions by a fictional eclectic therapist, Dr. Ellsworth. Dr. Ellsworth is no more than a figment of our imaginations, but the reader will recognize aspects of his work that bear some resemblance to approaches taken by the therapists who conducted the four demonstration interviews with Larry and Jennifer. The couple in our hypothetical case is meant to bear striking resemblance to Larry and Jennifer, the couple presented throughout this volume. Although we have had to speculate about their responses to Dr. Ellsworth, we have begun with what we have been told about their history, their personalities, and their relationship.

Dr. Ellsworth's Background

Dr. Ellsworth is a clinical psychologist in his mid-30s who completed his training a few years ago in another city. Since that time he has worked in Boston, half-time in a clinic and half-time in private practice. He sees individuals as well as couples and families. Immediately prior to coming to Boston, Dr. Ellsworth received training in family therapy with a focus on structural techniques. Although he is intellectually committed to family therapy and systems theory, he is still most comfortable with individual therapy. His graduate training reflected a strong psychoanalytic bias. A detached and reflective attitude always seemed to him to be the proper posture for a therapist; in fact, he finds the dramatic personal styles of some family therapists a bit disturbing and difficult to emulate.

As the youngest of three children in his own family of origin, Dr. Ellsworth was generally perceived to be the favored child. He often acted as a mediator in the conflicts between other family members and later jokingly referred to this role as his genesis as a family therapist. His personal experience as a client in therapy is limited to a brief course of psychoanalytically oriented psychotherapy that occurred during a period of career confusion in his early 20s. He is married with no children.

As a couple therapist, Dr. Ellsworth has a difficulty common among his peers: He is familiar with a variety of theories of couples therapy, yet there are times when he feels his application of these theories is random; he lacks an overview to organize his work. His work with Larry and Jennifer exemplifies this problem.

Dr. Ellsworth's Presentation of his Work with Larry and Jennifer

The following is a description of Dr. Ellsworth's work with Jennifer and Larry, as he might have presented it at a couple therapy conference. We have annotated this description with commentaries emphasizing key choice points, theoretical shifts, and the influences that shaped Dr. Ellsworth's choices. In the second half of this chapter we will catalogue these and other influences, referring to Dr. Ellsworth's work for illustrations.

My First Approach

Larry and Jennifer were referred to me by the therapist who had been treating Jennifer for about one year prior to the referral. She had been pleased by the therapy with Jennifer and considered it a sign of Jennifer's progress that she had "put some pressure on Larry to straighten out their relationship."

During the initial session I had with the couple, they identified several problems: Jennifer felt that Larry was too aloof and unemotional. She wanted to feel closer to him and stated that Larry, absorbed with television, resisted this. Larry agreed that their relationship could use improvement, but emphasized his desire for greater harmony rather than more closeness. He felt that Jennifer was too emotional and that things would improve if she would only relax, enjoy herself more, and accept that all relationships have imperfections. In addition, he pointed out that while Jennifer wanted closeness, she worked 16 hours a day, to which she responded that "quality, not quantity" was the issue. Both agreed that even though they had been together for almost 10 years, they were not prepared to marry. They told me this was not a major issue.

My initial formulation focused on the couple system, and attributed to Jennifer and Larry a pursuer–distancer relationship. Jennifer experienced Larry as remote, rejecting, and uncommunicative and told him so in order to feel closer to him. Larry experienced Jennifer as critical. Although he made efforts to satisfy Jennifer, Larry felt hurt, irritated, and mistrustful. He withdrew from her. Completing the cycle in their couple system, Jennifer became more upset by Larry's remote response and increased her efforts "to get through to him." Since Larry and Jennifer agreed that they would like to feel closer, I recommended that they turn off the television one full day during the week. Jennifer was pleased with the suggestion and Larry was willing. However, after a few weeks there seemed to be little difference in their interaction. They had followed the assignment but spent the time working separately. When I suggested that they not work either, they read separately. I felt that this intervention was not productive and decided to explore their resistance.

COMMENTARY

Dr. Ellsworth made a very reasonable initial systems formulation. This was a pursuer–distancer system, with a self-reinforcing repetitive cycle. His hypothesis led to a direct behavioral intervention: assignment of a task requiring that they spend time together without television. He persisted with this when they worked rather than interacted, but when they resisted again, he backed away from his formulation.

The couple's resistance, which was manifested by their saying that they wanted to be closer but ignoring opportunities to achieve intimacy, shook Dr. Ellsworth's confidence in his theoretical position. He failed to explore the option of persisting with the pursuer–distancer formulation, treating the resistance as further information about the nature of the system, and refining his intervention accordingly. He might have noticed, for example, that in assigning and reassigning the task he had become inducted into the system. He became the pursuer. Now his pursuit was met with resistance, and the therapy was beginning to reflect the couple's system.

Dr. Ellsworth might have tried a new therapeutic tactic before abandoning his initial formulation. For example, he could have told the couple, "I have made a perfectly foolish mistake in my first assignment. If the solution were so simple, you would have obviously thought of it yourselves. I have failed to consider the role of deeper fears. Larry, I have a hunch that Jennifer believes that you are afraid of her. Even though you see no direct evidence that she has this belief, it may still be true. It may be critically important for you to actively prove to Jennifer that you are not afraid of her by arranging to spend a significant amount of time with her. During this time you must probe for her dissatisfactions with the relationship and with you. Only in this way will you prove to her that you are not afraid of her."

This intervention would deal with the pursuer–distancer relationship by firmly installing Larry as the pursuer in order to alter the sequence. This is only one of the many possible moves with which Dr. Ellsworth might have remained consistent with his original theoretical position. Like many of us, when faced with resistance to our attempts to apply a model, he did not redouble his efforts or alter their direction, but blamed the theoretical approach and reverted to older, more familiar models (or turned to newer, more daring ones). Although there is nothing intrinsically incorrect about the next direction taken by Dr. Ellsworth, we do contend that he may have changed his viewpoint prematurely.

My Second Approach

Getting nowhere with a direct behavioral intervention, I decided to explore with Jennifer and Larry their families of origin. Larry's family was large, noisy, loving, and Jewish. His mother was an archetypical Jewish mother and proud of her role. Larry had established his pattern of distancing from an intrusive pursuer in relation to her. It was also clear that Larry identified with his quiet, stolid, and competent father, whom he said "spoke only as necessary." There was a loving feeling in this family, and neither the mother's noisy nosiness nor Larry's retreat from it alarmed anyone.

Jennifer's family contrasted remarkably. She experienced silence and distance everywhere within her family. She believed that she was an unwanted child and felt that her mother and sister had become pals after her birth, caring little for her. She was left, *de facto,* to her silent and distant father with whom she slept until age six. This relationship, although it apparently involved no incest, felt more like a burden than a comfort. I pointed out that Jennifer's loneliness and sense of being unloved by Larry was similar to her early experiences. She felt relieved by this insight, but she also felt blamed. Larry was relieved to discover that Jennifer's feelings "came from her childhood," and recognized that he too was repeating his childhood pattern, but in a context where it no longer had any value. He seemed willing to try to be more responsive to Jennifer's overtures.

COMMENTARY

Dr. Ellsworth's second approach rests on the premise that insight into early origins of current reactions can be a curative element in therapy. He has brought to the surface important information applicable to the couple's situation. Jennifer may now experience her pursuit of Larry as part of an old quest for love from her family, in addition to being an aspect of the relationship with him. Larry now understands that his reserve, which has a benign meaning in his old exchanges with his mother, may be quite painful in another context. This new information may lead him to consider new responses to Jennifer. In this approach Dr. Ellsworth is comfortable relying on a theory in which he is well-versed. His formulations are psychodynamic, although clearly applied to the couple's context. But there are pitfalls in this approach (as there are in any) to which Dr. Ellsworth will have to respond in the next session.

My Third Approach

While I felt that the rigorous examination of their histories had been informative to them, I nevertheless felt their new awareness would not be sufficient to generate substantive change. I speculated that my second approach would have little effect, because Larry and Jennifer had an intellectualizing response to the insights. They had a considerable faculty for speculating and talking about it without showing much impetus to change.

To deal more directly with the strong affective patterns each had established, I encouraged them both to participate in family of origin meetings in which these feelings would be aired and discussed. Although Jennifer initially felt threatened by this idea, both she and Larry agreed. I intended to explore Jennifer's loneliness within her family and Larry's traumatic encounter with cancer within his.

The meeting with Larry's family produced valuable information concerning death and misfortune in the family, stimulated by consideration of Larry's illness. The meeting resonated with themes important in the Jewish culture: themes of tragedy and persistence and of bonds across the generations. Intergenerational conflict was not prominent in this family meeting.

The meeting with Jennifer's family was more dramatic and affectively charged. She finally told her family how lonely and unloved she had felt growing up. She was able to absorb both explanations and expressions of caring from her mother and sister. Some specific agreements were made that the family would try to stay closer and share more with one another.

COMMENTARY

Family of origin meetings are dramatic and powerful tools for couple therapy. Old conflicts and behavioral patterns that were established during certain developmental periods are brought forward into new relationships, so that in family of origin meetings current problems can be confronted in their original interpersonal context. New possibilities can be sought out and adopted. This method seems wisely chosen by Dr. Ellsworth at this stage of the therapy. He had secured a strong working alliance with the couple and had identified significant themes, but felt the need to generate stronger affective involvement. In presenting these meetings, he strongly supported the optimistic views that risks are worth taking and that people can indeed change the quality of their relationships.

My Fourth Approach

Not long after the family of origin meetings, Jennifer and Larry took a summer-long vacation for the first time and traveled in Europe together. They felt very close during the trip. Upon their return they felt rejuvenated and optimistic. Once back, Jennifer established regular and very satisfying contact with her mother. Larry also felt closer to his father, with whom he now had occasional long talks, something unheard of previously. The couple seemed significantly more comfortable and flexible with one another.

In the fall, however, both Larry and Jennifer returned to their customary heavy work schedules. Jennifer again began to feel cut off from Larry. This time she found the experience all the more painful, since they had felt so close at the end of the summer, when they had been seriously discussing marriage and having a baby. She began to wonder if the closeness she had experienced during the summer was an illusion and if they would be better off to admit that they were incompatible and break up. Larry, on the other hand, felt that he needed an outlet (meaning watching sports on television) all the more since he was back to the pressure of his professional life.

This resurgence of the old conflict led them to contact me at the end of September. I thought then that there were several theoretical positions I could utilize. I could return to the psychodynamic approach I was following prior to the family meetings and try to challenge and bring out Jennifer's deep ambivalence about loving and being loved. Along the same lines, I considered trying to elicit Larry's deep self-doubt. It seemed to me that the psychological pain of losing his foot and having to give up the sports he loved so much had never been fully worked through.

However, because I felt there were limitations to insight-oriented approaches with this couple, another approach appealed to me more. I decided to make a major effort to reframe their conflict as essentially normal, growing out of the complementary roles in their relationship. This approach had the added benefit of offering the possibility of a shorter intervention. I pursued this option in two stages. Initially, I worked to redefine their return to therapy (which had irked Larry) as an act of generosity on Jennifer's part. I suggested that her extensive experience in individual therapy had been valuable to her and she wished to share this with Larry. Although she was not entirely pleased by this idea, she could not easily reject it. It allowed me to bring up her unspoken wish to change Larry, even though in a teasing way I suggested that this was unreasonable. I then strongly developed the idea that they were quite different from one another, forming a complementary system that had substantial benefits for them both. Larry was the solid, steady one; Jennifer was the expressive, imaginative one. I used the metaphor of amplifier and damper (which appealed to Larry), and of a rock and a helium balloon (which appealed to Jennifer). They both clearly understood this "normalizing" idea and were intrigued by it. I further suggested that they should reconsider the advisability of changing such an obviously well-balanced arrangement and asked if we could meet again in three weeks to discuss it.

COMMENTARY

Dr. Ellsworth has now moved to a more systemic/strategic approach. He has employed a reframing that delivers the message of his original interpretation in a new way, ascribing a positive connotation to the pursuer–distancer structure. In so doing, Dr. Ellsworth avoided the trap of accepting Jennifer's negative framing and being inducted into the system as Larry's pursuer. In employing a "restraint of change" prescription, he left it to the couple to recognize and take responsibility for the shortcomings in their arrangement and thus preempted the couple's previously observed resistance to change.

In selecting this approach, Dr. Ellsworth is dealing with a central concern of couple therapy, that of first-order change being stimulated without affecting the basic belief systems governing the relationship. Larry and Jennifer experienced their relationship as stronger and more intimate, but their propensity to fall back into old patterns of alienation indicated that more fundamental change was necessary. In order to accomplish this, Dr. Ellsworth used a systemic/strategic intervention.

Dr. Ellsworth will be faced with another choice point when the couple returns in three weeks. We imagine that the couple might be reluctant to accept his embracing the status quo. He has two general options for dealing with their skepticism. One option would be to remain doggedly with a "restraint of change" position. Certainly it can be argued that such an apparently paradoxical stance may have merit with this system. Larry and Jennifer might find themselves drawn into an alliance against the unreasonable therapist. They might jointly insist that some changes would be worthwhile.

A playful elaboration of this position would be to ask them to act out a ritual in which each overtly expresses the other's worst fears. For example, Jennifer might be asked to say, "You are so unloving and withholding that I am now going to flood you with my emotions until I get a lively and connected response." Larry would ritualistically respond, "All right, dear, but I understand that you are so emotional and unstable that I will be very calm and restrained so you won't go crazy."

A second possibility, one particularly worth considering if Larry and Jennifer return insistent that the status quo is unacceptable, is for the therapist to reluctantly show them how to experiment with new structures for the relationship during the session. This might be accomplished by means of role playing, but can also be approached indirectly through metaphor. Dr. Ellsworth can ask that they recreate their system in a context of fantasy and creatively solve the problem in that context. If instead Dr. Ellsworth had guided them in a step-by-step process through their restructuring, with assignments to practice what they learn in therapy at home, he would be returning to a more rigorous implementation of his original behavioral approach to intervention.

If at some point Dr. Ellsworth is given enduring evidence that he has helped Larry and Jennifer to achieve their goals, he may take pride in his eclecticism and feel he has shifted perspectives smoothly and effectively. If not, he may feel uncertain. In either case, why did he proceed the way he did? On what grounds did he make his choices?

UNDERSTANDING ECLECTICISM

Dr. Ellsworth's experience illustrates a problem common to many beginning couple therapists. We operate in a field of rich complexity where numerous theories, methods, and strategies inform our moment-to-moment decisions. Yet we often feel like media through whom the voices of teachers and authors speak and act in mysterious ways. Even when we are helpful, we may not understand why.

In response to this concern, we will attempt to define eclecticism in dynamic terms, not simply as any application of an aggregate of theories and methods, but as a process of assessing, acting on, and reassessing our shifting approaches with attention to variables that include our educational and personal background, the specific attributes of the couple, and the process of the therapy itself. Each of these factors interacts in a mutually influencing and evolving manner to produce effective therapy in practice (Colapinto, 1984).

Eclectic therapists are like master cabinetmakers using the various tools of their trade to produce a piece of furniture. Master cabinetmakers understand that their choice of a tool in a given situation depends not only on the product they are trying to create, but also on their level of skill and comfort with the tool, on the type of wood with which they are working, and on the specific problems they encounter at each point in the creative process. Certainly, they use a method, but they are also flexible, able, and willing to adjust their design and modify their plans during the course of their work.

In the following pages we will examine several factors that influence our choice of tools. We will consider how the particular couple we encounter can affect our choice of tools and how the process of the therapy can influence when we decide to change the tool. We will also refer to some emerging ideas for the systematic application of eclecticism, and, finally, explore some implications for the training of eclectic therapists.

We will begin with four assertions that we will develop in the rest of the chapter:

1. We know of no model for couples therapy that is demonstrably more valid than any other. We believe that many therapies, many theories, and many tactics offer something useful when employed by a particular therapist with particular clients at particular times in therapy.

2. Therapists, for the most part, do not follow theories as an amateur carpenter might follow a simple construction plan. Like master cabinetmakers, therapists make use of certain standard plans (theories) and tools (techniques), but their work involves a more complex process than the straightforward application of theories and techniques. The therapist develops his or her own set of models of therapeutic understanding and therapeutic behavior. These models are amalgams of behaviors, beliefs, and theories, consciously and unconsciously assimilated from training, from clinical practice, and from personal life.[1] It is preferable that our models be consciously apprehended and applied. Ideally, any therapist could stop at any moment in the therapy and relate his or her therapeutic decisions to some theoretical understanding. The more clearly we can identify our theoretical guides, the greater control we have over the direction of our work.

---

[1]Grunebaum (1988a) has described this phenomenon in a retrospective analysis of a single interview.

3. A couple's behavior will suggest certain hypotheses to the therapist. These hypotheses, in turn, shape what the therapist sees and does. The couple's reactions to an intervention will support the initial hypothesis or call another one forward. Thus, our models, the basic structures of understanding we bring to our work, both influence and are influenced by the very thing they seek to describe and explicate.

4. In the process of the therapy, events (often experienced as blocks or resistances to the therapy) cause us to re-examine our models. These moments often produce a kind of crisis of confidence for the therapist. He or she must decide whether to alter the model (reach for a new tool) or persist with renewed vigor with the model at hand.

What is a Model?

A "model," *as we are using the term here,* is not simply a theory that we read about or an approach observed in a workshop. A theory or an approach is an idea invented by others. It becomes a model as it is filtered through our own personal experience and expressed through our particular talents and abilities. Thus it is not the theories themselves that interest us, but the "tools" *as employed by* each particular "craftsperson." This system of tool-plus-craftsperson constitutes a model. Thus, in our definition of "model" there are as many models as there are therapists—even more, since therapists have a variety of models. The more we study and train, the longer we practice, the more models we incorporate into our repertoire. In addition, the greater our experience, the more complex each model becomes. In this way, the models of an expert clinician are like tools in the hands of a master woodworker; they can shape and create with a subtlety that the same tools cannot achieve in the hands of a novice.

We maintain that the majority of clinicians employ their models in the following way. The couple presents a variety of behaviors, affects, and interactions that form a recognizable pattern within the diagnostic framework of one of our models. An eclectic therapist possesses a variety of such frameworks, often associated with various schools of thought (e.g., behavioral) or an author's name (e.g., Jim Framo's or Norman Paul's theory). We employ the model that seems to explain the couple best, at least initially. That model provides us with a rationale for our initial therapeutic strategy and with a means of evaluating our efforts (de Shazer, 1984).

The process by which therapists apply a model to a couple is analogous to the Piagetan process of assimilation (Piaget with Inhelder, 1969). We begin with our own private repertoire of models and then attempt to assimilate our experience with the couple into one or more of the models, just as a child attempts to assimilate a novel object into his repertoire of cognitive–behavioral schemes. Sometimes assimilation proves impossible, and we must synthesize several models or learn a new one in order to accommodate to the specific couple system with which we are engaged.

Factors That Influence the Use of Models

In this section we will review some of the factors that reside within the therapist and influence his or her choice of a model for treatment. In developing our models we are influenced not only by the books we read, but by our personal style, individual history, and as Hare-Mustin and Lamb (Chapter 13, this volume) point out, our fantasies. We will briefly review some of these influences, using the fictional work of Dr. Ellsworth for the purpose of illustration.

Training

For the most part, we learn to practice couple therapy apprenticed to, or supervised by, senior clinicians from particular schools, and our biases tend to reflect the biases of our teachers. Dr. Ellsworth's first teachers and most influential role models were practitioners of individual psychodynamic psychotherapy, not systems theory. Therefore it is not surprising that when he was faced with client "resistance" to his initial systemic intervention, he returned to a more psychodynamic theory of therapy.

We are often strongly influenced by the most recent training we have undergone. Most of us have had the experience of returning from a workshop or conference filled with enthusiasm for some new perspective. Suddenly we see our clients from an entirely new point of view. Over time we digest new theories and absorb them into our personal repertoire of models, incorporating what is useful and discarding what we cannot use or understand.

One of the strongest influences on trainees is the *personal style* of our teachers. Both Carlos Sluzki and Peggy Papp are systems therapists. Yet we experience them quite differently. We learn the nuances of their behavior as much as their theoretical constructs. Couple therapists find themselves trying to "do a Framo move" or "do a Sluzki move" as if it were a new dance step. In such instances the concept behind the move (or intervention) may not feel important. The practice of therapy is a *behavioral–cognitive* scheme; intervention involves a complex sequence of verbal and nonverbal behaviors, which senior therapists appear to undertake with an ease that is the envy of their protegés. We learn from Jim Framo, for example, not only how to structure a family meeting, but how to engage the patient's resistances with empathic understanding while pursuing with a kind of paternal firmness one's explicit therapeutic goals. From Peggy Papp one learns not only the technique of metaphorical representation of underlying structure, but how to implement this technique with a sense of gentle playfulness.

Personality

Imitation enhances our skills best when our own personality is consistent with the personal style of the teacher. Watching Peggy Papp interview Larry and Jennifer, for example, may remind us of our own playfulness and allow us to creatively employ capacities we have previously not felt free to use. On the other hand, if we are not easily playful, our efforts to mold ourselves to Peggy Papp's methods may have the unfortunate effect of making us clumsy and unnatural. Similarly, if the confrontational message of Carlos Sluzki is delivered in a weighty, pedantic, or humorless style it is far less likely to be effective than in Sluzki's somewhat avuncular, joking manner (even though it may rest on the same theoretical premise). The smoothest fit occurs when the theory is attractive and stimulating on the cognitive level and when the style of one of its practitioners suits the trainee's personality.

Every theory we explicitly or implicitly promote leads to a range of interventions. How we choose among these interventions will depend in large part on our own personalities. Some salient personality variables include the following:

Active versus Reactive. Some therapists are characteristically quiet and reflective, and therefore most comfortable, when they can observe the spontaneous enactment of a couples' conflict before they react. Other therapists, perhaps less patient or reflective by nature, may learn more and feel more at ease initiating action and "making things happen." A reactive therapist may be more comfortable with a psychodynamic theory and practice, while an active therapist may prefer structural or strategic approaches.

Authoritative versus Empathic. Although these qualities are not polarities, they are often inversely related in personal styles. "Close versus distant" represents a similar distinction. Some therapists are most comfortable when they can take a relatively distant and authoritative stance. These therapists may feel more comfortable than their more "empathic" counterparts using certain interventions (e.g., giving paradoxical prescriptions), and may work particularly effectively with clients with boundary confusion and a tendency toward enmeshment. Other therapists, however, may feel that they can only work effectively when they feel "close" or in empathic resonance with the couple. For them, their own emotional experience of the couple may be the most valuable source of information for the therapy. These therapists may gravitate toward what Chasin and Grunebaum (1980) call the "experiential" perspective.

Affective versus Cognitive. Again, these qualities are compatible, but they often vary inversely with one another. Some therapists are most comfortable and effective when they communicate in a cool and reasoned manner, while others are most at ease or most alive in a strong emotional field. A reflective, intellectual sort of person may feel most effective when able to develop and prescribe strategic assignments. A more affectively inclined therapist may accomplish the same therapeutic goals with an emotionally powerful family meeting like those described by Framo and Paul (Chapter 4 and 5, this volume).

Cognitive Style. A therapist's cognitive style, his or her manner of thinking about and understanding the world, will be more congruent with some schools of therapy than others. Systems theorists have argued that to achieve a systems perspective one must maintain a sustained and disciplined effort to shed the cognitive habit of linear causality. A common shortcoming of novice couple therapists is the tendency to think in a linear fashion while trying to practice systemic therapy. Dr. Ellsworth encountered this difficulty in his initial pursuer–distancer formulation. His formulation had a static, linear quality, rather than the active flowing quality that accompanies a thorough circular hypothesis in which beginnings and endings are illusions of perspective. His cognitive style was not sufficiently congruent with his guiding theory.

Family of Origin

Just as couple therapists pay careful attention to the couple's families of origin as determinants of their own model of being a couple, we as therapists must be aware of how our own families affect our model of therapy. As an active mediator in his own family, Dr. Ellsworth was comfortable facilitating conflict resolution. It was natural for him to move very quickly toward a behavioral resolution of Larry and Jennifer's problems with intimacy. Only later in the therapy did he choose to employ a strategic intervention that might exacerbate rather than quiet the conflict at hand. Examining this sequence in light of Dr. Ellsworth's own family background, we can well imagine that a strategic model might reawaken his own childhood anxieties, thus making it more difficult for him not only to use this model in the first place but to persist with it when painful conflict emerged. While we do not wish to imply that Dr. Ellsworth acted improperly in his sequence of interventions, we are suggesting that his choices might have been influenced by family patterns that affected him unconsciously.

Previous Experience in Therapy

Most therapists have been in therapy and most would agree that having been "on the receiving end" exerts a significant beneficial influence on their work. Dr. Ellsworth's experience with individual therapy may have predisposed him to working individually with Larry and Jennifer and shying away from more interactive approaches.

Clearly, a therapist's experience as a client in therapy can be positive or negative. A poor experience may influence us to avoid a certain therapy; a good experience may be a beacon to us. A positive experience is most significant because it can generate a sense of conviction about the therapy which will enhance the hopefulness and optimism of the clients. However, like any other influence, personal experience may constrict a therapist's viewpoint or generate unreasonable dogmatism.

Client and Process Factors That Influence the Choice of Model

Diagnosis

In any given case, choosing a model based on diagnostic consider-ations generates an interesting dilemma: The way in which one diag-noses a couple is itself determined by the model one employs (Gurman, Kniskern, & Pinsof, 1986). In couple therapy, diagnostic theories range from individually based theories of psychopathology, in which the functioning of each partner may be assessed independently of the other, to rigorously systemic theory, in which individual functioning is only understood within the context of the family system. There are few incompatibilities among the variety of diagnostic frameworks. However, each one may be more or less useful for any particular case. For example, it is probably futile to try to comprehend a couple with a psychotic spouse using only a psychodynamic model. Similarly, many therapists believe that in cases of substance abuse, physical abuse, or incest, a broad systems model *must* be employed. Lack of theoretical clarity on diagnostic issues can lead to ineffective therapy (Grunebaum, 1988b).

Some people avoid both individual and broad systemic formulations and look only at the couple dyad. In such cases, it is helpful to diagnose the level of couple dysfunction. Alan Gurman (1978) has developed a useful framework for this task. This system assesses levels of functioning. Clients may range from quite functional couples, for whom a psychoeducational theory may be most useful, to severely embattled couples, for whom combined individual and couple treatment is employed. (For the most conflicted couples, Gurman suggests that the therapist take a very active facilitating role.) According to Gurman's criteria, Larry and Jennifer were a relatively low-conflict couple. Dr. Ellsworth's early shift to a family of origin theory made sense in this context.

The Couple's Learning Style

A consideration that may influence the choice of therapy is the couple's learning style. How do they best assimilate information? Some couples are able to translate intellectual understanding into behavioral changes. For others, such interpretations may be wasted. They may learn best through experience (e.g., through behavioral prescriptions). Some couples may be more accessible through affect, others through meaning. Some may respond well to interventions that encourage playfulness, but others may find "artificial" exercises too threatening. When the partners have different styles, an eclectic therapist may have an advantage if he or she can manage to shift fluidly between two models, each suited to one spouse. Through the activity of the therapist, each spouse may be gradually involved in the metaphors and perspectives of the other. Dr. Ellsworth's use of cognitive and experiential interventions was especially useful to this couple as it mirrored Larry's more intellectual style and Jennifer's more affectively charged style.

Feedback

After we have evaluated the couple and determined an initial direction, we then remain attentive to the couple throughout the therapy for feedback (both verbal and behavioral) as to the effectiveness of each approach. We take a pragmatic stance, looking for clues as to what works with the couple and what falls flat. We must, however, be cautious in our judgments regarding success and failure. We must discriminate between normal resistance[2] to a potentially useful intervention and totally "missing the mark" with an incorrect model. And we must consider the factors beyond the therapy that might influence the couple's direction (e.g., the way Larry and Jennifer's vacation and subsequent return to full-time work schedules seemed to undo much of Dr. Ellsworth's good work).

---

[2]We use the term "resistance" here both to absorb the psychoanalytic idea of resistance against the therapist, and to include the broader and richer meaning of the homeostatic properties of all systems.

The feedback between couple and therapist is a complex process to which we should never react reflexively. We cannot respond to every sign of resistance or every lull in the progress of therapy with a shift in our model. Because every successfully employed model promotes in the clients new patterns of behavior, some inertia is to be expected. On the other hand, we cannot ignore the signals coming from the couple that our approach is simply not working. It is a matter of critical clinical judgment to distinguish an unsuccessful implementation of our models from incomplete or slow progress.

Paradigms for Systematic Eclecticism

There are critical times in the process of therapy that require the therapist to review his or her choice of a model. In the beginning of therapy, the couple presents to the therapist not only a sample of their behavior, but in most cases a description that may imply a particular model of their own (e.g., "The problem is that we can't stop fighting"). They may present conflicting descriptions (e.g., "The problem is that he won't talk to me," and "The problem is that she won't stop nagging me"). Since the therapist is there to treat the system, his or her first task is to understand the couple's own description while retaining a more comprehensive view. It may be that the therapist arrives armed with a model he or she will use regardless of the information the couple presents. But as this is rarely the case, the initial interview becomes the first choice point, as the therapist's first interventions present the couple with a new perspective which coordinates, elaborates, or challenges their own point of view. Their response to this challenge sets up the next choice point for the therapist.

Occasionally the couple will embrace the therapist's new model, follow his or her prescriptions, and find relief from distress. More frequently, they will struggle with the model or its derivative interventions and issue a challenge, implicitly or explicitly, to the therapist: "Your ideas do not work," "I can't do it," "We tried but all hell broke loose," and so on. Dr. Ellsworth encountered such reactions early in his therapy with Larry and Jennifer.

Temporary ineffectiveness or slow progress obviously does not *require* a theoretical shift, but it always challenges our understanding. Sometimes making a theoretical shift is helpful to the therapist: For example, Dr. Ellsworth undoubtedly felt freed to operate more forcefully when he moved away from his initial posture.

Circumstances in the couple's lives may also create choice points: "How can we sit here talking about our families of origin when he has just told me he is having an affair and wants a separation?" Finally, the process of change itself leads to choice points. As the couple changes, new issues may arise that require the therapist to re-evaluate the couple and the therapy. The decision to terminate is the final such re-evaluation in the therapeutic process.

In Dr. Ellsworth's therapy with Larry and Jennifer, every shift in model occurred in response to the process of the therapy. We can imagine from our own experience the soul searching and lapses of self-confidence Dr. Ellsworth may have had during each of his attempts to achieve a creative re-evaluation. This leads us to wonder if there might not be a system, a kind of metamodel, that could allow us to anticipate and prepare for these shifts.

Many therapists employ rules of thumb to guide model shifts. For example, some therapists begin work with a couple using a structural model, and then, if unsuccessful, shift to a strategic intervention. Another common sequence is from a communications model to a psychodynamic or family of origin model (Norman Paul's or Jim Framo's theories). Such sequencing of models can be of great value. They allow the couple to proceed gradually from a conceptual framework congruent with their own understanding of the situation, to one that is less readily assimilated. They also promote efficiency, helping us comply with what we might think of as a therapeutic Occam's razor: that the most parsimonious use of the clients' and therapist's time is to be preferred; the most economical intervention should be considered prior to a more complex or lengthy one.

A few authors (e.g., Garfield, 1986) have attempted to construct such metamodels. One that we find particularly useful is William Pinsof's "integrated problem-centered therapy" (IPCT; Pinsof, 1983). IPCT is a metatheory: a theory for integrating a variety of theories. Pinsof summarizes his model in eight steps.

In the first two steps, the presenting problem is identified and previous attempts to solve the problem are discussed. In the third step, the therapist engages the couple in efforts to identify the emotions they experience in connection with the problem, and then to understand how they use or fail to use their emotional reactions to facilitate resolution of the problem. "Rules" or assumptions associated with emotions (e.g., a good husband is never angry with his wife) are identified and discussed. In the fourth step, the therapist works with the couple to formulate a new solution to the problem, but one that remains consonant with the couple's understanding of the problem as it has evolved through the second step. If the new solution is successfully carried out and the problem resolves, the therapy may either end or focus on another problem.

The first four steps, in essence, test the hypothesis that the information provided in the second step was the critical ingredient in successful problem resolution. Frequently the hypothesis is not supported; more therapy is required. In such cases the fifth step introduces "block identification." "Immediate" causes of problems (such as biological, interpersonal, or other local causes) are initially examined; the search expands to include "remote causes" only when immediate causes are not sufficient. The sixth step involves identification of "catastrophic expectations." "Every nonbiological block," Pinsof writes, "is directly associated with one or more *catastrophic expectations*" (p. 29). The seventh step involves exploration of these catastrophic expectations (e.g., Are they realistic? What would happen if the block were overcome? etc.). Pinsof comments that this step frequently uncovers other problems initially hidden by the presenting problem. These "secondary problems" become the explicit focus of the therapy only when the contract between therapist and client is specifically renegotiated to include them. Termination is the final step.

A particular strength of this metatheory, in our view, is its orderly and rational means of moving from one model to another. It is also efficient, looking first for the simplest solutions and those in most harmony with the couple's experiences and beliefs. If such a solution fails, the therapist and the couple can move with more confidence and commitment to alternative conceptions of the problem and its possible solutions.

Implications

The emergence in recent literature of metamodels such as Pinsof's, and of other attempts to integrate a variety of previously distinct theories and systems of therapy, points to a growing acceptance of the eclectic approach. This is a development that we welcome, as we believe that it is valuable for therapists to take advantage of the many different tools at their disposal. However, a commitment to multiple theories brings with it the task of developing the means to know when and how to choose among them. This choice is usually undertaken within the subjective confines of the therapist's mind. When a therapist feels sufficiently perplexed, unable to formulate a useful approach, or anxious about how to proceed, there is generally good reason to consider whether he or she is using the most effective model. In our view, therapists must also learn to understand and respect the nuances of their own personal reactions. When confronting a block in therapy, therapists must have the tools to analyze the impasse, not only "objectively," in terms of their assumptions and observations about the patient system, but also "subjectively," questioning their choice of model and its adequacy for the use at hand.

Dr. Ellsworth's problem with Larry and Jennifer was not that he failed to maintain constancy in the use of his therapeutic model, but that he was not adequately trained to be an eclectic therapist. He had been trained to use a number of distinct models, each one of which was represented to him as a comprehensive perspective on couple functioning and couple therapy. He became an eclectic therapist out of necessity in the heat of the therapeutic encounter. Like most of us, his conversion to eclecticism was private and pragmatic, a personal synthesis wrought amid anxiety and self-doubt. Perhaps the most important lesson we can learn from his experience is the necessity of including training for eclecticism in every curriculum for teaching therapists. Students need to learn various theories of therapy, and must receive guidance in how to integrate these theories with their individual personalities.

Our purpose in this chapter has been to discuss the difficulties, pragmatic and conceptual, that arise when the practitioner is confronted with the variety of theories that characterize our field. We have described how each therapist transforms theories, through his or her own personal experience, into operational models for couple therapy. We believe that it is to our advantage as practitioners to make our own models as conscious, clear, and coherent as possible.

We have argued here that there is no such thing as a correct model of couple therapy. There are too many complex variables relating to the couple, the therapist, and the circumstances of therapy for any one model to dominate the field. Nor are we likely to observe the emergence of some sort of metatheory that will serve as a final and simple guide to the use of all the ideas populating our profession. Each practitioner is therefore left with the task of evaluating and selecting among the remarkable number of theories and techniques available, and with them charting a course for each therapeutic voyage.

REFERENCES

Chasin, R., & Grunebaum, H. (1980). A brief synopsis of current concepts and practices in family therapy. In J. K. Pearce & L. J. Friedman (Eds.), *Family therapy: Combining psychodramatic and family systems approaches.* New York: Grune & Stratton.

Colapinto, J. (1984). On model integration and model integrity. *Journal of Strategic and Systemic Therapies, 3*(3), 38–42.

de Shazer, S. (1984) . Fit. *Journal of Strategic and Systemic Therapies, 3*(3), 34–38.

Garfield, S. L. (1986). An eclectic psychotherapy. In J.C. Norcross (Ed.), *Handbook of eclectic psychotherapy.* New York: Brunner/Mazel.

Grunebaum, H. (1988a). The relationship of family theory to family therapy. *Journal of Marriage and Family Therapy, 14*(1), 1–14.

Grunebaum, H. (1988b). What if family therapy were a kind of psychotherapy? A reading of the *Handbook of psychotherapy and behavior change. Journal of Marital and Family Therapy, 14*(2), 195–199.

Gurman, A. S. (1978). Contemporary marital therapies: A critique and comparative analysis of psychoanalytic, behavioral and systems theory approaches. In T. Paolino, & B. McCrady, (Eds.), *Marriage and marital therapy.* New York: Brunner/Mazel.

Gurman, A. S., Kniskern, D. P., & Pinsof, W.M. (1986). Research on the process and outcome of marital and family therapy. In S. L. Garfield & A. E. Bergin (Eds.), *Handbook of psychotherapy and behavior change* (3rd ed.). New York: Wiley.

MacKinnon, L., & Slive, S. (1984). If one should not marry a hypothesis, should one marry a model? *Journal of Strategic and Systemic Therapies, 3*(4), 26–39.

Piaget, J., with Inhelder, B. (1969). *The psychology of the child.* New York: Basic Books.

Pinsof, W.M. (1983). Integrative problem-centered therapy: Toward the synthesis of family and individual psychotherapies. *Journal of Marital and Family Therapy, 9*(1), 19–35.

15

Toward a Theory of Marital Bonds, or Why Do People Stay Married?

HENRY GRUNEBAUM

It's love that makes the world go round.
—W. S. GILBERT, *Iolanthe*

Most couples in the Western world marry for love. And love is poetry when it is going well. Interestingly, while there are innumerable volumes of poetry on love, there is almost no poetry of marriage.[1] Therapists, however, rarely think about love or why couples stay together. On one side of the consulting room we find people who feel love and anger, desire and boredom, companionship and loneliness. On the other side of the consulting room we find therapists thinking about projective identifications, unresolved griefs, unbalanced structures, and dysfunctional systems.

How can we hope to develop effective therapies for couples if we ignore what they believe brought them together, and what still holds them together, even in the face of hurt and disappointment?[2] Perhaps therapists would be more helpful if they approached couples with ideas and language that more closely reflect the couples' experience. But our way of thinking about what keeps couples together must be in accord

---

[1] An exception is the tradition of the epithalamium. These, however, celebrate the ceremony of marriage but are silent about what follows.

[2] This chapter is based on a schema first described earlier (Grunebaum, 1976). It is primarily about heterosexual couples who are considering getting married, are married, or are divorcing. This is the group of couples with which I have had the most clinical experience. However, much of what I say about bonding between individuals is also true for other kinds of long-term, committed, adult relationships.

with our current state of knowledge about human bonding. The theory proposed in this chapter represents an attempt to accomplish this task while also honoring the experience of couples and the knowledge of therapists.

Probably all therapists intuitively evaluate what they believe holds couples together. We assume that partners who love one another are easier to help than those who do not. We believe that joyful sexuality holds a marriage together, while an unhappy sexual relationship is a source of discontent. And we think that a couple with many shared interests enjoys each other more than a couple with few shared interests. We also believe that people who act thoughtfully and who are true to their commitments are likely to have better marriages than those who act impulsively and are inconsistent. Although these assumptions are part of our practical wisdom, they merit closer examination.

The theory I present in this chapter has implications for how we evaluate and intervene with couples. It enables us to understand better the rich diversity of marriages that work and the equally rich diversity of marriages that fail. In addition, it enables us to assess the bonds of couples falling in love as well as those married for many years. The core of the theory is the proposition that in marriage there are multiple bonds between the partners, each of which has developmental precursors and each of which is associated with a fundamental mode of human relating. Five bonds are posited: the bond of attachment and caring, the bond of friendship and partnership, the sexual bond, the bond of decision/commitment, and the bond of social networks.

Using this theory of multiple bonds, we can view marriage as an effort to maximize success in each of these modes of relating in a long-term relationship with one person. Many strong marriages, in this view, will manifest strength in a number of these bonds, but not necessarily in every one. Many weak marriages will exhibit a weak profile of bonds. In between, however, are a great number of marriages, some weak and some strong, which exhibit uneven profiles (i.e., strength in some areas of bonding and weakness in others). For a variety of reasons, some marriages can tolerate or even require an uneven profile while others cannot. For example, some couples with a strong bond of intimate friendship can tolerate serious difficulty in the area of sexuality, while for other couples disturbances in the sexual realm usher in the demise of the marriage in spite of other strong bonds.[3]

---

[3]The use of the word "bond" is suspect among some family therapists, as it smacks of 19th-century physics and the language of force and attraction. However, couples do, in fact, describe their attraction to each other as a force and their continuing need as an attachment or relationship. The language of forces and bonds is phenomenologically true. For the purposes of this chapter an experience-close language has much to commend it, just as 19th-century physics is useful for designing houses, roads, cities, and other human

INTRODUCTION TO A THEORY OF BONDS

> Every sentence I utter must be understood not as an
> affirmation, but as a question.
>
> —NIELS BOHR

Clearly, there are an infinite number of perspectives from which one can think about what holds a couple together, and also a considerable number of ways in which one can delineate separate bonds. Before discussing in detail the five bonds I have posited, I will present the criteria I have used to delineate the five bonds, and suggest desiderata for a theory of bonding.

1. A bond should be describable in terms of some combination of affect and behavior. Thus a strong sexual relationship is not identifiable strictly by the frequency of intercourse (behavior), but requires some desire and passion (affect) as well. On the other hand, desire and passion (affect) without any sexual activity may be somewhat empty and signify a weak bond.

2. Each bond should be distinguishable from the others, and each should vary independently of the others. Covariance of two bonds would constitute strong evidence for combining them into one.

3. Each bond should represent an appropriate level of generality. A concept such as intimacy is too broad, as it fails to capture the independent variance among its components (e.g., sexual intimacy and the intimacy of friendship). The attribute of shared musical tastes is clearly too specific. While music may be of importance to some couples as a component of their companionate relationship, it is totally irrelevant to others for whom athletic interests or religious values may be far more important.

4. A theory of bonds should enable us to form a couple profile that captures differences within a single couple relationship over time and differences among couples. It should also be helpful to us in describing differences through history and across cultures. This is not to say that this delineation of bonds would apply to all cultures; that would be a "category fallacy" (Rogler, 1989). Other cultures may delineate the components of human bonding differently. However, the theory will be validated by the extent to which it can help us to characterize couple relationships in times and places other than our own.

5. A theory of bonds should be buttressed by studies of humans as well as other species, especially primates.

---

structures. Twentieth-century physics can then be employed for the purposes for which it was developed: particle and nuclear physics and relativity theory.

6. Most importantly, a theory of bonds should be experientially valid. The theory should be comprehensive enough to reflect the ways ordinary people talk and think about strength and weakness in couple relationships—whether in common discourse, in surveys of marital satisfaction in popular magazines, with best friends on the golf course, over a cup of coffee, or with therapists. It should cover the range of emotions couples feel, including passion, comfort, protection, caregiving, and enthusiasm for common goals.

The bonds that meet these criteria (in the order that they arise developmentally) are as follows:

1. The attachment/caregiving and care-receiving bond. This bond is developmentally rooted in the parent–child relationship.

2. The friendship/partnership bond. This bond is rooted in the peer and play experiences of childhood. It usually exists between members of the same generation and involves chosen intimacy and/or shared enterprises.

3. The desire/sexual activity bond. This bond involves sexual attraction and the satisfaction found in sexual activity. It usually involves members of the same generation and becomes an important force during adolescence.

4. The decision/commitment bond. This bond involves the cognitive aspect of giving a relationship thoughtful consideration and having made a decision to be committed to the relationship. While the human qualities of reflection and commitment begin in early childhood, they are the hallmarks of maturity.

5. The social network bond. This bond differs from the others in that its origins are less clear. It may be a derivative of the bonds of attachment, friendship, and decision/commitment, or it may be a wholly independent bond. It is meant to encompass the relationship between an individual or a couple and significant others, including children, families of origin, extended families, neighborhoods, congregations, and the like.

Each of these bonds will be discussed following a review of the literature.

REVIEW OF THE LITERATURE ON BONDS AND MARITAL INTIMACY

How do I love thee? Let me count the ways.
—ELIZABETH BARRETT BROWNING
"Sonnets from the Portuguese"

This section is not intended to offer a comprehensive literature review on the subject of bonding and intimacy, but to cite work that has influenced me in the development of this theory, particularly work with which some therapists might not be familiar. I will briefly review studies of bonding in higher primates and psychological studies of human bonding and then describe some recent work on intimacy that bears on marital satisfaction and stability.

Primate Studies

While we can never know if animals experience love, we can learn much about attachment and bonding from studies of other species. Certain bird species, for example, are monogamous and apparently grieve for the loss of a partner. And among the four highest primates, we find many of the varieties of adult male–female relationships seen in humans cross-culturally. Monogamy is seen in the gibbons; polygamy in the gorillas, which have harems; promiscuity in the chimpanzees; and single mothering in the orangutans, where the adult male has almost nothing to do with his offspring (Wilson, 1975). These observations suggest that the primate sexual bond can take many forms. While we are not totally like any one of these, our nearest animal neighbors, their styles of female–male relating are not foreign to us.

Suomi and Harlow (1975) have conducted a particularly illuminating series of studies with rhesus monkeys. They observed that rhesus monkeys manifest six different types of bonding: mother–child, child–mother, adult male–child, child–adult male, adult male–female and peer–peer. They emphasize the developmental importance of two bonds in particular, those between mother and child and between childhood peers. Adult males interact intensively with children only in the absence of adult females!

In mother–child relations, care-seeking and caregiving behavior of the type that Bowlby (1969) has so eloquently described in his book on attachment are most salient. Monkeys reared by mothers but without peer contact suffered from severe problems as adults in peer relationships, including the inability to deal with hierarchies, unsocialized aggression, and sexual problems. Many therapists will remember the pathetic behavior of infant monkeys clinging to wire mesh surrogates. Such wire-mesh-reared infants grew into severely impaired adults. Suomi and Harlow found that these monkeys could be resocialized by a younger peer, the so-called monkey therapist.

Most clinicians understand the importance of attachment and the mother–child relationship for adult development but rarely take seriously the essential influence of peers. The primary form of peer interaction is play. In play, monkeys learn to socialize aggression, to find their place in the tribe, and to play at sexual behavior, which leads to the ability to perform adequately as an adult. In the absence of peer play, all of these capacities are severely impaired.

Human Studies of Love

Psychological studies of adult human love have been reviewed in a recent book, *The Psychology of Love*, edited by Sternbach and Barnes (1988). Sternbach (1988), in one chapter of this book, posits a triangular theory of love involving three components: intimacy, passion, and decision/commitment. This theory was developed from a factor analysis of questionnaires asking subjects to rate what they believed entered into their feelings of love.

Sternbach illustrates how different types of couple relationships result when different legs of the triangle have greater salience. Thus, intimacy alone leads to "friendship," passion alone to "infatuation," and decision/commitment alone to "empty" love. Combinations of the components have yet other outcomes: Intimacy and passion together lead to "romantic" love; intimacy and commitment lead to "companionate" love; and passion and commitment to "fatuous" love, which by definition lacks intimacy.

While Murstein (1988) agrees that Sternbach's theory is useful, he emphasizes that the salience of each of the three components varies over the courtship period. Typically, courting couples begin by feeling passion for the other, go on to feel romantic, and in time come to feel conjugal (companionate). In the first stage, Murstein (1976) found that a "person is drawn to the other because of his perception of the other's physical, social, mental, or reputational characteristics" (p. 175) (i.e., the other serves as a stimulus). In the next stage, individuals assess whether they and the other share similar values, and in the final stage the couple attempts to ascertain whether they can function in compatible roles.

The theory I propose is like Sternbach's in that it involves component bonds, but my theory differs from his in that it is based on clinical and developmental perspectives rather than a factor analysis. For example, I separate intimacy into two components with separate developmental tracks having their own courses and vicissitudes: one arising from the relationship with the parents, and the other derived from experiences with peers.

Currently there is considerable interest in the similarity between adult romantic love and the infant–caregiver attachment, which includes caregiving, care receiving, and intimacy. Shaver, Hasan, and Bradshaw (1988) have described how in both infant attachment and adult couples the presence of the other leads to happiness, proximity seeking, physical contact, touching, smiling, sharing, prolonged eye contact, singing, baby talk, and experiences of the other as all good. If the bond is disrupted, both the baby and the romantically involved adult feel loss, cry, and become hypervigilant. Just as Ainsworth found that infant attachment can be secure, avoidant, or anxious, these characteristics are also present in adult descriptions of love relationships (Ainsworth, Blehar, Waters, & Wall, 1978). Particularly interesting is Shaver et al.'s finding that adult styles of relating appeared to correlate with remembered childhood experiences of parents. Certain types of addictive love, what Tennov (1979) has called "limerence," may be the result of certain early attachment experiences.

Frances Givelber (Chapter 9, this volume) and Lyman and Adele Wynne (1986) have discussed the importance of intimacy in marriage. Givelber believes that the components of viable intimacy are "separateness, mutuality, acceptance of self and other, empathy, and collaboration." The Wynnes note that couples frequently seek therapy "to achieve intimacy" and describe their problem as "we cannot communicate." Intimacy, as the Wynnes describe it, is not a bond, but rather a consequence of many other aspects of a relationship. Their epigenetic model involves four "major relational processes which unfold in sequence":

1. Attachment/caregiving, complementary affectional bonding, prototypically manifest in parent–infant relatedness;
2. Communicating, beginning with the sharing of foci of attention and continuing in the exchange of messages and meanings;
3. Joint problem solving and renewable sharing of day-to-day tasks, interests, and recreational activities; and
4. Mutuality, the flexible, selective integration of the preceding processes into an enduring, superordinate pattern of relatedness. (1986, p. 385)

These various efforts at understanding marital intimacy are useful. They are not, however, an examination of marital bonding, and their authors did not intend them to be. As they well understand, intimacy is not a bond but rather a desideratum. It may be salient for some couples and not nearly so for others. Certainly, there are couples that stay together without intimacy. These schemata are useful in understanding an aspect of the marital relationship that may be of clinical significance, but do not explain the bonding that brings or keeps couples together.

A CLINICAL AND DEVELOPMENTAL THEORY OF THE COUPLE BOND

The theory I present is predicated on the axiom that different developmental lines lead to different kinds of bonding in couples. Each of the bonds and their developmental precursors will be discussed. Aspects of each bond will be illustrated with cases. Finally, I will offer a number of questions that can help the therapist investigate couples from this perspective.

The Bond of Attachment/Caregiving and Care Receiving

I want a girl just like the girl that married dear old Dad.
—*Popular song*

Attachment, caregiving, and care receiving are part of what is sought in marriage and are derived from the human characteristics most prominently seen in the parent–child relationship as described in the classical work of Bowlby (1969). Object relations psychoanalytic theorists, most notably Balint (1968), Fairbairn (1952), Winnicott (1965), and Guntrip (1969), have placed at the center of their theories the fundamental need of each human being for others. This perspective was first applied to couples by Dicks (1967).

Most therapists share the view that adult relationships (object relations) are shaped by childhood experiences with parents. The quality of the parent–child bond, whether it is empathic and permits separation and individuation or not, will influence what individuals expect in marriage (Shaver et al., 1988). Couple relationships offer an opportunity for individuals to re-experience and improve on what occurred with the parents. This has been called by Sager (1976) the "unconscious contract." Therapists generally attend to the adverse effects of projective identifications upon the couple's relationship (see Givelber, Chapter 9, and Low, Chapter 12, this volume). Methods for influencing this dynamic in therapy, such as the family of origin interview (see Framo, Chapter 4, this volume) and the examination of unresolved family grief (see Paul, Chapter 5, this volume), have been developed. Because projective identification is well discussed elsewhere in this book, I will review it only briefly.

Projective identification involves the projection of aspects of the self (e.g., being critical, sexual, spontaneous, or organized) onto another person. The other is then viewed as having those attributes and the subject no longer needs to experience himself or herself in these ways. The other is partly chosen to fit in with what the subject needs to project. Finally, although this was not part of the classical definition, the spouse is often induced or even coerced to act in ways that accord with what is projected (e.g., to be critical, sexual, defensive).

Projective identification is probably a normal and necessary process in marriage. In fact, some amount of projective identification may serve to make a spouse seem familiar and known. Otherwise, the spouse may not fit into important lifelong psychological needs and patterns that one does not seek to change.

But, of course, individuals do seek to change some aspects of themselves and their lives when they marry, and they tend to marry a partner whom they imagine will facilitate that process. People say things like "I married him because he would help me be neat" or "I married her because she was so fun-loving and I'm inclined to be quiet." Thus are sown the seeds of both positive change and negative conflict. Gender issues involved in these common styles of projective identification are discussed by Low in Chapter 12 of this book. It is not the absence of projective identification that makes for a satisfactory marriage. Rather, it occurs when the parent–child aspects of a marriage fit the needs of both partners, permitting empathy, regression, childish play, and complementarity where appropriate; it occurs when the projected aspects of the relationship are not dominant or skewing, but rather are compatible with the needs of each partner.

Projective identification is typically viewed as a process that arises in an individual's relationship with his or her mother and father. However, individuals also experience their parents as a couple, and they project that relationship onto their own marriage. For instance, even though your father did not bully you, you may believe that he bullied and dominated your mother and may seek to prevent that from recurring in your own marriage. Napier (1971), in a fine paper, has described how this was the case for two couples he studied.

People do not simply ask themselves if they are as happy as their father or mother; they compare their whole marital relationship with that of their parents. They wonder if their parents had as much sexual enjoyment or enjoyed their adult children as much. Did they fight as much? These questions are often difficult to answer since most of the observations were made when one was a child, but answers are sought nonetheless in discussions between siblings who often compare their necessarily different experiences of their parents' marriage.

Useful questions to ask couples in order to learn about the attachment, caregiving, and care-receiving bond are as follows:

1. Tell me something about your relationship with your father, your mother, or other important caregivers. Did you feel close to them? Were you a favored child?
2. How did you relate to your siblings? How did they get along with your parents?
3. What was your parents' marriage like? How do you want yours to be different?

4. What are the things you don't like about yourself?
5. What are the things you most admire, most dislike about your spouse?
6. What changes did you hope your marriage would make in you? And what personal deficiencies did you hope it would make up for?

The Friendship/Partner Bond

It is not lack of love but lack of friendship that makes unhappy marriages.
— FRIEDRICH NIETZSCHE

Probably the marital bond that is the least attended to by therapists is that of friend and partner—two major forms of peer bonding.[4] This is surprising, since these words are commonly used by spouses to describe one another. The ability to relate to peers, to have friends, and to be a colleague has its developmental roots in childhood peer relations.[5]

Much has been written by therapists about the influence of the family of origin on individual development and on marriage; precious little about peer relationships and marriage. This may be because children tend to keep their peer relationships private from adults and later may remember little about their early peer experiences. In addition, mental health professionals always have focused major theoretical and clinical attention on individuals and more recently on the family. After all, who comes to therapy with their childhood chum or present best friend?

Adults usually find that the relationships that allow for the greatest mutuality, empathy, and collaboration are those with peers (Grunebaum & Solomon, 1980). The capacity to engage in both the intimacy of friendship and the shared work of partnership is developed in early peer relations through the medium of play.[6] As discussed earlier, the importance of childhood peer relations is supported by studies of

---

[4]The word "partner" is used in the sense of business partner, meaning someone with whom one shares tasks and divides labor. Other equally valid terms are "teammate," "helpmate," and "colleague."

[5]This section of the chapter owes much to Leonard Solomon, who was my collaborator on a series of four papers on the subject of peer relations, in which we reviewed the literature and applied our findings to an understanding of self-esteem and group psychotherapy (Grunebaum & Solomon, 1980, 1982, 1987, and Solomon & Grunebaum, 1982).

[6]The capacity for both friendship and partnership is developed during childhood through experiences with peer relationships. For this reason, I have considered them as aspects of the same bond. Friends often collaborate well on tasks, and often colleagues at work become good friends. However, this is not always the case and some couples are good friends but poor partners, while for others the reverse is true. Because these aspects of the friendship/partner bond can vary independently, other theorists may find advantages in considering them as separate bonds.

animals; all animals who are social in adult life have peer relationships during childhood characterized primarily by play. As E. O. Wilson (1975) states, "Play, virtually all zoologists agree, serves an important role in the socialization of animals. Furthermore, the more intelligent and social the species, the more elaborate the play" (p. 164).

Through social play, the child learns to create and conform to rules and regulations, and thus gains membership in a social group and support in dealing with natural out-group threats. Peer relationships offer an alternative source of support to that provided by the family and vice versa. But the need for a social group also makes the child vulnerable to rejection and ridicule from peers since his or her self-image is now anchored to peers as well as family.

Among the social skills children learn with peers are how to participate in group play and accept group pleasures and pains. But children also learn how and when to be independent, to stand on their own, and to defend themselves against the pressures or scapegoating of group members. If development proceeds in a healthy manner, children will learn when and how to seek privacy and freedom from group exposure or interaction (Grunebaum & Solomon, 1982; Solomon & Grunebaum, 1982).

In human beings, as Piaget (1932) has described, moral development arises largely in the context of peer relations. Children learn in peer play how to take turns and they come to appreciate the importance of fairness among equals. The child's ability to be fair can be damaged if he or she is scapegoated, whether by parents or by peers.[7] Today, most partners approach each other expecting to be treated as an equal. This was not always so, nor is it so everywhere. And even today many couples have acknowledged areas of differences where one or the other is in charge. This can be experienced either as just or imbalanced.

Couples are peers,[8] and the capacities and experiences of each spouse in peer relationships have a vital impact on their relationship with each other. Research shows that both men and women rate the most valued characteristics in a spouse as follows: good companion, considerate, honest, affectionate, dependable, intelligent, kind, understanding, interesting to talk to, and loyal, in that order (Buss & Barnes, 1986). These sound like the attributes of a good friend. Many spouses refer to their partners as their "best friend," and they hope for an I–Thou dialogue with them (see J. Grunebaum, Chapter 10, this volume). A review of the

---

[7]Having been treated unfairly as a child by parents or peers can lead to "destructive entitlement," which can have a major impact on one's marriage. This is discussed by J. Grunebaum in Chapter 10, this volume.

[8]Even when they differ greatly in age, there is some expectation that they will treat each other as peers rather than as parent and child.

literature found that satisfactory peer relationships correlate with self-esteem, and adequate self-esteem requires good peer relationships (Grunebaum & Solomon, 1987). Both self-esteem and good peer relations are important in the successful selection of a partner, in courtship, and in marriage. An example of friendship in a marriage—a second marriage—is seen in the following case. Unfortunately for the client, it also illustrates the frustration that can result when marriages are characterized by marked deficiencies in certain bonds.

> A 45-year-old man left his first wife. She had been quite undependable and exploitative. He felt used by her both before and after their divorce. It had become his responsibility to take care of their two daughters' medical needs, their educational problems, and all other issues requiring parental decisions. This was true despite the fact that the daughters lived with their mother. In his second marriage, he wanted something very different.
>
> Soon after leaving his first wife, he moved in with another woman and eventually married her. He says that he and his second wife are "best friends." She is remarkably fair, unexploitative, dependable, and loyal. But he is dissatisfied that their sexual relationship is not nearly as exciting as it was with his first wife, which tempts him to have affairs.

Clearly, there are many different types of peer relationships. An intimate friend differs from a trusted colleague or partner at work. There is a continuum from pure emotional involvement to pure task-centered performance. Couples have to function, depending on the situation, at many points along this continuum, but are often better at one end than the other. Each partner may prefer one type of peer relating to the other. Men and women tend to have different developmental experiences and therefore evolve different standards in friendship or teamwork. Perhaps, until recently, men have had more experience with the sort of sharing that occurs among teammates while women have had more experience with intense and intimate twosomes (see Low, Chapter 12, this volume).

An individual may be very successful at work as a member of a team and yet have no close friends. The reverse also occurs, but is less common. Today many people regard their spouse as their most intimate friend. This was not always so; for most of the 19th century, same-sex intimate friendships were the rule (Smith-Rosenberg, 1979). For many individuals, especially women, their most passionate relationships were their friendships with other women. Today we may speculate that the growth of coeducational dormitories and the growing similarity between the lives of men and women have had a positive impact on friendship between the sexes. (Rubin (1985) has discussed the differences in friendship style between men and women). Yet it is noteworthy that men are still more likely than women to have their spouse as their sole or most important confidant. Women, even though friends with their spouse, more often than men have a same-sex friend with whom they feel more intimate. Men typically seek and develop less intimate friendships with each other, in part because of the greater importance of activity as opposed to emotional sharing in male bonding.

We should, however, be aware that we are using a "female" definition of "intimacy" here, one that emphasizes feeling rather than doing— affect rather than instrumentality. In our culture women have been regarded as both responsible for and expert in intimate relationships. However, as Cancian (1986) concludes, "Who is more loving: a couple who confide most of their experiences to each other but rarely cooperate or give each other practical help, or a couple who help each other through many crises and cooperate in running a household but rarely discuss their personal experiences? Both relationships are limited." (p. 709)

Many people seek in a marriage an opportunity to share their innermost self in a safe dialogue, yet failures in this area are a common complaint. This expectation is undoubtedly influenced by social class and by ethnicity. Nonetheless, couple therapists see many married individuals, wives in particular, who complain of being lonely.

A man comes for psychotherapy because his wife has had an affair. He has no one he can talk to about his pain. He is not close to his only brother. He has poker-playing companions and business associates, but no friends except his wife. She, on the other hand, has friends but complains that she feels alone in her marriage.

Marriage is not only a friendship, it is also a working partnership. It is an enterprise often involving cooperative juggling of the many demands on the couple's time, energy, and money. When children are involved, these demands intensify manifold and tend to lead to an asymmetrical division of labor with the woman more responsible for child care and the man more responsible for economic support. The couple has to decide whether to divide up each of the tasks of life in a symmetrical or complementary way. The more complicated the tasks and the less custom dictates who does what, the greater the interpersonal skills they will need to negotiate task distribution. Thus isolated farmers along the fjords of Norway need to and do talk very little (Hollas & Cowan, 1973), but dual-career couples in urban America have to do a lot of negotiating and problem solving. They typically engage in complex complementarity with specialization by the more skilled or motivated partner, who performs certain roles exclusively. However, since they rarely live in extended families where other family members can pitch in, they are wise to develop the capability to substitute for one another; they should not allow themselves to become too specialized.

One common symptom of failure in the bond of partnership is difficulty in managing finances. All therapists are familiar with couples who could enjoy each other if they were not constantly squabbling about money. In fact, talking about financial problems is one of the more common tasks of couples and their therapists. Money troubles are often not merely a displacement. Here issues of problem solving, power, and values are joined. There are couples who know how to manage their feelings but not their dollars, and vice versa.

Inquiring about experiences in peer relationships will prove invaluable to couple therapists. They should ask about issues of friendship and partnership in the couple:

1. Are you friends? Companions? What interests do you share?
2. Do you tell each other intimate details about your inner lives?
3. Do you collaborate well on joint projects? Household tasks, child-care tasks, planning vacations, or financial matters?
4. How do you divide these tasks? Do you experience the division as equitable?
5. Tell me about your experiences with friends, beginning with your first memories.
6. What was it like for you in school with classmates?
7. Did you have a best friend?
8. How did you begin dating? Did you have a boyfriend/girlfriend?
9. Do you have friends now? How close are they?

The Bond of Sexuality

> Sex is the work of our ability to imagine, which is no longer an instinct, but exactly its opposite: a creation.
> —JOSE ORTEGA Y GASSET

> Sex is an emotion, set in motion.
> —MAE WEST

The importance of the sexual bond in the couple relationship may appear to be obvious. For most couples, sexual desire is part of what led them to marry. However, we all know that most lovers who desire each other sexually do not get married, and that some couples marry without desire as a significant part of the relationship.

A woman had been separated for four years from her husband, having left him to have a passionate affair. Sex had never been important in the marriage, but she could not seek a divorce even after the affair had ended. She explained "He is my best friend. How can you divorce your best friend?" (This case also illustrates the importance of the friendship bond.)

On the other hand, there are couples for whom desire and sex are so central a bond that they continue their sexual relationship even after divorcing.

The salience of this bond tends to vary, depending on the stage of the relationship and of the life cycle. Sexual attraction is usually most important in courtship. Marriage itself often leads to changes in the intensity of sexual desire; the direction of the change depends on whether the marriage is experienced as an increase or decrease in freedom. The birth and care of children tend to lead to a decline in a couple's sex life, the emptying of the nest to its renaissance. If sexual desire is not adversely influenced by illness, sexual activity, while changed in form, often continues into old age. Some couples remain passionately involved with each other for years. Naturally, the importance of sex and feelings of passion may differ in men and women.

The significance of the sexual bond between members of a couple would seem to require no proof. However, there are cultures in which sexual pleasure with a spouse is of secondary importance to producing children. Marriages are arranged by the extended family to serve the economic and social ends of the family rather than the individuals, and often involve a dowry.

Even in our own country, over the past 200 years, there have been great changes in the perceived importance of the desire/sexual bond in marriage. We are all familiar with Victorian strictures, but are less aware that around the time of the American Revolution and in the early 19th century attitudes toward sex were fairly liberal (Rothman, 1984). Recently, in the 1960s and 1970s, the variety and frequency of sexual expression increased, as did public attention to sex. The "sexual revolution" not only affected the generation coming to adulthood at that time, but also apparently had a liberating effect on their parents as well. The 1980s and the beginning of the 1990s seem to be characterized by a more restrictive attitude to sex due to concerns about AIDS, sexual violence, and pornography; moreover, sexual activity is surely dampened by the pressures experienced by dual-career couples.

It is useful to think about desire and sexual behavior separately. Desire seems to be quite an ineffable "chemistry." People cannot will themselves to desire partners who are in all other ways suitable, nor rid themselves of the desire for highly unsuitable people. The following case illustrates this regrettable state of affairs:

A couple sought therapy to create sexual desire between them. They had married a few years ago, and their sexual relationship had become so unsatisfactory that they gave it up. He was frustrated by her lack of flexibility, and she was angry that he would want her to do anything she did not desire. They began living apart but did not date other people. They talked to each other every day and were each other's most trusted confidant. All therapeutic efforts were fruitless, love potions being unavailable. Neither of them could initiate or permit the slightest affectionate overture. They agreed that neither experienced any desire for the other, but they could not divorce.

The case cited above illustrates that therapy was of little use in helping an otherwise compatible couple to experience sexual desire for each other. The following case shows that therapy may help a marriage and still have little impact on passionate desire.

A man in his 40s seeks therapy because during a passionate affair he has feelings that he had never thought he could experience. He now wants to have these same feelings with his wife of 15 years. They have had a rather boring sex life and he has never felt much desire for her. The therapy led to considerable improvement in his hitherto unsuccessful professional career. It also led to a more harmonious relationship with his wife, but to little change in his desire for her. He continues to dream about his lover.

A couple's sex life may be profoundly affected by nonsexual events, such as a betrayal of trust or a success in life leading to greater self-esteem. The following case illustrates how another kind of experience can influence the sexual relationship of a couple in surprising ways.

A man desired his wife, but she had little desire for him as he was "unexciting." She had arranged to have relations with him once a week in a rather perfunctory way. She also had many affairs, which he knew about. He believed that he could not object to the affairs because if he and his wife parted, no other woman would ever love him. He had been a lonely misfit in school peer groups and had never dated. When their child suffered a tragic and ultimately fatal illness, he was so deeply affected that she concluded that he was a more passionate person than she had previously thought. She began to experience desire for him, which led to their seeking therapy at her insistence to improve their sexual relationship. (This case also illustrates the profound effects of childhood peer experience on marital relations.)

While therapy usually has little impact on desire, it can sometimes help a couple to return to the level of desire they experienced at an earlier time. It can also lead to changed behavior which can in turn lead to significant shifts in sexual satisfaction. This has been well known since the pioneering work of Masters and Johnson (1970) and is well described by Offit (1976) and Kaplan (1974). Couples who have specific neurotic barriers to certain aspects of sexual behavior can also be helped (for instance, couples who desire each other and enjoy foreplay but are fearful about sexual intercourse). Often what appears to be a sexual problem involves other issues, such as inequality in the relationship, questions about who takes the initiative, fears of being rebuffed, or fears of pregnancy. All of these can be dealt with in therapy. However, the basic chemistry of sexual desire is difficult if not impossible to change.

The potential for destructive impact of passion on both men and women is well known and illustrated by the fate of Emil Jannings in the famous Marlene Dietrich movie *The Blue Angel.* Sophie Freud (1988) has described the harmful effects of passion in women and notes that the object of the passion is sometimes a therapist.

Couple therapists should explore the sexual bond in some detail with their clients and show interest in feelings, thoughts, and, most importantly, behavior. If the therapist does not take the lead, the couple is likely to believe that the therapist finds the topic too threatening. It is striking that beginning therapists, in particular, often do not inquire at all about a couple's sexual relationship. Even experienced therapists frequently do not take an adequate sexual history and omit the behavioral information necessary for evaluation and therapy. In addition, today it is vital to ask about extramarital relationships because of the dangers of AIDS. Here again, the couple may think that the therapist avoids this area because it is too anxiety-provoking.

Often, initiating a discussion about desire and sex seems difficult. I sometimes introduce the subject by inquiring what the couple does for fun. Couples will take their cues about discussing sex from the therapist's willingness to do so.

Useful questions to ask couples about the sexual bond are as follows:

1. Do you desire your partner? What is the history of your desire for each other?
2. How do you decide to have sexual relations? Who takes the initiative? Always?
3. What is the usual course of your sexual relations? (Get behavioral details if there are problems.)
4. Do you enjoy your sexual relationship? Do you have an orgasm?
5. Is your partner satisfactory to you? Does he or she respond the way you would like?
6. How has your sexual relationship changed?
7. How could your sexual relationship be improved?

The Decision/Commitment Bond

Harry, Harry, here is my answer true.
I'm not crazy over the likes of you.
I want a fancy marriage. I also want a carriage.
And I'll be damned if I'll be jammed on a bicycle built for two.
—HARRY DACRE, "Daisy Bell"

Embarking on a marriage, even in this age of divorce, is considered a serious commitment; it is a decision usually made after much reflection. In the past, as in many cultures today, it was parents and marriage brokers who made the decision about who would marry. Today, even in our culture which values romantic love, people do not simply fall in love, get married, and live happily ever after. We are also pragmatic. Individuals considering a date, a relationship, or a marriage evaluate what kind of a person they are getting involved with. This evaluation begins early and is ongoing. At the same time, they evaluate themselves and their own readiness for marriage and for the particular kind of marriage that they would have with this partner. Clearly, criteria for suitability are influenced by the urgency of the desire to be married, to leave the parental house, or to have children.

There is evidence that both men and women use what has been called "balance theory" in deciding to marry. They assess what they have to offer, what they are receiving, and strive for an equitable balance. Thus we are not as surprised that the famous and beautiful Jackie Kennedy married Aristotle Onassis, a very wealthy man, as we would have been had she married someone of modest means. At the other end of the socioeconomic spectrum, one of the findings of research on psychotic women has been that their partners are usually poorly functioning individuals as well. It appears that "Like attracts like."

Murstein (1988) has emphasized this aspect of courtship, pointing out that after initial attraction, individuals evaluate one another's relative assets and liabilities. Clearly one of the important tasks of a marriage broker was to assess partners to insure that each family felt justly treated. Men appear to be more influenced by physical characteristics and women more by economic ones (Buss & Barnes, 1986). Sociobiologists believe this reflects men's concern with what will be inherited by their offspring (genetic qualities that can be evaluated from the outside) and women's with how they and their children will be provided for (survival in a potentially dangerous environment) (Kenric & Trost, 1989). Inquiring about what was involved in a couple's decision to get married is often useful. This is particularly important if certain real assets were expected that were not forthcoming, violating what Sager (1976) has called the "explicit contract."

Many people are very careful about whom they date, wary of falling in love with a nice person of the wrong religion, race, or ethnic group. When this happens it is often extremely painful for the couple to part. For instance:

A middle-aged Jewish delicatessen owner and a former nun fell passionately in love with each other, having met in a year-long painting class. They were profoundly attached to their respective cultures, and neither of them fit comfortably into the life of the other. What linked them was their shared passion. Painfully and reluctantly they parted, as they could not find a way to reconcile their differences.

Other couples in this situation might find ways to resolve such differences. I recently treated a married couple, each of whom belonged to a different persecuted minority group to which they were intensely loyal. They took over a year of painful psychotherapy (painful for the therapist as well) to decide in whose religion they would rear their child.

While decision making is necessary for commitment, commitment requires more than decision. People differ in how seriously they take their commitments. Some individuals consider their marriage to be for life even when the facts that determined the original decision have changed. They will not go back on their promises. Others constantly re-evaluate their commitment even when there are no problems. Today we Americans have great difficulties in articulating the importance of commitment in language which goes beyond the language of the self as Bellah et al. (1985) have described. We believe in the values of an enduring shared life but cannot say why loyalty to others, historical continuity, and common memories are virtuous and fulfilling, why we should not simply seek to optimize the realization of our individual needs.

Marriage requires a long-term commitment to solve problems, to care, to be a companion, and to be a sexual partner despite the inevitability of change. The spouse one marries in young adult life is no longer the same in middle or old age, nor is one the same as one was. Each has changed and been changed by the other. The culture in which one is living also changes.

Spouses evaluate each other's ability to commit. We think differently about a marriage in which both prospective partners have maintained lifelong commitments to friends, religion, career, and family of origin than we do about a marriage where each partner has moved often, abandoned old friends, experimented with a variety of religions, and lacks consistent goals in life.

The bond of decision/commitment requires more self-examination and thus is more cognitive than the previous four. The decision to marry is perhaps the single most important decision that one makes in life and the most difficult. It requires that one know oneself and one's feelings.

One must ask what kind of a person one is marrying and what that person will be like many years hence. Is the person trustworthy, and what sort of a parent will he or she be? Will the person really care about me and our children "for better or worse and in sickness and health"? If I suffer financial adversity, will he or she stick with me? Will he or she still love me "when I'm 64" and am not as attractive? Does the person have the will to do this? These questions are far more difficult to answer than assessing what adjustments one will have to make because of differences in age, education, religion, and ethnicity.

Perhaps the main reason why commitment is so important in marriage is that luck or fortune plays so large a role in how individuals and couples fare. As Marx (1898/1963) said, "Men make their own history, but they do not make it just as they please; they do not make it under circumstances chosen by themselves, but under circumstances directly encountered, given, and transmitted from the past."

> A couple, for each of whom this was the second marriage, consulted me because of marital strife. They had been married only a few years, and each was a moderately successful artist. She earned some money working as a nurse, and he was a teacher in a public school. About six months prior to the consultation, she had had a show in a major museum in New York City and was now selling her work at a major New York gallery for what seemed to be astronomical sums, given their prior economic situation. This break in her career altered the dynamics of the relationship in terms of both power and relative acclaim.

It is the unpredictability of life that makes commitment to a marriage so vital. The outcome is determined in large measure by the circumstances with which the couple is confronted, their commitment to the marriage, and the competence of each of the partners separately and together to cope with the vicissitudes of fortune.

In making a commitment to marriage, couples make an agreement— usually implicitly—as to how decisions will be made during a marriage. Until recently, women promised to "love, honor, and obey." This clearly implies that one partner, the man, was the decision maker. The inequality of this arrangement is obvious and much, although not nearly enough, has been done to redress this imbalance. Not unexpectedly, many decisions are still made according to customary role definitions, and the couple has to learn how to make them in terms of their own abilities and interests.

Increasingly, couples have to negotiate and renegotiate every decision. There is a fascinating illustration of this in Pruett's (1985) study of fathers who, either through choice or necessity, parented infants full time. The fathers became very involved with their infants and good at caring for them, and the infants thrived. But the fathers experienced child care as tiring, arduous, and boring. Interestingly, when there was a second child in the family, responsibility for child care was usually renegotiated. The mothers sought to stay home, and child care became their task.

Every marriage has to face and deal with the injustices each partner has experienced in the past (J. Grunebaum, 1987; see also Chapter 10, this volume). The commitment to "rescue" the other is often a factor when one partner has had more advantages in the family of origin than the other. While the influence of past injustices involves a confusion of contexts in which the present is experienced as the past, the need for current redress of past injustices makes sense to most people; it seems justified.

> A couple came for therapy because of sexual problems. While at first he was delighted with her shy and hesitant interest in sex, gradually they got into difficulties as he desired a more ardent sexual relationship and she experienced his approaches as aggressive. Therapy revealed that she was an incest survivor, and this made it extremely important to her that she be sexually passive. Her partner had to take responsibility for sex, but was then often experienced as repeating the earlier trauma.

In the course of life, the balance of equity, of who has done more for the other or for the marriage, will never be even, but most couples seek some assurance that the efforts of both partners will be to strive for long-term fairness. They both hope and expect that their contributions will be recognized and at some time rebalanced by their spouse.

> A couple gradually were getting to know each other when she was diagnosed with a treatable form of cancer. Because of problems in her family of origin, he undertook to care for her. She felt grateful and indebted to him and was deeply committed to working so that he could go to graduate school. The caring each had done for the other was one of the bonds that held them together and enabled them to manage other crises in their relationship.

Certain questions are useful in assessing the decision/commitment bond:

1. What did you know about your spouse that made you decide to marry him or her?
2. What did you expect he or she would be like as a partner?
3. How is he or she different from what you expected?
4. What kind of a life did you expect to have? How is it different from what you had hoped for?

5. Do you think you have been, and are, fairly treated?
6. How much of this did the two of you talk about then? Now?
7. How committed are you to this marriage? Has your commitment changed? If so, how much and when?
8. How do you explain this change to yourself? To your mate?

The Family and Social Network Bond

> In my own very self, I am part of my family.
> —D. H. Lawrence, *Apocalypse*

The final bond differs from the others, first of all, because it reaches beyond the couple to include other people such as children, extended families, friends, neighborhoods, tribes, religions, and nations. Second, it is unclear if this bond is simply a combination of the bonds of attachment, friendship, and decision/commitment and hence derivative, or if it is a unique and independent bond. Nevertheless, couples have powerful bonds of love, commitment, and loyalty to their children, their mutual friends, their extended families, and their wider social networks. These loyalties can either support or divide the couples. While during courtship this bond may appear less salient than the others, it often becomes clear in planning a wedding how deep the ties are to each family of origin.[9]

It is difficult to describe the developmental precursors of a social network bond. While everyone is born into the larger social networks of a family, a neighborhood, a religion, and an ethnic group, it is not clear how and when the bond to these groups evolves. As people mature, they chose to become involved in schools, workplaces, and other organizations. The strength of ties to these networks varies greatly; some individuals uproot themselves with ease and others only with great anguish. Rootedness can be seen in the common statement, "I do not date people outside my religion."

The importance of this bond can be seen during courtship. When a couple moves beyond the initial stages of their relationship, they often introduce each other to their friends. This is an important test, because people become friends through shared interests, beliefs, and compatibility. It is affirming to find that one's friends like one's beloved; one does not have to choose between them. In our society, this test usually precedes introducing the other to one's family.

Most people remember the anxious moment when they introduced their loved one to their family of origin. In the movie *Annie Hall*, we see

---

[9]The influence of this bond is seen in the marriage vows, which usually include "God and this company." "This company" are the friends and relations who have come to share the occasion and who will share in the couple's good and bad times.

Woody Allen at the dinner table of Annie's Midwest family, meeting them for the first time. It is a total mismatch and the meal a fiasco. On the other hand, people are often influenced in the choice of spouse because they believe that their potential in-laws will provide the parenting for them that they did not receive at home. A man recently said to me, "Since I couldn't have the mother, I married the daughter." What has been said about friends and families applies also to broader social networks. We want the other person to fit in where we fit.

> After many years of unsuccessful dating, a young Christian man, a mathematician, fell deeply in love with a Jewish woman, a physician, who loved him and introduced him to sex. He was reluctant to do anything that she did not agree to, but felt he had to go to his family's Christmas celebration even though she said she would not come. She was quite angry, but as they worked on the issue in couple therapy they both came to see that their going together still allowed them to acknowledge and even live by her religion as a couple.

This bond becomes stronger as the couple's networks increasingly merge. But networks can also be divisive, and strife within the family of origin can severely stress a marriage. The couple may be forced to take sides or mediate the split. If one loses a spouse by divorce or death, one often loses a significant part of a shared social support system, some members of which one has come to love and depend on. This clearly is one of the major stresses in a divorce. Will my children still love, respect, and visit me? Which of our friends will remain true and which will defect to the other? Will our neighbors take sides? Can I continue to go to the same church or temple?

Useful questions for eliciting information about a couple's social bonds are as follows:

1. Who are the other people—children, friends, colleagues, family members—who are important to you? Are certain organizations—churches, clubs—important to you?
2. Tell me about your children. What sort of relationships do you each have with them? What do you feel about the other as a parent?
3. Do you have separate friends or do you have friends in common?
4. Whom do you feel you can depend on now? As individuals? As a couple?
5. Were you accepted readily by the other's friends and family?
6. How do you get along with his or her friends and family now?

APPLYING THE THEORY: JENNIFER AND LARRY

Let us apply the theory of marital bonds to the case of Jennifer and Larry. While they had been together for 10 years at the time of the conference, we know little about several of the bonds between them. In fact, their therapist's case report and the interviews do not even tell us if they are now in love or ever were in love. We do know that, early in the relationship, Larry pursued Jennifer, who felt she could count on him. He was probably in love with her, but we cannot be sure.

1. *Attachment.* Because other chapters in this volume discuss the couple from the point of view of object relations and projective identification (see Paul, Chapter 5, Framo, Chapter 4, and Givelber, Chapter 9), I will be brief. We are told that Larry felt Jennifer needed to be taken care of. He would wait outside her house until she returned from dates with other men. During this period she was the one who could not make a commitment. We never learn why she moved in with him.

Larry's and Jennifer's relationship underwent a dramatic transformation when, due to his illness, he had to depend on her and she took care of him. We are told that after he had his operation for cancer, he felt he had to be "more self-centered." It would be important to know how this event affected their feelings for each other. One must wonder why the interviewers did not inquire more about this potentially tragic event in their lives.

At the beginning of their relationship, taking care of someone else was important for Larry, and being taken care of was important for Jennifer. However, Larry's operation and his need for care may have enabled them to enhance their commitment with a new appreciation of mutual caring and receiving.

In terms of closeness, it appears that it is Larry who requires more distance than Jennifer. He watches TV and she feels excluded from his thoughts and from his daily activities. On the other hand, she may feel more comfortable with a more distant man, given the fact that she shared her father's bed as a child. We also know that Jennifer works long hours; apparently Larry is not the only one who distances. Caring and closeness are often parallel aspects of attachment, but this case shows that they are not necessarily correlated.

2. *The bond of friendship/partnership.* Here we are given some useful information, although it is not used by most of the authors. Jennifer, we are told, "escaped" into music, art, and studying. At age 12–13 she started to "hang out with hoods" and enjoyed being two different people. Perhaps this scenario was repeated when she had a continuing relationship with Larry but went out with other men, as there too she was two different people. In addition, Jennifer remembered having many superficial relationships but no real friends. Since siblings often influence peer relating, it is significant that Jennifer depended on her older sister and felt terrified and abandoned when she left the family.

We may wonder if Jennifer has ever had any very good friends. In the enactment with Papp she rescues a lonely boy who, perhaps, represents aspects of herself. She is said to function well in group work settings, but she is also a workaholic, and this may not leave much time for friends. This information suggests that Jennifer may be a good partner, but may still have some problems with close friendship.

Larry, for his part, has a history of having friends, especially in connection with sports. This is portrayed in the drama he enacts with Papp. While we know little about his relation to his brother, we learn that he could not be seen as successful in his cousin's eyes, which may have influenced his expectations about peers as well. Finally, we are told that of the two, Larry is more talkative with his friends, while Jennifer often will not even answer the phone.

It seems that Larry has more peer supports than does Jennifer, and he uses them effectively. He has friends, but may be comfortable with them only in the somewhat less intimate setting of sports and activities. He may have initially experienced Jennifer as an unavailable woman, but gradually found her to be more interested in him and perhaps even intrusive like his mother. People like Jennifer, who are interested in exploring a partner's motives and feelings, are felt to be intrusive by individuals who are more action-oriented. Characterologically, he seems to be satisfied with less and she seeks more, in terms of both closeness and friendship in their relationship.

Despite these differences, Jennifer and Larry appear to be good partners. They both work very hard, do a little cooking, and split up chores, with Jennifer being more concerned about the house and Larry more concerned about the car. A particularly striking example of their mutual caring and their friendship/partnership was the cross-country car trip they took after Larry's operation during which he withdrew from painkillers.

Their partnership is important, since being good workers is so vital to both of them. While each of them has a history of competitive relationships, she with her sister and he in sports, they do not appear to compete excessively with each other. Rather, they appear to collaborate rather well.

3. *The sexual bond.* We are told that Larry and Jennifer consider their sexual relationship "not a major problem." Sex was initially terrific, but now is felt to be tepid and mechanical. For reasons of privacy, the case report does not provide additional material about the couple's sex life; nor did the four interviewers investigate this area further, doubtless because they were exercising the discretion appropriate for a conference.

Let us speculate that Larry may be fearful of a close relationship with a woman because he experienced his mother as intrusive. The effects of his surgery cannot even be guessed. Jennifer, having slept with her father and feeling "something fearful might happen if she fell asleep," may similarly be uneasy about closeness with men, particularly if that closeness involves loss of control. In addition, Jennifer's mother derided and scorned men. Sex was something horrible, which women occasionally permitted men to indulge in to keep their interest. Larry's and Jennifer's childhoods are not likely to be conducive to a good sexual relationship, but many couples overcome such obstacles.

While the couple is quite attached to each other, their tepid and mechanical sex life suggests that this bond is not strong. The couple might be missing a source of mutual happiness with which they could receive help. Improvement in this area might well strengthen the relationship. On the other hand, Jennifer and Larry may not consider sex particularly important, given their commitment to work. In terms of the sexual bond, a couple therapist would have many unanswered questions.

4. *Decision/commitment.* Once again, we know far too little. We know that Larry and Jennifer have been together for many years and gradually decided to live together and later to engage in couple therapy. We are told that they dealt together with the crisis of Larry's surgery, which suggests a strong commitment. We must be impressed with the courage and fortitude with which they faced this crisis in their lives together.

However, we do not know how they decided to make any of the decisions along the way nor what they each believe their commitment to be. We are not told whether they experience their relationship as one of equals. We do not know why they have not chosen to get married yet, or whether they have decided to do so, but simply postponed the act.

5. *Family/social network bond.* We know that Jennifer feels safer with Larry's parents than with her own and has come to confide in them. This may well be an important social support to her. It has the additional advantage for the couple of relieving Larry of having to relate as closely with his family as he might otherwise. We have learned little about Larry's relationship with his brother.

How the couple relates to Jennifer's parents is only hinted at when, before the Framo interview, Larry suggests that he does not believe that Jennifer's mother is as fragile as Jennifer believes (see Chapter 4). We know that Jennifer's relationship with her older sister involved conflict and distance before the Framo interview, and we may wonder if the apparently conciliatory effects of that interview endured. In addition, Larry and Jennifer have visited her extended family in Holland and she found them welcoming and warm, quite different from her own nuclear family (see Chapter 18). Here, once again, we would be interested in further information, especially about the nonfamily social network.

In summary, we have a couple who are quite strongly attached, who are good partners—perhaps complementary in the way that Sluzki suggests—and who may well have significant relationships with each other's parents as well as with extended family. On the other hand, they may not be as good sexual partners or intimate friends as might be rewarding to them. We know they have been committed to each other for a number of years, but we do not know what hopes they have together for the future; no one asked.

A therapist looking at the couple this way would consider various approaches to their sexual relationship, which would probably involve learning more about barriers to intimacy between them. In addition, the issues of peer relatedness presented may suggest that a group therapy format might have much to recommend it.

One of the problems with the conference as a whole and the four demonstration interviews is that everyone assumed that the couple is bonded, and strongly so. In a sense, then, therapeutic interventions were made in an affective vacuum, decontextualized from real life. This occurred even though all therapists know that the success of intervention with a couple depends on the desire of each member to have a good relationship and on how good their relationship is now. In large measure, these distortions of clinical practice are an inevitable result of the skewing nature of teaching conferences (Grunebaum, 1988; Zinberg, 1987).

ON LOVE

Love—bittersweet, irrepressible—
loosens my limbs and I tremble
—SAPPHO, "To Atthis"
(transl., Willis Barnstone)

They are struck in extraordinary fashion by friendly feeling (*philia*) and intimacy (*oikeiotes*) and passion (*eros*), and are hardly willing to be apart from one another even a little time.
—PLATO, *The Symposium*

When couples speak of why they are together, they usually speak of love. Whatever else love is, it is not a particular combination of bonds. We would, of course, be surprised if people could love each other in the absence of most of these bonds, and we would expect that if they felt firmly bonded in all five ways they would probably feel love. Nonetheless, one cannot add up what does or could hold two people together and call that love. For instance, a person can be "perfect" for you, but you may not love him or her. Similarly, the person with whom one is most intimate is often a friend, not a spouse. Even good sex does not necessarily lead to love.

Often people "know" on meeting another person that that person is "special." As Martha Nussbaum (1986) says about Aristophanes' myth that we were male and female once united, but have been severed from our other half: "It is mysterious what does make another person the lost half of you, more mysterious still how you come to know it" (pp. 173–174). We call this "love at first sight," but it can occur at other moments in a relationship. One can view this transformation in one's perception of another as an unusual and inexplicable happening, and explain it as "chemistry." Or one can simply believe that every story has a beginning,[10] noting that there are many momentary infatuations that go nowhere. Of course, people can also fall out of love with startling suddenness.

It appears that for the kind of love I have been discussing to occur, certain conditions must be present. In particular, the individuals involved must have the opportunity and ability to choose each other. Both cross-culturally and historically, marital choice has not been an option for most people. For this opportunity to exist among the prerequisites, private space must be available, the lovers must regard each other as equals, and they must be able to survive economically as a couple on their own. These conditions have only been met at certain times in history and in certain cultures.

Not all love leads to lasting relationships, but we all know of long and loving marriages. People can love in many different ways. For instance, I recently saw a 50-year-old business executive who had been widowed after a long and happy marriage and then had a disastrous although passionate second marriage. After divorcing his second wife, he contacted his college girlfriend whom he had loved many years before. She had thought him too immature then, but now they resumed their relationship as passionately as when they parted, regretful of the lost years.

Individuals can love different people in different ways, they can love the same person in different ways over time, and they can fall in and out of love. They consult therapists when they have fallen out of love with a spouse, have fallen in love with an inappropriate person, or cannot get over a irretrievably lost love. For instance, I was consulted by a couple after the woman had fallen in love with her employer and did not know

---

[10]The beginnings of relationships often illuminate characteristics that pervade the entire relationship. For instance, a woman described how, on their first date, her husband could not make up his mind which movie they should go to. She took the matter in hand and decided for them. Twenty years later she had gotten tired of deciding for them and divorced him.

what to do, as she still cared deeply about her husband and they had three children and a life together. Another couple sought consultation when they felt their love for each other had been driven underground by the stresses they had been experiencing. Only the individual can decide what is "good enough" love to make a relationship worth having and working on. The therapist cannot decide for them. The therapist can help people understand some of the reasons why they stay together or are forced apart, but cannot adequately explain why they love each other or why they fall out of love.

While it is useful for the therapist to look at a marriage from the perspective of bonds, it is also essential to find out if the couple one is seeing love each other. Useful questions are as follows:

1. Did you ever fall in love? Under what circumstances?
2. Do you still experience romantic love? Other kinds of love? When?
3. If you have lost your love for each other, do you believe it can be rekindled?

A PERSONAL EPILOGUE

Marriage . . . is a damnably serious business,
particularly around Boston.
—JOHN P. MARQUAND, *The Late George Apley*

Generally, therapists (and probably other people) believe that it is best to have attachment, sex, friendship, and commitment in one and the same relationship—that this is a mature relationship. But why? Cuber and Harroff (1965/1976) have made it eminently clear that one couple's marriage may be another's recipe for boredom and vice versa. There may be as many kinds of good relationships, Tolstoy's contrary opinion in *Anna Karenina* not withstanding, or bad ones as there are kinds of people. A fair portion of all the bonds could be a recipe for a marital stew—a little of this and a little of that, which might result in not much of anything or something absolutely delicious. Perhaps it is the extreme that is most exciting. Like Edna St. Vincent Millay's candle burning at both ends, intense love may not last, but it does give a lovely light to a life.

Even though the unusual and the skewed relationship may be the most exciting and memorable, I suspect that many women and men will attempt to find love, sex, companionship, and commitment in one and the same working relationship. Such a combination is probably most efficient, saving time and energy, and thus has survival value. I also believe that there is a basic human tendency that manifests itself in our admiration of synthesis. In art and literature this is reflected in our esteem for great artists like Rembrandt and Shakespeare, for instance, and the same holds true for our evaluation of relationships. We may envy a passionate love affair, but we admire two people who have integrated many facets of their life together over time.

Acknowledgments

I am delighted to acknowledge the critical assistance of my friend, Dick Chasin, and of Maggie Herzig, editor extraordinaire. The words of this chapter are mine; many of the experiences described and the thoughts expressed are an outgrowth of the dialogue, discourse, and love I have shared with my wife, Judy.

REFERENCES

Ainsworth, M. D. S., Blehar, M. C., Waters, E., & Wall, S. (1978). *Patterns of attachment: A psychological study of the strange situation.* Hillsdale, NJ: Erlbaum.

Balint, M. (1968). *The basic fault.* London: Tavistock.

Bellah, R., Madsen, R., Sullivan, W., Swidler A., & Tipton, S. (1985). *Habits of the heart: Individualism and commitment in American life.* Berkeley: University of California Press.

Bowlby, J. (1969). *Attachment and loss: Vol 1. Attachment.* New York: Basic Books.

Buss, D.M., & Barnes, M. (1986). Preferences in human mate selection. *Journal of Personality and Social Psychology, 50*(3), 559–570.

Cancian, F. M. (1986). The feminization of love. *Signs, 2*(4), 692–709.

Cuber, J. F., & Harroff, P. B. (1976). *Sex and the significant Americans: A study of sexual behavior among the affluent.* Baltimore: Penguin Books. (Original work published in 1965)

Dicks, H. V. (1967). *Marital tensions.* New York: Basic Books.

Fairbairn, W. R. D. (1952). *Psychoanalytic studies of the personality.* London: Tavistock.

Freud, S. (1988). *My three mothers and other passions.* New York: New York University Press.

Grunebaum, H. (1976). Some thoughts on love, sex and commitment. *Journal of Sex and Marital Therapy, 2*(4): 277–283.

Grunebaum, H. (1988). The relationship of family theory to family therapy. *Journal of Marital and Family Therapy, 14*(1), 1–14.

Grunebaum, H., & Solomon, L. (1980). Towards a peer theory of group psychotherapy. I: On the developmental significance of peers and play. *International Journal of Psychotherapy, 30,* 23–49.

Grunebaum, H., & Solomon, L. (1982). Towards a peer theory of group psychotherapy. II: On the stages of social development and their relationship to group psychotherapy. *International Journal of Psychotherapy, 32*(3), 283–307.

Grunebaum, H., & Solomon, L. (1987). Peer relationships, self-esteem, and the self. *International Journal of Group Psychotherapy, 37*(4), 475–513.

Grunebaum, J. (1987). Multidirected partiality and the "parental imperative."

Psychotherapy, 24(3), 646–656.

Guntrip, H. (1969). *Schizoid phenomena, object-relations, and the self.* New York: International Universities Press.

Hollas, M., & Cowan, P. A. (1973). Social isolation and cognitive development: Logical operations and role-taking abilities in three Norwegian social settings. *Child Development, 44,* 630–641.

Kaplan, H. S. (1974). *The new sex therapy.* New York: Brunner/Mazel.

Kenric, D., & Trost, M. (1989). A reproductive exchange model of heterosexual relationships: Putting proximate economics in ultimate perspective. In C. Hendrick (Ed.), *Review of personality and social psychology.* Newbury Park, CA: Sage.

Marx, K. (1963). *The eighteenth brumaire of Louis Bonaparte.* New York: International Publications Company. (Original work published in 1898.)

Masters, W. H., & Johnson, V. E. (1970). *Human sexual inadequacy.* Boston: Little, Brown.

Murstein, B. I. (1976). The stimulus–value–role theory of love. In H. Grunebaum & J. Christ (Eds.), *Contemporary marriage: Structure, dynamics, and therapy.* Boston: Little, Brown.

Murstein, B. I. (1988). A taxonomy of love. In R. J. Sternbach & M. L. Barnes (Eds.), *The psychology of love.* New Haven, CT: Yale University Press.

Napier, A. Y. (1971). The marriage of families: Cross-generational complementarity. *Family Process, 10*(4), 373–395.

Nussbaum, M. C. (1986). *The fragility of goodness: Luck and ethics in Greek tragedy and philosophy.* Cambridge, England: Cambridge University Press.

Offit, A. K. (1976). Therapy of sexual dysfunction. In H. Grunebaum & J. Christ (Eds.), *Contemporary marriage: Structure, dynamics, and therapy.* Boston: Little, Brown.

Piaget, J. (1932). *The moral judgment of the child.* London: Kegan Paul.

Pruett, K. D. (1985). Oedipal configurations in young father-raised children. *Psychoanalytic Study of the Child, 40,* 435–456.

Rogler, L. H. (1989). The meaning of culturally sensitive research in mental health. *American Journal of Psychiatry, 146*(3), 296–303.

Rothman, E. K. (1984). *Hearts and hands: A history of courtship in America.* New York: Basic Books.

Rubin, L. (1985). *Just friends: The role of friendship in our lives.* New York: Harper & Row.

Sager, C. J. (1976). *Marriage contracts and couple therapy.* New York: Brunner/Mazel.

Shaver, P., Hasan, C., & Bradshaw, D. (1988). Love as attachment: The integration of three behavioral systems. In R. J. Sternbach & M. L. Barnes (Eds.), *The psychology of love.* New Haven, CT: Yale University Press.

Smith-Rosenberg, C. (1979). The female world of love and ritual relations between women in nineteenth century America. In N. F. Cott & E. H. Plect (Eds.), *A heritage of her own.* New York: Simon & Schuster.

Solomon, L., & Grunebaum, H. (1982). Stages in social development: Friendship and peer relations. *Hillside Journal of Clinical Psychiatry, 4*(1), 95–126.

Sternbach, R. J. (1988). Triangulating love. In R. J. Sternbach & M. L. Barnes (Eds.), *The psychology of love.* New Haven: Yale University Press.

Sternbach, R. J., & Barnes, M. L. (Eds.). (1988). *The psychology of love.* New

Haven, CT: Yale University Press.

Suomi, S., & Harlow, H. F. (1975). The role and reason of peer relationships in rhesus monkeys. In M. Lewis & L. A. Rosenblum (Eds.), *Friendship and peer relations*. New York: Wiley.

Tennov, D. (1979). *Love and limerence: The experience of being in love*. New York: Stein & Day.

Wilson, E. O. (1975). *Sociobiology: The new synthesis*. Cambridge, MA: Harvard University Press.

Winnicott, D. W. (1965). *The maturational processes and the facilitating environment*. New York: International Universities Press.

Wynne, L. C., & Wynne, A. R. (1986). The quest for intimacy. *Journal of Marital and Family Therapy, 12*(4), 383–394.

Zinberg, N. E. (1987). Elements of the private therapeutic interview. *American Journal of Psychiatry, 144*, 1527–1533.

PART V

RETROSPECTIVE REPORTS BY THE COUPLE AND THE EDITORS

16

Introduction to the Retrospective Reports

THE EDITORS

This series of extensive retrospective reports, largely authored by the couple, is the most distinctive feature of this book. In general, such reports by clients are rare, and no similar clinical demonstration, such as the Hillcrest series, offers a detailed follow-up.

The first report was produced by the couple,[1] on their own initiative and with no direction from us, one day after the last of the four interviews. The second report presents transcript material from a videotaped follow-up interview that we conducted with the couple six months later. Six years later, a third report was written by the couple, following only general suggestions from us regarding overall length and subject.[2]

The content of these retrospectives is distinctive. In the first and third, the couple had wide latitude in what they addressed and how they framed their statement. Unlike most follow-up reports, the couple's responses were not structured by a clinical or research protocol. The topics covered were of the couple's own choosing, reflecting their own interests. Even in the second retrospective, which was guided by the interviewers' questions, the couple's experiences and opinions are expressed in their own words.

In the introduction to this volume, we explained that the demonstration interviews were not intended as therapy *per se*, but as illustrations of different approaches and techniques. A good demonstration of therapy prepared for a conference, and effective therapy as it naturally

---

[1] The report was written by Jennifer in consultation with Larry.
[2] References to our work at the time of the conference and the six-month interview are to the work of Chasin and Grunebaum only. All three of us worked with the couple at the time of the six-year report and in preparing this volume.

occurs in the consultation room, can look very similar; they may in fact be one and the same in a particular case, if the demands of the demonstration and the needs of the clients are in harmony. However, there can be no guarantee of such harmony, as will be evident from some of the data presented in this section of the volume.

If we believed that the interviews should be considered solely as demonstrations (i.e., if we believed that they would have no impact on the couple), we would not have conducted any follow-up work with the couple at all. Our follow-up for the conference exercise would have consisted only of the course evaluations that we asked participants at the conference to complete, evaluations of the exercise as an educational experience. As for the couple, we would have thanked them for their time, like subjects in a perception experiment, and sent them on their way. Obviously, this is not what we did. We were in contact with the couple by phone, and we conducted a six-month follow-up interview with them, because we knew that the four demonstrations would be experienced by them as therapy; we wanted to know how they had been affected by those experiences. We were interested in knowing whether they had found the sessions helpful, and also whether the sessions had had any negative consequences.

We did not have any special concern at the time about the family of origin sessions, even though they were compressed and Jennifer's family was obviously quite vulnerable. This will be discussed in some detail later. We mention it here because the information in the retrospective reports has prompted us to examine with greater care and concern the dilemma inherent in "demonstrations of therapy": How do you conduct a good, time-limited demonstration without running the risk of going too fast or pushing too hard, especially when the technique to be demonstrated requires as much care and preparation as family of origin work? (See Appendix, this volume, for a detailed consideration of this issue and other therapeutic and ethical aspects of making and using videotaped demonstration interviews.)

As indicated in the introduction to this volume, we designed this exercise to approximate "real" therapy more closely than the exemplary cases we typically read about in the clinical literature. We selected the one case rather than allowing each of the four presenters to select his or her own case; the couple that they were to work with was to be like the one that might have walked through the door on any particular day of any week. The case would not be the one that, after months of work, elegantly validated the therapist's dearly held beliefs about clinical theory and practice. One "natural" element that we did not preserve in our exercise, however, was flexibility of time. We scheduled one session for each interview, leaving it up to these skilled clinician-teachers to strike a balance between the needs of the couple and the needs of the demonstration. Striking this delicate balance was a lot to ask.[3]

The retrospective reports presented here are even less like typical clinical or experimental follow-ups than the demonstrations were like typical therapy. These reports are not only unsystematic, they are indeed highly idiosyncratic. This is particularly true of the six-year report. In order to insure that we had adequately fictionalized the details of the case to protect the couple's privacy, we asked the couple to read each of the chapters of this volume in draft form. They happened to do that before they decided to write the six-year retrospective report. How much were their comments simple appraisals of an event long past? How much were they responses to the fresh experience of reading about the interviewers' clinical evaluations and strategies for intervention?[4] We never can know. Furthermore, the couple, on their own initiative, reviewed all 12 hours of the original videotapes in their entirety immediately before drafting their six-year report.[5] How much was their report like an ordinary follow-up, in which the focus is primarily on current functioning and only secondarily on a backward glance through the mists of time, and how much was it influenced by their re-experiencing of old events from the vantage point of a new maturity?

Given all of these considerations, we urge that the retrospective material be read with an eye not to comparing the effectiveness of the four sessions, but to understanding the couple's experiences of the four demonstration interviews. The reader should view these experiences as those of a unique couple at particular times in their lives — experiences recollected, re-experienced, and reconsidered three times, in unusual circumstances, at varying intervals from the original interviews. We recommend that the reader focus not so much on the ratings that the couple chose to include in their reports, but on the quality of the impressions and reactions that they convey so directly and authentically in their own language.

We believe that these retrospective reports, in spite of the limitations we have outlined, constitute important and unusual clinical documents: They allow us to explore questions that therapists often ask, but cannot find the data to answer, either in their own experience or in the literature. Consider, for example, the variability of recollections of past experiences both across time and across individuals. When we look back on an experience in our past, some of our initial images and evaluations

---

[3]This is especially true for the family of origin therapists, but true also of Papp, who, as described in her chapter, typically uses two meetings to conduct an assessment.

[4]One can imagine, for example, that a feeling of being manipulated would be more likely to emerge after reading about an interviewer's covert strategies than after experiencing the interview itself.

[5]They also reviewed the tapes before the six-month follow-up interview. They now guess that, at that time, they watched only the 45-minute edited tape of each interview.

appear unchanged, but others may be radically different. Indeed, each time we look back we may appraise some aspect of an experience differently. We can only guess at the reasons for the differences, or lack thereof. To some degree they may reflect a relatively stable element of personality; some people may tend to be loyal to their original impressions, while others typically change their minds. For example, at a college reunion, when two roommates discuss their recollections, one of them may continue to uphold her original perceptions of her teachers, while the other has a revised opinion of all of them. We were not terribly surprised that Larry and Jennifer, Sluzki's "rock" and "balloon," differed in the way that they did: Jennifer (the balloon) shifted her opinions more dramatically than Larry and energetically explored and explained her reactions and feelings about the sessions as therapeutic events; Larry (the rock) changed very few opinions and staunchly kept in mind the couple's status as volunteers for "demonstrations."[6]

As important as character, in accounting for variability of recollection and shifts in evaluation, are the experiences of intervening years. For example, most of us revise our evaluations of our parents after we have raised children. Change also arises from forces in our current contexts. An individual undergoing marital separation develops a revised account of the marriage that is not only different from the one he or she first had and the one once shared with his or her spouse; it is also likely to be markedly different from the version that the spouse now holds (Weiss, 1975). With the loss of the shared context of the marriage comes the loss not only of a shared vision, but also of the ability to create shared revisions.

The shifts in the retrospective reports presented here are most apparent in Jennifer's reactions to her sessions with Papp and the Framos. With regard to the Papp interview, in the report that Jennifer wrote one day later (in consultation with Larry), she said that Papp's interview left them "feeling cold," as though there was no "hope for improvement." She wrote that Papp's technique "stressed problems . . . and might be more suitable for divorce therapy." At the same time, she acknowledged that Papp's technique had the positive effect of helping them "to *more clearly see* each other's conflicts, as well as those of which [we] were never even aware before." (Italics in quotes are Jennifer's.)

Six years later, Jennifer's positive reactions were more strongly stated and her negative ones completely dropped out. In the six-year report, she described Papp as "warm, genuine, and highly empathic" and wrote

---

[6]It should be borne in mind, however, that the balloon was not always a balloon and the rock was not always a rock. Larry's expression of admiration and love for Jennifer in the six-year report was not very rock-like, and Jennifer's detailed and somewhat technical approach to critiquing the clinical methods was not very balloon-like.

that Papp's *"astute and insightful interpretations* helped allay much of my anxiety and feelings of hopelessness regarding the seemingly insur-mountable nature of our situation." Far from thinking of Papp as best suited for "divorce therapy," Jennifer described her as one of the best suited of all four therapists for the couple over the long run.[7] (We have no evidence that Jennifer envisioned the "long run" of her relationship to include divorce. Rather, we have much evidence to the contrary!)

There are any number of possible explanations for this shift in perception about the value of Papp's techniques for the couple. One explanation might point to the sharply different contexts in which Jennifer first experienced and later re-experienced the session. Jennifer was scheduled for a family of origin interview on the afternoon of the day that she and Larry met with Papp. Could it be that, dreading the later meeting, she felt particularly vulnerable? Six years later, when Jennifer reviewed the videotape of the session with Papp in the comfort of her own home, was she more open to the warmth and hope communicated by Papp? Did she have a greater appreciation of Papp's relatively modest agenda for the single session, as compared with the Framos' much more ambitious agenda? Another possible explanation would take into account gender issues. To what degree was her new appreciation of Papp a reflection of her own increased self-esteem as a woman? We might wonder whether it was an extension of her positive feelings about her current female therapist.

A shift in the opposite direction occurred in Jennifer's feelings about her family of origin meeting with the Framos. Jennifer's initial feelings, as expressed in her letter to Jim and Mary Framo and her first follow-up report, have a quality of euphoria. In spite of the fact that she reported feeling "tremendous anxiety and fear," she said that the "direct confron-tation" with her family was *"extremely positive"* and broke through "impenetrable barriers." She felt "extricated from the shackles of a very dark and terrifying past." She described Jim and Mary Framo as utilizing an approach including *"empathy, sincerity, and honesty."* Six months later she characterized the interview as very powerful, catalyzing "tremen-dous change" in her relationship with her mother. She said, "I feel a lot closer to her now. I feel a lot less threatened by her. I feel a lot safer talking to her." She then explained that she had carried forward the work on her own initiative by making a very positive and "necessary" (though "frightening") visit to her mother to continue to explore the truth about the past.

In the six-month interview Larry concurred with Jennifer's assess-ment of the dramatic change in her relationship with her mother, referring to a quality of friendship he heard in Jennifer's voice during a

---

[7]The other therapist she felt would be good for the couple was Paul.

phone call to her mother. He was very surprised to discover later that it was indeed her mother on the other end of the line and not a good friend: "I've known both her and her mother for ten, for eleven years. It was the first time I heard them communicate on that level. . . ." In addition, he felt that the new openings carried over to the couple relationship (the "floodgates" opened) and even to Jennifer's extended family in Europe.

In both the first report and the six-month follow-up, Jennifer mentioned the anxiety she felt in her family of origin session, and in both, she criticized Jim Framo for validating the feelings of her family without sufficiently validating her own. However, in those early reports, this criticism seemed to be overshadowed by Jennifer's feelings of liberation and hope. Six years later, the negative aspects of Jennifer's experience overshadowed the positive. She acknowledged that the Framos may have influenced the "intermittent" more open relationship with her mother, but wrote that "It's difficult to assess whether this change (and, if so, to what degree) resulted from the interview, or whether it occurred because my mother and I felt 'safer' sharing our respective hurt and sadness with each other as we grew older." Moreover, she described the interview as "traumatic" and even as a "violation."

We believe that the time constraints imposed on the Framos, and the conflicting roles of therapist and theory presenter, contributed significantly to this outcome. The lack of follow-up work may have contributed as well.[8] Nonetheless, this dramatic shift, and the fact that it occurred when it did, raises many questions about the case and the Framos' approach to it, only a few of which we will address here. The reader will, no doubt, have other perspectives and explanations.

A therapist accustomed to taking a psychoanalytic perspective might hypothesize that Jennifer initially idealized Jim Framo, hoping that he could satisfy her longings for an empathic parent. Then when the "liberation" coming from a single intervention wore off (after several months), she became disappointed in her liberator and ultimately transferred onto him the unexpressed rage she had accumulated over the course of her painful childhood. As some analysts say, "What transference giveth, transference can taketh away." In this regard, we

---

[8]Framo strongly believes that family of origin work should be followed up by work with a systemic therapist, preferably one with a good deal of experience with family of origin sessions. He offered to provide such follow-up to Jennifer and Larry. We, the editors, also offered to provide or arrange for follow-up service, and in the six-month follow-up, initiated by us, inquired specifically about negative consequences and about the possibility of setting up family sessions to attend to "unfinished business." However, the couple acted independently, and virtually all of their subsequent therapy was with therapists who do not routinely work with families of origin. We cannot know to what degree their retrospective was affected by their later therapeutic experiences.

might note that she exempts Mary Framo from the shift, and instead applauds Mary's empathy in the session. This is especially interesting since there appears to be no striking difference between the stances of Mary and Jim. Is this an instance of split transference?

Some therapists might question whether the short-term effects that Jennifer and Larry so clearly acknowledge—the deepened communication between mother and daughter, and the consequent opening of the "floodgates" in other relationships—might have had long-term benefits that Jennifer (negatively disposed, six years later) did not acknowledge. One such benefit may have been the deepened commitment that Larry and Jennifer experienced as a couple in the few months during which Jennifer and her mother were exploring their pasts and their feelings toward each other. This may have been a step in the direction of their ultimate marriage. Could Jennifer's work with her family have loosened old bonds of pain just enough to free her for deeper commitment to Larry and to their future together? We cannot know, but it is reasonable to so speculate.

An equally persuasive explanation comes to mind if we take into account the fact that Jennifer is a recovering victim of abuse.[9] Perhaps her increasing awareness of past abuse (partly through discussions with her sister) helped her to identify more clearly other experiences in which she was persuaded to set aside her pain or to move too quickly into an experience that she was convinced was over her head. Perhaps Jennifer's initial idealization of the Framos reflected a readiness on her part to behave as do many victims of abuse: to sacrifice her own needs for the sake of others, and cover up that sacrifice with demonstrations of loyal appreciation.

We might also wonder whether Jennifer's shift in her reaction to Jim Framo might, to some degree, reflect a broader shift in her responses to men in general. Her mother had admonished her to be suspicious of men. Early in her relationship with Larry, Jennifer resisted commitment to one man, looking to several men to fill her needs. Over the years, she became more trusting of and committed to Larry. She also became more appreciative of other women and of herself as a woman. In addition, Jennifer has seen some hope for improving her relationship with her mother (or at least feels "ambivalent"), but has never expressed hope of communicating with her father.

Finally, a feminist perspective might attribute Jennifer's shift neither to transference nor to her specific history of abuse. Rather, it might focus on the gender-role training that kept Jennifer from asserting her needs more forcefully in the interview. In this account, Jennifer, as an

---

[9]In our opinion, this is a well-justified assumption, if not an established fact. Jennifer certainly believes it to be so.

individual, is depathologized. She is seen as a recovering victim of sexism who has, over a six-year period, found her own voice and her anger at the stressful therapeutic agenda that was carried out despite her protests—an agenda that asked of Jennifer much more empathy and understanding than it gave her.

Yet another perspective from which to view Jennifer's intensity of feeling in the six-year report—one that is consistent with any and perhaps all of those offered above—suggests that Jennifer's viewing of the videotape of her family session may have reminded her of old feelings of powerlessness, feelings with which she now felt she could do battle. She chose to do battle with Jim Framo, which could be seen as both directly "valid" and as fueled by transference. She expressed her anger rather than sinking into despair.

Perhaps the simplest explanation for the shift in Jennifer's reaction is that the positive effects of her work with the Framos did not last over the years. It is not surprising that one family of origin consultation failed to reverse nearly three decades of painful family relations.[10] (In fact, it could be argued that the transient effects were quite impressive!) Nonetheless, Jennifer was disappointed that her hopes for sustained closeness with her mother were not met. Her hope and excitement created a positive mindset; her disappointment, a negative one.

It is worth noting that Larry's responses, both to Jennifer's initial euphoria and her later anger, were those one might expect of a complementary partner. When Jennifer was singing the Framos' praises in the six-month follow-up, Larry agreed that things had changed, but portrayed the Framos as having merely provided a setting in which they got out of the way to let something happen that was ready to happen anyway. Six years later, when the valence of Jennifer's feelings had shifted, he agreed with her criticism about inadequate follow-up, but acknowledged the value of a family of origin approach: "I thought (and still do) that if she worked out the many serious problems with her family, especially her mother, our lives would be better for it."

Clearly, Jennifer would agree. Even though she was critical of Jim Framo, Jennifer made perceptive distinctions between the value of his general approach and its specific implementation in stressful circumstances. "I realize that Framo had a difficult task to accomplish in a short period of time," she wrote, "and I believe his motivation was well intended."

By contrast with the Framos' interview, Jennifer's reaction to the family of origin session that Paul conducted with Larry's family was consis-

---

[10]This is not to say that the positive effects of single consultations are always doomed to dissolution. Single consultations (whether using family of origin approaches or other approaches) sometimes do have sustained mutative effects.

tently favorable, from the first to the last report. In fact, when we met with the couple shortly before they wrote their six-year report, Jennifer mentioned that if she and Larry were to now choose a couple therapist from among the four interviewers, she might choose Paul. To this Larry responded, "That's because it was safer with *my* parents!" Jennifer found the Paul interview to be very useful, as it revealed striking similarities between Larry and each of his parents. This helped her to feel more understanding of and less responsible for Larry's style of interaction with her. In the six-month follow-up interview, she described a marked improvement in Larry's relationship with his father. Larry acknowledged that he learned from the Paul interview ("I understand more now"). Specifically, he said that he was surprised to hear from his father that his (Larry's) bout with cancer was "the worst thing" that happened to his father. But when Jennifer described the increased communication that she saw between Larry and his father since the Paul interview, Larry said, "It's not a big deal." In the six-year report, Jennifer retained her appreciation of Paul's work, but Larry said that he didn't feel particularly good about himself in that interview; he felt "awkward."

It appears that both family of origin meetings, the one with the Framos and the one with Paul, were experienced quite favorably by the partner relieved of the "hot seat" position, the partner who had much to gain and little to fear. Perhaps with more time for preparation and more follow-up, the clients who worked with their own families would have reacted as favorably as their partners did. In this regard, it is noteworthy that the Paul interview was criticized in the one-day report as too long and tiring, but this criticism dropped out later. Perhaps with the passage of time, the couple came to appreciate the greater ease that was made possible by the extra time Paul spent with them.[11]

With regard to the couple's interview with Sluzki, there was little change in the couple's evaluation over time, and little difference in their viewpoints. Both Larry and Jennifer felt that Sluzki's portrayal of their relationship as complementary (as a relationship between a rock and a balloon; damper and an amplifier) was helpful, and both appreciated Sluzki's acknowledgment of the positive qualities in their relationship. In the six-month interview, Jennifer appeared to be more open than Larry to Sluzki's suggestion that they "each become more like the other." When Jennifer suggested that they "reverse roles," Larry ob-

---

[11]Because Paul practices in the Boston area, he had more flexibility in scheduling his interview than any of the others. In fact, he spent almost four hours with the couple and Larry's family. The Framos and Papp had to schedule their interviews during a one-day trip that the couple made to New York City. Sluzki, who had to fly in from California for the interview and the conference, met with the couple *for an hour* the afternoon before the conference.

jected that that wouldn't be "real . . . it wouldn't be us." Nonetheless, Larry said that he found the image helpful: "I've sort of fooled around with the game," he said.

It is interesting to note that Jennifer never criticized Sluzki, as Low does, for his use of the balloon metaphor or for his "devaluing Jennifer's ability to express her feelings in therapy" (Chapter 12, this volume). In the six-year report, which was written after Jennifer had read drafts of the book chapters, Jennifer explained her acceptance of this treatment. "At least superficially, Sluzki appeared to be 'poking fun' (with a bit of sarcasm) at . . . my pedestrian knowledge of psychotherapy. His subtle teasing or playfulness served to maintain a constant dynamic in the 'therapeutic triad.' I believe it enabled Larry to be more involved and expressive in what was being discussed." Was Jennifer too willing to accept what she experienced as a bit of sarcasm or was her flexibility and good humor a sign of strength? We leave these questions for the reader to ponder.

*****

We are very grateful to the couple and their families for their participation in this exercise. We led them on a voyage into unfamiliar waters, and they stayed with us even when the waters were a bit rough. We admire them not only for the courage they demonstrated through their participation in the interviews, but also for the thoughtfulness they brought to the task of conveying their experiences to us as accurately and honestly as they could. We are also enormously grateful to the four therapists for their courage and openness. The therapists were sailing on familiar waters, but some of them were not at all accustomed to the time constraints imposed on them. More importantly, the therapists, unlike the clients, enjoyed little protection from exposure. After the four public conferences were over, the couple could control their personal exposure; in the book, they have been given every opportunity to achieve total anonymity. The therapists have had no anonymity at any time. They were well known before the project. During the conferences, they were watched at work by audiences who had heard about them. In this book, they permit a level of exposure and evaluation that few expert clinicians are requested to undergo. Perhaps we should compare the courage of all the participants, the couple and the therapists, not with that of each other but with that of the vast majority of clients and experienced therapists who only work in private. We hope that the readers of this book will benefit from their courage.

REFERENCE

Weiss, R. (1975). *Marital separation.* New York: Basic Books.

17

One Day Later: A Report from the Couple[1]

"LARRY" and "JENNIFER"

BACKGROUND

We (Chasin and Grunebaum) invited Jennifer and Larry to attend the conference and they did so. Due to time constraints, they decided to come to only one of the two days, choosing to come on the first day, the day on which the family of origin meetings were discussed. We alerted the audience to the possibility that the couple might be present on either or both days. We would have expected the audience of clinicians to treat the clinical data respectfully without the announcement, but out of concern for the couple, we felt that we should specifically solicit such treatment (which was, indeed, forthcoming).

At the end of the day, Jennifer asked us if we would be interested in hearing from her and Larry about their impressions of the interviews. We said that we would very much like to hear from them and asked if they would be willing to write something about the experience for us. We hoped to conduct a follow-up interview at a later time, but felt that an earlier report would provide an interesting point of comparison for their later recollections. We offered no direction or structure for their report, as we were interested to hear about their experiences as they construed them in their own minds. What follows is the report that Jennifer wrote that night in consultation with Larry. They gave it to us the next day. It is presented here, edited only in very minor ways for ease of reading.

---

[1]Editors' note: This report was given to us after the first day of the first conference. Some of the more positive comments were read at the conference the next day. Thus, the interviewers know that a retrospective report had been written. They did not see the full report, however, until the summer of 1989, after they had either completely finished writing their chapters or were making only minor revisions to them.

RESPONSES OF JENNIFER AND LARRY TO THE COUPLES CONFERENCE

February 10, 1983

Dear Henry and Dick,

Enclosed are the critiques you asked us to write. We hope you will find them useful and self-explanatory. Please feel free to use them as you wish for the conference. We divided each interview/technique into positive and negative aspects. . . . We realize that our comments are valid only pertaining to our special needs as a couple and that another couple with totally different needs and problems might feel very differently. This critique, therefore, should not be seen as "representative."

Feel free to call us if you have questions.

Best regards,
Jennifer and Larry

Overall Impression

The experience was very useful and informative, and provided new insights into existing problems in the relationship. We wish to thank both Alice and Alexandra[2] for their concern, encouragement, and support which helped in giving us the necessary courage and confidence to participate in this workshop. Jennifer would never even have considered doing this a year ago.

On a scale of 1–10 (10 = highest) for *helpfulness*, we would rate the techniques as follows:

	Jennifer	Larry		Jennifer	Larry
Papp	7	6	Framo	10	9
Paul	8	5	Sluzki	6	7

Peggy Papp

On the positive side we found:

1. Fantasy is a novel, interesting method for *restating* problems in a relationship because (a) it feels *safe* (i.e., no one can criticize or make a value judgment about a fantasy), (b) it is *unadulterated* by the confusion

---

[2]Editor's note: Alice was their couple therapist. Alexandra was Jennifer's individual therapist.

of reality, and (c) it allows the "fantasizer" to reveal his or her *wishes* regarding resolutions of the problems.

2. It enabled both Jennifer and Larry to *more clearly see* each other's conflicts as well as those of which they were never even aware before.

3. It emphasized the usefulness of *compromise*, which is helpful in reducing anxiety and guilt about satisfying either "your" or "my" wishes, and *role reversal* (being in the other person's shoes), which is helpful in understanding the other's needs and feelings and, consequently, feeling closer.

On the negative side:

1. Her technique may not have general applicability because it requires complete spontaneity and honesty, as well as a lack of inhibition about appearing "silly" in order to be most effective. (For instance, Jennifer changed one of her original fantasies because she felt hurt and humiliated by one of Larry's and wanted to retaliate. Realizing this later on, however, was very useful.)

2. It stressed problems or negative aspects of the relationship *more than* solutions or reconciliations. We were sometimes left feeling cold, as if our problems were insurmountable, change was not feasible, and we are two very different people who will never be able to meet each other's needs. The technique, therefore, lacked positive reinforcement and hope for improvement. It might be more suitable for divorce therapy.

3. It was a bit too theatrical, contrived, and predictable.

Jim Framo

On the positive side we found:

1. Many problems of a couple do indeed stem from *unresolved conflicts in the families of origin.* Jennifer believes that a lot of her problems with Larry are really problems with the members of her family (especially her mother). Jennifer looked to Larry for the things she felt she didn't get from her parents and, paradoxically, expected not to get those things from Larry either. Jennifer also "transferred" a lot of her feelings toward her parents onto Larry.

2. Direct confrontation between the members of Jennifer's family (which might never have taken place without the intervention of an objective yet empathetic therapist) resulted in her being extricated from the shackles of a very dark and terrifying past. Having heard both her parents' (especially her mother's) accounts of their own emotionally unfulfilled childhoods and having voiced her own feelings regarding her own, Jennifer feels *"freer"* with her emotions now, as if she has finally

somehow acquired a *license* to actually have these feelings. Larry also felt absolved from his "responsibility" to mother Jennifer and to worry about her feelings, a task which always made him feel uncomfortable and burdened. Larry was surprisingly very supportive of Jennifer's distraught state after the interview and Jennifer felt much *more trustful and closer to him* as a result. Larry felt that he was no longer to blame for keeping the distance between Jennifer and her mother.

3. The therapists (Jim and Mary) utilized an approach which included *empathy, sincerity, and honesty*, which Jennifer felt were *instrumental* in getting her family (which she always viewed as incapable of feeling, extremely private, well versed in denial and shifting the blame, and terrified of being exposed or criticized) to open up communication and break through impenetrable barriers which had evolved over 25 years. Having Mary there was a real consolation, as she provided a neutral backdrop when discussions threatened to become too heated and served as a focusing device when discussions tended to digress. She was also able to verbalize and translate some of the important unspoken messages which were being transmitted *all too quickly* during the barrage of emotions.

4. We all (including Larry) feel that this cathartic experience was an *extremely positive* one, one which will leave an indelible mark on us. It will hopefully serve as a *beginning* for establishing a real relationship (which only superficially existed before) between the members of Jennifer's family. Jennifer, her parents, and her sister already feel *a lot closer* and have expressed their feelings regarding one another in various ways since the interview, something which was never done before.

On the negative side:

1. There was tremendous anxiety and fear on all our parts (except Larry's) regarding confronting one another. Reassurance and encouragement *prior* to the meeting would have helped to assuage those feelings.

2. Jennifer experienced being alone and emotionally unsupported during the interview, doubting that anyone would believe her story, as the past was re-enacted. She felt she was once again the powerless, troublesome, unwanted child who was always in the way, and her parents' and sister's behavior toward her was justified. The therapists got what they wanted; her parents were left alone to deal with the tremendous emotional upheaval.

3. The aftermath was somewhat anticlimactic. Although Jennifer felt relieved and elated by the experience, she felt as though she had been stripped of something in the process. (Holding onto all these feelings over the years had led her to believe that their release would move

mountains, etc., and when wishful expectations and reality clash . . .) Follow-up is therefore very important in this type of therapy.

Norman Paul

On the positive side we found:

1. *Sharing one's vulnerabilities and inner feelings* (especially the *sad* ones) with one another is extremely important in a good relationship, and *patterns* which emerge may in part have their origin in previous generations.

2. This technique, employing videotapes, enabled Larry and Jennifer to see each other as they really are. It disclosed *striking similarities* between Larry and his parents which made Jennifer aware of how much Larry is like his father (i.e., "emotionless") and how much she, Jennifer, is like his mother (i.e., controlling, frustrated, emotional, and unable to "connect" with or share with the other). The point that his inability to communicate may have been transmitted to Larry from his uncommunicative parents was *well illustrated*.

3. Larry and Jennifer heard *for the first time* Larry's parents' accounts of their own parents' deaths. Larry's father never cried; neither did he ever tell Larry about his feelings of hurt and loss at never having his real father around. Larry's behavior (inability to allow himself to feel and discuss "sad" matters, including the loss of his foot) was explained. This was very *revealing and informative* for Jennifer.

On the negative side:

1. There was not enough effort made toward resolving the issues or tying information together. Is awareness of the root of these problems enough? Can parents who have been "educated" not to show emotion and have trained their children along the same lines suddenly exhibit emotion and undo the "damage"? It would make more sense to understand why it is taboo to share "bad" or "sad" feelings.

2. The therapist was too biased by his own views. He had a set hypothesis and extracted information which fit this hypothesis. He also misunderstood our reasons for going into couple therapy.[3]

3. Larry felt threatened by this technique and consequently was very resistant throughout the interview.

4. This interview will probably not help the relationship, but will help Jennifer to better understand Larry's behavior.

---

[3]Editor's note: Some of Paul's questions pertained to the making of a decision about marriage, not an issue of salience for Larry and Jennifer at the time.

5. The interview was too long and tiring. It could have been better organized and more coherent.

Carlos Sluzki

On the positive side we found:

1. He didn't delve into the past or require information about our respective backgrounds. He had a very *practical, unbiased,* and *direct* approach to our problems.

2. He *emphasized the positive aspects of the relationship* and reasons for the present situation (i.e., complementarity and equilibrium can be obtained with two very opposite personality types). It was quite refreshing!

3. He made potentially helpful suggestions for breaking the "vicious cycle" which has existed for so long via behavior modification.

On the negative side:

1. The interview was somewhat disjointed and it was sometimes difficult to understand what the therapist was driving at.

2. It was not as informative as some of the other interviews.

18
Six Months Later:
A Follow-up Interview

"LARRY," "JENNIFER," CHASIN, and
GRUNEBAUM

BACKGROUND

While planning the second conference, we (Chasin and Grunebaum) asked the couple if they would be willing to participate in a videotaped follow-up interview. They readily agreed, and a date was set for an evening in October of 1983. For reasons of convenience, the interview was held in the home of the filmmaker who had produced the videos for the conference, where the couple had met with Carlos Sluzki six months before. Our agenda for the interview was very simple. First and foremost, we wanted to hear how Larry and Jennifer were doing, individually, as a couple, and with their families. We also hoped to hear from them about their experiences as participants in the conference exercise and about any impact they felt the interviews may have had on their relationship. The interview lasted about one and a half hours. An edited videotape, 45 minutes long, was presented at the second, third, and fourth conferences, held in Boston, San Francisco, and New York. The transcript presented here represents about 90% of the full interview; it is edited primarily to eliminate repetition and discussion of logistical details.

JENNIFER: This might be of interest to you. We've actually had some time to view the tapes and we learned a lot just from looking at them. It was a very interesting experience to see ourselves.

GRUNEBAUM: What did you learn?

JENNIFER: Oh, well, lots of different things, I guess . . . about my reactions towards situations, Larry's reactions. I can go into specific details, but I'd say generally it added more information to what I already had. It was very, very helpful.

GRUNEBAUM: Can you think of anything specific, either of you?

JENNIFER: Um . . .

LARRY: Well, you don't usually see yourself react to a situation and that was interesting, for me. I see how other people see how I react during situations, and I think that there was a lot to learn from that in one way. And viewing again how everyone interacted in the family session was very interesting to see. My parents . . . it was like replaying a memory, only it was clearer because it was in color.

GRUNEBAUM: Um hm.

JENNIFER: Well, it really happened. It was, you know, reality and . . .

LARRY: It was five months . . . how long ago was it?

JENNIFER: Well, I think that the interesting thing is how we changed too. I mean . . .

LARRY: . . . or we thought we changed.

JENNIFER: (*Mildly laughing*) Well, I think that we did. I mean individually and as a couple. Given the same questions now, I think I would have answered them differently. I *would* answer them differently.

LARRY: I think you definitely changed, in your relationship with your parents.

JENNIFER: Oh, yeah, for sure.

LARRY: I remember, Jennifer has a friend in New York and the phone bill is about $25 each time she calls her. One night, soon after the conference, I walk into the house and I hear her talking on the phone and I know it's long distance, and I just assume it's her best friend in New York, and I say, "Jennifer, you're talking to her again? You just spoke to her last night!" and Jennifer says, "No, it's my mother." And that was an extremely big surprise to me because in person she's never talked to her mother in that way. From how she was conversing and communicating, I just assumed it was her best friend in New York, and in fact, it wasn't; it was her mother! That was very strange for me since I've known both her and her mother for ten, for eleven years. It was the first time I've heard them communicate on that level, and that was . . .

JENNIFER: Things have changed.

LARRY: . . . very important.

CHASIN: You've said a number of times that things have changed. Our biggest hope for tonight was to find out how things are with each of you, separately, how things are between the two of you, and how things are between each of you and your families.

GRUNEBAUM: And within the families.

CHASIN: Yes, exactly. Be as specific as you care to be.

JENNIFER: Well, I would say that the biggest change for me, really, individually, came with my parents. I mean, I think that the session with Jim Framo was very helpful in starting communication, in opening up communication between my parents and myself, especially my mother. My father and I are still a bit distant and it's a problem in the relationship that I think needs a lot of work. But I would say there's been a tremendous change in the relationship between my mother and myself. I feel a lot closer to her now. I feel a lot less threatened by her. I feel a lot safer talking to her. As a matter of fact, it wasn't too long ago that I went home and spent a weekend just talking to my mother, with the specific purpose of finding out answers to certain questions that I had about what actually happened during my childhood, things that were unclear to me. Was it just my perception or did these things really happen? And what was her perception of what happened? I needed to know that. It was a very frightening thing to do. I remember being terrified about going home, but I felt like at that point I could do it, and it needed to be done. The result was a very positive one. We both started crying and we opened up to each other. She never knew that I thought a certain way about her and I never knew that she thought certain things about me, and it really helped clarify a lot of issues that were continually bothering me all my life, and also perhaps interfering with my relationships with other people. I felt a sense of relief afterwards in knowing the truth and finding out at least what she felt about these things. I needed to know her side of the story, which I was too scared, in the past, to even pursue. I didn't want to know. I mean, I was too afraid of finding out that she really didn't want me and she really didn't like me. And as a matter of fact, it turned out that a lot of that was just my perception, how I perceived it. And it was a very positive thing. So I would say that my relationship with my mother, specifically with my mother, has changed because of what happened. My sister, that's another story altogether (*laughs*). There wasn't much change there. But then again, I haven't actively pursued working on that relationship. I might have to do one at a time. But I think the session that I had with Jim Framo was instrumental in enabling me to do this.

LARRY: In my opinion, I think it was ready to happen for a long time.

JENNIFER: That was the catalyst though.

LARRY: I think what Jim did was he sort of didn't get in the way. And he got them in the same place to talk about what they should talk about. He didn't prevent them from doing it and he might have helped somewhat. But I think they were ready, both of them. They just didn't know how to go about it.

JENNIFER: But we might have postponed this talk that we needed to have for many, many years. Both of us were scared. I obviously sensed her fear.

LARRY: Yeah, you needed the setting, with someone objective around, a safer environment. Her mother doesn't do things that would be too threatening. But in this case I think that she was ready and Jennifer was ready and it really worked out well.

JENNIFER: Sure. I'm not taking credit away from my mother or myself. You're saying that maybe I'm giving too much credit to the therapist. But he might have been the catalyst. I think it required a third party.

CHASIN: (*To Larry*) I wonder if you would like to say something about yourself. How are things different within yourself now, perhaps as contrasted with the period of time during these interviews?

LARRY: Well, I don't know how much I've changed although I have realized recently that I feel more confident in our relationship. I don't know if that's due to the interviews or the conference or just the time that's passed. Or, I think, more importantly, that Jennifer feels better about her origins, especially with her mother. Of course there are my sides of the problem. But one of the problems was that Jennifer was very unsettled in terms of her family. So that affected our relationship. In terms of me personally, I think that I just feel more confident in our relationship. We went on a vacation to Holland for three weeks, and one of the problems we were trying to work out was my television watching or, according to Jennifer, my ignoring her. And luckily, I guess, I didn't understand much Dutch so I couldn't watch the television. So she saw that I wasn't really ignoring *her*, because I was able to get along with her very nicely on this three-week trip with no television at all. So that helped. There are a number of things that have helped since that time. So, if anything, I personally feel better about our relationship. I don't know how much I've individually changed—it's hard for me to gauge that—but one more example comes to mind. Jennifer has an opportunity to go to Kenya for two months. A few years ago that would have been like, terrible, *the end*, that she'd be leaving, that she'd consider leaving for that long. But now I realize that it's a career opportunity and the opportunity to see new places and do interesting things, and I think we feel confident in each other enough to say, "OK, it's two months but that's fine." It's part of what we have to do. And it isn't like, you know, *death*, that she has to—that we have to be apart that long.

JENNIFER: You don't feel as abandoned as you would have in the past.

LARRY: Right. We feel more confident in each other.

GRUNEBAUM: Have you changed in some ways that he feels more confident in you?

JENNIFER: I think I'm a lot more open than I used to be. I used to have a terrible time getting angry; I used to repress it all the time. I think now, if I'm upset or angry I'm more open about it and I can express those feelings and not feel like he's going to leave if I get angry. I also feel that the openness is important. I think he senses that I'm more open about things and I think he's been a lot more open about things, too. The two of us have been a lot more, I would say, confident in each other's feelings and I guess more trusting of each other, which is important. And the other thing, too, that I wanted to mention was I think Larry learned a lot from viewing his parents on tape, you know, after the session with Norman Paul. I don't know why he didn't bring it up now, but I remember when we were viewing it together it seemed like he was going through a horrendous educational experience watching this tape. I was too, actually. But I picked up a lot the first time because I was more the observer of that particular interview and he was the active participant. And I think he saw a lot of himself in his father, you know? (*To Larry*) You said you didn't realize that until you looked at the tape and you saw his reactions to certain situations, and you could see how similar your reactions were to his reactions. And I think it made you more aware of interactions in your family that you weren't aware of before, that your parents don't really communicate that well.

LARRY: Well, I . . .

JENNIFER: I mean, I think they're very close . . . but they don't communicate very well. That's not to say they don't care very deeply for each other, but there's a communication problem there. I think that was very clearly illustrated.

LARRY: That's not to say that we wouldn't have gotten to this point without any conference or couple therapy. Also, we're not perfect. I mean we're sort of presenting the ideal couple. I think we have a ways to go. And I think we will forever.

JENNIFER: There can always be improvements.

CHASIN: What would you now say about your relationship with your own family? How is it now?

LARRY: Well, my relationship with my family has always been pretty good. There are definite problems like with any family, the same kinds of problems. I understand more now. It isn't usual that my father gets to talk about *his* childhood—very rarely—or *his* family. It was always my mother's family. We all grew up in the same small area in New York. Also, as Jennifer mentioned, seeing my father in that kind of environment and seeing me at the same time, as a viewer, there are definite correlations — which is not surprising, he's my father. You know, it's not a revelation.

JENNIFER: Don't you think you're closer to your father now? I sense that. Maybe it's just, you know, before you were very distant.

LARRY: Well, one thing that surprised me and it shouldn't have because I didn't really think about it, but at one point my mother was asked, "What was the worst thing that happened to you?" and my mother said, "Well, Larry got sick." And I assumed that was always true. Then he asked my father, and my father says, "Yeah, Larry got sick," and it never occurred to me that that was the worst thing that happened to him. . . . It occurred to me that it was the worst thing that happened to my mother because she constantly tells me about it, but it never occurred — I mean, now that I think about it, it's an obvious thing. His son was very sick. But it surprised me at that instant and I remember it surprising me. And so when I thought about why it surprised me, I sort of learned something. . . . Also, I was always sort of sociable and louder than most of my friends, so I always assumed I was more like my mother than my father, but there are definite aspects that move me more towards my father than I had previously thought. Like any child, I'm some combination. But I always figured my mixture was more toward my mother and it's actually more towards the middle than I thought.

JENNIFER: Well, you see more of your father now, in yourself.

LARRY: Yeah.

JENNIFER: Yeah.

LARRY: I don't know, I was always close with both of them, and I don't know if we've gotten closer because . . .

JENNIFER: I sense you've gotten closer with your father. Like you'll call him up now and talk with him for more than two minutes. Before, it was just sort of, "Hi, how you doing? Everything's OK, yup, yup." It was very superficial. Now you get into deeper conversations. You know, you might talk about how you're feeling, or what's going on.

LARRY: Yeah.

JENNIFER: I mean, that's something I've noticed.

LARRY: It's not a big deal.

JENNIFER: You've noticed differences in my relationship with my mother.

I've noticed differences in your relationship with your father. It's like you almost want to talk to him sometimes. You'll come home and you'll call him up on the phone and tell him about something that happened during your day or something exciting that's going on at work. Before it used to be your mother, I think, that you would talk to about those things and then she would relay the message to your father. That's how he got the information. So now it's a lot more direct. I mean, I think you feel like you can just directly approach your father now without actually having to go through your mother first, which is kind of interesting.

GRUNEBAUM: I noticed one thing. When you talked about being more open with each other, you mentioned that you were able to be more openly expressive of things when you are angry. I wondered, does that also apply to affection?

JENNIFER: Yeah, it does. I think it works across a whole spectrum of feelings and we're also more open with affection. As a matter of fact, we went to Maine not too long ago, you know, for a weekend, and we had a really nice time there. I mean, we were a lot more openly affectionate than we used to be. And even when we were in Europe it seemed to be a lot easier to do. It was more spontaneous.

LARRY: I remember what I wanted to say. Jennifer's family, her parents, are in the United States. They've been here for 30 years. But, really, no one else in her family is here. They're all in Holland. When we went over to Holland I met her family for the first time. And I think that really helped her, too. She was used to growing up without very much of a family outside of her parents and sister. Whereas there, she has family all over the place and they're very close. They all live in very close proximity and they come over every night and they're warm people, and . . .

JENNIFER: Very much like Larry's family.

LARRY: It reminded me, in fact, it was exactly like my family in the sense that everyone wanted to talk over everyone else. And what was good about that was, Jennifer felt when we were there like a different person because she was right in the middle of all this support. They obviously care about her. She's been there six other times, so they know her quite well. And I think that helped, too, to know that she has some roots, a family.

JENNIFER: You understood how much I miss that here, because I don't have it here.

LARRY: Which is why you were attracted to my family, because they're very similar types.

JENNIFER: Very close, very warm, you know, very responsive in many ways. I think that you benefitted from that, too, because you never realized how close I could be in a family setting like that. Or how happy I was in that particular environment.

LARRY: But I think that the advances you made with your mother helped in your dealing with the rest of your family there.

JENNIFER: Well, because I feel more open now, in general.

LARRY: I think that the floodgates just sort of opened.

JENNIFER: Yeah.

CHASIN: I wonder, if you look back on the interviews that you had with the four therapists, if you can identify in addition to what you've already talked about, anything that stands out in your mind. Particularly anything that you think may have had some kind of enduring impact, whether it was intended or not. Anything that is highlighted in your memory and seems to have been worked over by you in some way, that you have made use of for yourselves.

LARRY: Well, I can quickly go through the four. Sluzki, I think, brought up a point that remains with us, that I'm sort of the attenuator and Jennifer is sort of the amplifier, and that image, I think, is a very good one.

JENNIFER: And you're the rock and I'm the balloon (*laughter*).

LARRY: Right, and I think I have become much more of an attenuator than I would have been if she weren't an amplifier. It's sort of a non-linear system, you know, who came first? We don't know, but we were in, sort of.

JENNIFER: But the point he made was to exchange roles for a while and . . .

LARRY: . . . it's impossible! (*Laughter*) We tried that for about three minutes.

JENNIFER: But he gave us an option. I mean, you don't always have to be the rock, and I don't always have to be the balloon. I mean . . .

LARRY: But his point was that we're both afraid that if I don't start out attenuating, that she's going to sort of blow up and the resonance will create an explosion. If I don't attenuate, right off the bat attenuate it, and . . .

JENNIFER: He says we sort of complement each other in that respect, but he also—I mean, it's good to remember that you can reverse roles if you want to. I mean, just knowing that you can be something different, it's important to know that you don't always have to . . .

LARRY: Yeah, but playing a role isn't real because, by definition, you're playing a role. So, if we would switch roles it wouldn't be us.

GRUNEBAUM: I noticed that you didn't bring up the alternate possibility that if she didn't sort of lift things, you'd be sitting there as a rock (*laughter*).

LARRY: Well, I didn't bring that up because it isn't as complimentary.

CHASIN: But what I was also curious about is how you have utilized that imagery? I think you've (*to Jennifer*) put it to use in assuring yourself that you aren't ordained forever to be in a certain fixed position . . .

JENNIFER: Exactly.

CHASIN: . . . but I wonder how you (*to Larry*) have used it?

LARRY: Well, there have been a few incidents when she said, "Oh, I can't believe this one did this to me," and I said, "Yeah, that was really rotten." Previously, I would have said, "Ah, it's no big deal." It's sort of on a minor level. That's how I've used it. And she says, "Yeah, you agree with me, then." See, what I'd thought was that it would make her worse because I had confirmed that she should really worry about it.

JENNIFER: But you found that if you agree with me and get just as worked up about some things as I do that might just stop for a while; I mean, it might have sort of a positive effect.

LARRY: Maybe. I think most of the time, though, things don't . . .

JENNIFER: It doesn't necessarily exacerbate my reaction, if you say "Yeah, that was horrible."

LARRY: It doesn't necessarily, but it could, still.

CHASIN: So you've experimented with variations and found out that the system didn't go completely out of control if you stopped being a perfect rock for a few seconds.

LARRY: That's right, that's right. Of course, you know, most things that you worry (*to Jennifer*) about would not bother *me*. Truly, you know. So I've experimented with different approaches to that. I've sort of fooled around with the game, the feedback system.

JENNIFER: But you realized that your worst fears weren't realized by changing. I mean, in other words, if you did feed into my anxiety about something, it wouldn't lead to, you know, a state of trauma for both of us.

LARRY: That's true now, maybe because you've changed. It might not have been true when I first formulated the strategy eight years ago. I just didn't change my strategy fast enough to meet your changes.

Um, so that was Sluzki. With Peggy Papp, it was interesting . . . what I chose as my fantasies. I was always trying to do something great and women were sort of necessary diversions . . .

JENNIFER: But sometimes in the way . . .

LARRY: . . . and sometimes in the way. Right. Which was an interesting perception on my part.

JENNIFER: And it also brought out how competitive the two of us are in a lot of situations. That's why we reach certain impasses in our relationship, because we're competing, whether it's consciously or subconsciously, I don't think it really matters. But those game-playing scenes really brought out precisely how competitive we really are in our everyday life.

LARRY: That's true.

JENNIFER: And I think that's something we have to watch out for because it can be very detrimental to the relationship. If you're always competing, you're not going to really make any significant gains in the relationship; you're going to always reach a stalemate or worry about who's going to win this situation and who's going to lose in the situation. You know, it doesn't matter if somebody wins or loses. No winning or losing, we're just going to have a good time. It sort of detracts from the real feelings and the spontaneity if you're always worrying about competing and winning and losing. And that was something that we were made aware of because of those sort of fantasy/game-playing sessions.

LARRY: I think if you are open to learning you will learn . . .

JENNIFER: But it brought a lot of problems to our attention that we weren't even aware of. So I think the main thing is that we could derive information about ourselves from the sessions and then at least we have the option to work on it. If you don't have any information it's kind of hard to know where to start.

GRUNEBAUM: Did you continue with some of that work with your couple therapist?

JENNIFER: Actually we didn't, because as it turned out, we went off to . . . oh, let me backtrack a little bit . . .

LARRY: We went to Europe.

JENNIFER: We did have a few more sessions with her. Then once we went off to Europe we just stopped.

GRUNEBAUM: Um hm.

JENNIFER: Then she went on vacation, so the summer was practically gone, and then we never resumed therapy again. But I think we're at a point now where we can do a lot of our therapy by ourselves. But I think at the time we started we really needed a third person for a therapist. But now I think we're at a point where we can talk to each other about problems, and I also feel that it's not just talking about it, I think that we're in a position where we feel that we're going to act on it, which is the important thing. We can go one step beyond just talking about problems.

CHASIN: I wonder what's next on the agenda with each other? What's in front of the two of you right now?

JENNIFER: Well, I would say in the immediate future it's to continue to work on the relationship and continue to improve things. Like I said, I think we've come a long way from, let's say, a year ago, but I think we have a ways to go and I think we're still . . . we've made a commitment to stay together.

GRUNEBAUM: You did?

JENNIFER: Yeah. Whether or not it's getting married, I think that it's not really a particularly relevant issue, but we feel emotionally committed.

CHASIN: When did that happen?

JENNIFER: I think it just happened with time. I mean, it wasn't a particular day or hour or—you know, I think it was just a feeling that we developed over a period of time. We feel a lot closer and a lot more committed to the relationship than we did in the past. And more secure about the relationship. (*To Larry*) Don't you think so?

LARRY: Yeah. We also are planning for children.

JENNIFER: (*To Larry*) That's after I come back from Kenya (laughter).

CHASIN: Do you have a sense, roughly, of when that shift occurred to feeling committed to the point of planning for children?

JENNIFER: Probably in Europe.

LARRY: I would say during the trip to Europe when we were sort of . . .

JENNIFER: We were just forced to be close, just by proximity. Because we were either in the car together or in the hotel together. I mean there was no TV. And I wasn't in the lab. And it was positive.

CHASIN: It gave you a lot of information, sort of a test . . .

JENNIFER: Yeah, it was. And we were terribly anxious before this vacation, like, "Oh my goodness, we're going to be alone together."

LARRY: Well, it wasn't "we" who were anxious.

JENNIFER: You were anxious too.

CHASIN: You obviously had a good time with each other in Europe. Has that led to some change in the amount of distance you keep between you?

JENNIFER: I think it's changed. I don't think you watch as much TV, and I'm not in the lab as much. I think we make more of an effort to do things together.

LARRY: Well, we do, but that can also be because I finally got out of school . . . and we have a little bit more money.

JENNIFER: So we have more flexibility. Like we can go to a play, for instance, which we hadn't been able to do before.

LARRY: I think money helps. I mean it's never the absolute yes or no, but it helps in a relationship. We were just in the Bahamas last weekend. We've been going places.

JENNIFER: And doing more things.

LARRY: It's not that we have more time. It's just that we have more money so we make the time.

JENNIFER: But I think you've changed. You don't watch TV as much. I've seen you reading books more, like you did in Europe. I mean, I don't feel as threatened by TV watching. Before, it used to really bother me. I mean, it used to be sort of the bane of my existence, you know. If only I could smash the TV set (*laughs*), you know? I wasn't competing with another woman, I was competing with a TV set (grins).

GRUNEBAUM: What does he compete with?

JENNIFER: I guess my lab work.

LARRY: I tell my friends that Jennifer is . . .

JENNIFER: A workaholic.

LARRY: . . . what I used to tell my friends is that Jennifer complains that I watch too much TV and they say, "You're a graduate student and you're running a company at the same time, and she complains that you watch too much TV?" So . . .

JENNIFER: You're just very efficient, Larry, that's all.

LARRY: But I think that was sort of a symbol of other problems . . .

GRUNEBAUM: Uh huh.

LARRY: . . . and I think even if I watched the same number of hours, I think she'd be threatened by it less. Probably because both of us have done work to allow her to be threatened by it less.

JENNIFER: I also feel more comfortable with you. I know now that if I say, "Look, I've got to discuss a very important problem and it's pretty urgent," that you would turn off the TV set and you wouldn't be so upset about doing it now. Or you'd say, "Well, maybe not now, but how about two hours from now?" And I could accept that now.

LARRY: Like I said, it's sort of the whole structure of the relationship that has improved so we've been able to work things like that out better.

GRUNEBAUM: We wondered also, the four interviews certainly covered a lot of areas, but were there things you felt were important that didn't get tapped?

JENNIFER: Um hm. I do. I think the major objection I had with the four interviews was that nobody really emphasized any of the positive things in our relationship. Obviously you're going for therapy because you're working out problems and, you know, you're dealing with negative things, so to speak, things that are upsetting to you or disturbing or whatever. But I don't remember any of the therapists, except for maybe Carlos, emphasizing any of the positive things in our relationship, and that was upsetting to me. You know, because obviously in any relationship there's a combination of both.

LARRY: In watching the tape . . .

JENNIFER: It made me feel a little bit empty and insecure afterwards, because they were always emphasizing, "Well, what are the problems in the relationship?" And then you go through the whole list: lack of communication, this and this . . . and it'd lead to a reiteration of all the problems.

LARRY: One of the things that struck me was why didn't anybody ask us if we love each other? You know, that never came up.

JENNIFER: Or why we'd been together for ten years . . .

LARRY: . . . or why we'd been together for ten years. I understand . . .

JENNIFER: There has to be something positive going on.

GRUNEBAUM: Maybe you'd like to say something about that now.

LARRY: Well, I sort of did, just now. Of course you can't show couple therapy in a conference with a couple that has only positive things to say about each other. But I think that could have been stressed more than it was. That was one point.

GRUNEBAUM: It would certainly set the problems in a different perspective if people knew that you cared about each other as much as you do.

JENNIFER: Sure. And I think that was neglected in pretty much most of the sessions that we had.

CHASIN: It's also true that both of you will do a great deal with a small amount of information or recognition. And the way you do things is so energetic and industrious and deliberate and intelligent. It's not as if you're the kind of people who throw away information or have an allergy to recognition.

JENNIFER: Right. If anything, we were looking for things.

LARRY: There was another thing. There was just limited time, so I understand, but I think that Jim Framo could have gotten at the relationship between her and her sister a little better and seen how phoney it all was. I think he should have nailed her more.

JENNIFER: I think Mary Framo nailed her. She was very perceptive. She saw exactly what was going on.

LARRY: Maybe he made a conscious decision not to delve into that one because there was so much going on with the mother.

JENNIFER: He obviously went after the relationship with my mother because he knew that that was probably the most important.

CHASIN: You mentioned at the beginning that you ought to get around to improving the quality of the relationship with your sister. That it's not something that you are undertaking at this minute.

JENNIFER: I would find that too overwhelming, even at the session. I mean it was hard enough to break the ice with my mother. I mean I was terrified before the session because I was afraid of what would happen, that there would be some sort of fiasco.

LARRY: Jennifer and her mother were ready. Her and her sister, you know, who knows?

JENNIFER: I think we have a lot of work to do.

LARRY: I also think it would have helped with my family if my brother were there. Unfortunately, he just couldn't make it. And it would have been informative to see him, because he and I are similar in some respects and not in others.

JENNIFER: But he was brought up on several occasions.

LARRY: Yeah.

GRUNEBAUM You know you've talked about feeling more solid in your commitment and your affection toward each other has changed. Has your feeling of desire for each other changed at all?

JENNIFER: The need is stronger. I mean I feel I need Larry more than I did before.

GRUNEBAUM: It also sounds like you're better friends to each other. You have more fun playing around. But money helps a little bit too.

LARRY: Yeah.

GRUNEBAUM: But you've got to want to play. The money can sit there in the bank too.

JENNIFER: That's right.

GRUNEBAUM: You can buy a full room of television viewing equipment with money.

JENNIFER: Or a brand new laboratory. So it shows that our priorities have changed. You know, we care to spend the money with each other.

GRUNEBAUM: Do you have any thoughts about the impact, for you and your families, of going through this conference? I would like you to be specific about the families' thoughts about it first, then give some sense of the impact for you.

JENNIFER: Well, his family, for instance, although (*to Larry*) you can speak for your family, but his mother was just so thrilled by this whole thing. I mean, she was probably the most excited person by all this.

LARRY: She wanted to know the audience's reactions to everything on the tapes.

JENNIFER: Your father, I think . . .

LARRY: My father enjoyed it.

JENNIFER: Everybody, I think, thought it was a positive experience. I don't think there were any negative reactions. My mother thought it was a good idea. My father was, you know, I don't talk too much to him about this. I think he was a little bit confused by the whole thing. He was a little bit . . . he didn't know, really, what to make out of it, and I think that's what my father's reaction was. My sister thought it was a wonderful opportunity to psychoanalyze everybody in my family (*laughs*). Let's see, what else can I say . . . but, I would say my mother thought it was great because, again, she benefitted very much from it and so did I. So I think that the families in general had a very positive response to it.

CHASIN: Do either of you have any inclination, if we could arrange it somehow, to have another session? You with your family and you with yours? I mean you say that there is some unfinished business.

JENNIFER: Well, that's something to think about. Certainly I would have to think about it.

LARRY: It's possible, it's just a question of logistics. I'm sure that my family would love to do it, it's just a question of getting together.

JENNIFER: My family, I don't know. Especially because of my relationship with my sister more than anything else. I mean, it was very, very traumatic for me to go through that. I remember having severe anxiety attacks.

GRUNEBAUM: Of course it could just be with you and your sister if you felt ready to do that. There's no set schedule for this sort of thing.

CHASIN: I think it's evident that you both have a good sense of what you can accomplish on your own and have done very nicely. So I think it would not be hard for you to spot those places where, despite confidence and motivation, you are running up against a snag that you might want assistance with at the time. I'm impressed by the amount of strength and confidence you have in your capacity to be working on these personal and family issues by yourselves.

GRUNEBAUM: What was it like for you? You were both at the conference, also.

JENNIFER: I really enjoyed it immensely. I thought it was interesting, you know, to see ourselves, and it gave us the opportunity to take a step back and look at our responses as sort of a viewer rather than a participant. You always get different information that way and it's sort of interesting to see how the people reacted to us, too. And we got a lot of responses, you know, people were coming up to us and talking to us. I felt like . . . you know, we made a useful contribution, somehow, and it was a good feeling. I like helping out.

GRUNEBAUM: Um hm.

JENNIFER: Part of my personality, I guess, but I felt very good about it. I was a little bit—at first, I mean, I was a little bit apprehensive about going to the conference because I just didn't know how the material was going to be handled. If it was going to be purely analytical and cold or if it was going to have some sort of personal element associated with it. But I found it was sort of a combination of the two, maybe even a little bit more of the latter. And I didn't feel like an object that was being analyzed and studied and probed and picked at, or anything like that. I mean, I felt like a person. And I think people reacted to us as people.

CHASIN: We were concerned about the kinds of difficulties that were engendered in you or your families, stresses, problems, by the whole process, by the interviews, by the conference. We worry about things like that and this is an opportunity that we have to learn about what kind of . . .

GRUNEBAUM: Adverse effects . . .

CHASIN: Adverse effects and problems may have been created either temporarily or for a longer time.

JENNIFER: I think the only very transient adverse effect was with my family. I think my mother, after the interview, was sort of a bit horror-stricken and upset and she didn't quite know what to make of it, and—you know, because it sort of came up so unexpectedly and out of the blue. But I mean the overall effect was a very positive one because we were able to talk about it and work out some of these conflicts that we had, and everything. But I think the immediate effect was a bit upsetting for her. My father too, I think, was a little bit confused by all this and felt that he was being somehow manipulated into a situation. He had no idea what he was getting himself into. Nobody had explained to him beforehand what this was going to be about and it turned out to be a very emotional experience for which he was not prepared. I think he was a bit confused by the experience more than anything. Again, I think my sister went into it with a sort of cold, analytical approach and she realized she wasn't going to be affected by this one way or the other. I was terrified, basically, before the interviews. Afterwards I felt a bit upset, too, because I wasn't sure what was going to happen.

CHASIN: So although your terror, your father's bewilderment, your mother's being overwhelmed, were part of the cost, which it sounds like—in the final analysis, you felt it was worth it?

JENNIFER: Oh, yeah. I would say definitely! I would say it was a good tradeoff. It was worth going through the very short-lived, but acute, stress.

CHASIN: I think the question that I wanted most to ask is really what you would like to say beyond the things we've specifically asked you. And perhaps most of all, what you want us to know. What should we be learning from you?

JENNIFER: It was a learning experience for everyone involved, and again, we're just an example of what can be done in couples therapy. I think that your approach, at least for us, was a very interesting one, having the same couple being interviewed by different therapists. I think it is a learning experience for you too. And we would like you to know, at least from my point of view, that it was a very educational approach and a very interesting one, a very good one, very beneficial. I'm talking as to how I would view it from your aspect. I want you to know that I think it was a reasonable approach and that we enjoyed it.

LARRY: Well, now that you asked (*laughter*). I don't really know much about psychiatry, but the way I viewed this was that each had their own point of view, their own style, and school of thought and we were more or less used as examples for each, for their style. But we didn't fit in each style equally well. I think that given each style, there are couples who do fit in each of those. We were just one example and we couldn't have been expected to fit in each of those styles.

JENNIFER: Different set of circumstances and different people.

LARRY: Right.

JENNIFER: Again, I would say it was a very, very beneficial experience for us and I'm glad to hear that you, on your end, benefitted from it and that pleases us too.

19

Six Years Later:
A Report from the Couple

"LARRY" and "JENNIFER"

BACKGROUND

In the summer of 1988, we (the three editors) contacted the couple in California to let them know that we were actively engaged in editing this volume and would like to start sending copies of manuscripts to them for their review. We asked if they would read each manuscript, paying particular attention to the ways in which we had disguised their true identities to protect their privacy, and let us know if they felt additional fictionalization was in order. They were pleased to hear that the book was in preparation and happy to review the chapters. (Knowing that they were both busy professionals with many demands on their time, we offered compensation for their time.) After they had read all but two of the chapters, we had an opportunity to arrange a meeting with them to discuss their thoughts about the book and to explore the possibility of a six-year follow-up. That meeting took place during a visit the couple made to the East Coast in the fall of 1988.

During the meeting, both Larry and Jennifer said that they would be willing to write a six-year retrospective and joked about the likelihood that Larry would be content to write two pages, while Jennifer would undoubtedly want to write at least 10. We asked them to address three questions in their writing:

What has happened over the past six years in your lives, individually and as a couple?
How do you feel about the four interviews, in retrospect?
How do you feel about having participated in the couple therapy conference, in retrospect?

We explained that educational ventures like the one in which they participated might be undertaken in the future, and that their honest feedback about their experience would help teachers and investigators design such ventures with heightened sensitivity.

Before writing this report Larry and Jennifer viewed all twelve hours of the original unedited tapes of the interviews. What follows is the couple's writing, reproduced here with no editing of content; only minor changes have been made in punctuation, spelling, etc.

THE PAST SIX YEARS: OUR LIVES AND OUR RELATIONSHIP

Jennifer: Personal

Since the conference, I believe I've changed in many ways, yet have remained the same in some ways, too. With respect to change, my perceptions of my intrapsychic world and its relation to the external world have expanded in becoming more self-reflective, insightful, and aware of my own psychic processes (i.e., in becoming more introspective). This was largely accomplished through a rather intensive four years (1985–present) in therapy (mainly psychodynamic in orientation) with an accomplished, astute, and empathic psychotherapist with whom I've developed a very stable therapeutic relationship over the years. Individual therapy has enabled me to "work through" much of the disturbing affect and conflict associated with dysthymia,[1] resulting from "post-traumatic stress syndrome" (the diagnosis I've been assigned throughout my life). Although I still struggle with considerable depression and anxiety (manifested by numerous symptoms), I am better able to identify, experience, and understand (without being so self-chastising) the feelings of anger, hurt, helplessness, and sadness, most often underlying the depression and anxiety, which revert back to a much earlier time when I wasn't allowed to "have" these feelings. I am still learning how to grieve for the lack of a nurturing and emotionally supportive childhood (stemming from both my parents' emotionally deprived childhoods) and plan to continue working with my current therapist on feeling more in touch or connected with my feelings. By owning my feelings and claiming my past (as painful as it has been and will be), I've been more able to understand and be empathic with others. For example, since the couples conference, I've developed several extremely close relationships with women, in which mutual and unconditional love and trust are the most vital components. I also feel I've

---

[1]Editors' note: In the *Diagnostic and Statistical Manual of Mental Disorders; third edition* (DSM-III; dysthymic disorder is parenthetically referred to as depressive neurosis. Its definition includes: "The essential feature is a chronic disturbance of mood . . . not of sufficient severity and duration to meet the criteria for a major depressive episode. . . . The impairment in social and occupational functioning is usually mild or moderate because of the chronicity rather than the severity of the depressive syndrome."

become more accepting of Larry's differences (and of that of the human race in general), by no longer having the burning need to change him (i.e., "*If only* Larry would be more . . . , then I'd and we'd be happier"). My relationship with my family is for the most part, the same, with some (perhaps, important) exceptions. My feelings toward my mother have become more mixed and ambivalent. I often find myself simultaneously experiencing anger, hurt, and sadness (for both of us). The sadness, however, appears to be the most prevalent emotion. Over the last several years, we've had intermittent conversations that resulted in both our mutually feeling more connected and understood, as well as in my feeling more estranged, enraged, and defensive. Consequently, I find myself feeling conflicted between still wanting and hoping to establish some sort of mother–daughter bond and maintaining a healthy distance (to avoid subjecting myself to yet another round of feeling hurt, misunderstood, and rejected).

My relationship with my sister, Beth, has remained superficial in nature with 6- to 12-month lapses between communications (most always in writing and in the form of birthday and holiday greeting cards). When Larry and I were married (to be discussed in more detail later), she never responded to our invitation, was "unable" to attend several parties, and gave us (via our parents) a wedding present one and a half years later. I think we were probably both maintaining some kind of healthy distancing (based on unresolved fear and resentment).

Recently, however, we had brunch together. Beth invited me, and I accepted with the hope, if nothing else, she'd at least be able to shed some light on haunting memories and terrifying flashbacks, (re: my childhood) manifesting themselves in recurrent nightmares, anxiety, and other symptoms. Beth said she "didn't remember what happened behind closed doors" when I slept with our father, but proceeded to tell me about some incidents she remembered about her childhood, strongly suggestive of her physical (i.e., sexual) abuse by our father. She also offered "Mom only wanted one child" as a plausible explanation as to why I "always had to be with Dad."

Finally, *my relationship with my father* has remained the most unchanged over the last six years. We've always had difficulty communicating with one another. I understand why we've had problems in this area, as I've never felt that we've had the necessary "facilities" to fully explore the problem. He keeps saying that if I would just tell them what my problem is, maybe they can help me solve it. It is difficult to explain (if not impossible) that it isn't only my problem.

Larry: Personal

Since I am not as "psycho-eloquent" as Jennifer (in more ways than one), I am afraid I will have to discuss changes in me on a more lay level.

I had always felt comfortable with myself as a child, whether I had a right to be or not. I had a "good" childhood with plenty of family and friends. There is not much doubt that my past was not perfect, but whose was? My goal, however, is to investigate and learn about those imperfections. This should be done not from an academic interest, but with the goal of understanding what is causing problems today so that it can help lead to a better future. This is probably an overly simplistic view, but if it works for me (thereby helping my relationship with Jennifer) I'll be happy. What else matters?

I have learned that parents are a lot like us kids, only older. This helps me understand the things they did when they were my age, and the things they do today. From this I understand that parents are people too. They have their faults and good qualities. I understand that their faults are probably not due to me, but more due to their parents. So if I were to blame anybody for the problems I have as a result of their imperfections, it should probably be my grandparents and not my parents (or should I blame my great-grandparents, or great-great, etc.). Or maybe I shouldn't blame anybody. Maybe it is understanding I should concentrate on, and not blaming. I have started this process while engaged in a short stint with a personal therapist. It is not that I necessarily believe in the "science" of therapy, but given the right individual, who does not come armed with the emotional baggage somebody closer to the situation has, it can be quite useful. Human beings are far too complicated and multidimensional for there to be a rigorous "science" presently, but the "art" of therapy can and has been quite useful.

The times I have not been so comfortable with myself mainly centered around the experience with my foot (10–12 years ago). It was not always easy to maintain positive self-esteem at those times. In the last six years, however, I've been trying to continue the adjustment one must make to a changed self-image. It has not always been easy. These dynamics are intertwined with my ongoing struggles with communicating my feelings at the proper times with the proper people (mainly Jennifer). True communication, however, takes more than one. It takes at least two, but there must be a minimum trust providing the foundation for that channel. We as a couple are working on that and I expect to always be working on it.

My relationship with my parents has not changed very much since the couples conference. My mother is a "Jewish mother" and will always be one. She will never be accused of thinking of herself before her children, or after her husband. Any time I want to hear a high opinion of myself, I will call her. In almost complete contradistinction to Jennifer's upbringing, I seemed to always be "wonderful" and the "best." My father is retired now, and has more time to enjoy life. They have a "conj-aminium" in Florida and are there for most of the winter. My brother and I are getting along better than ever. The five-and-a-half-year age difference between us doesn't seem as large as it did when I was 12. We think alike about most things (I guess the common-parent theory holds for us). This is not to say we as a family don't have problems. Of course we do. They center mainly about our ability to express emotion at the appropriate times, and communicate our feelings (sound familiar?). I think we will also work on this as we all get older.

Jennifer: Professional

Since the conference, I've undergone a major career change, a transition from theoretical scientific research to clinical medicine. My feelings of frustration with the isolation and lack of human interaction in research led me to the decision to become a physician. This allowed me to pursue a career in which I could more directly (in a "hands-on manner") help people than in basic research. Having been in medical school at Stanford for several years now and exposed to a variety of specialties, including psychiatry, I am leaning towards two major areas at the moment—- general practice and pediatrics. I am genuinely very satisfied with my career change and only regret that I hadn't initiated this transition sooner.

Larry: Professional

I also have undergone somewhat of a career change. I have changed the relative proportion of my time from private commercial pursuits to academic ones. Both Jennifer and I have always been drawn to that end of things. Whenever we travel, no matter the city (or the country), we always visit the local campuses because we seem to feel more at home there. It has only been recently that we've been able to afford to do it. I've been a little disappointed with respect to the time it takes to achieve certain milestones. This is from one who seriously thought, when in college, that a Nobel prize would be awarded by the time I was 30 (we have such an inflated opinion of ourselves when we're in college). I enjoy my work, however, and really have always enjoyed it.

Our Relationship Six Years Later
(Written by Jennifer in Collaboration with Larry)

When I was accepted to Stanford, Larry had already been looking to move with his career change (expanding from the private sector to include the academic) and began searching for professorships in the Bay Area of California. Larry decided to accept an assistant professorship in computer science at Berkeley. Subsequently, we bought a "Yuppie-type" upper-scale condominium between Berkeley and Stanford. Despite the fact that I was going back to school, we had achieved a substantial improvement in our financial status (from both of us being impoverished students most of our lives, it was not hard to do) resulting mainly from Larry's successful company back East. This was our first real home after many years of "schlepping" from one apartment to another as students. We still lead extremely busy lives, but find the time to relax together during the weekends. We now have a cleaning service, and eat out whenever we don't have anything that's microwaveable.

The *most significant change* in our relationship (and a surprise/shock to most of our family and friends who gave up on us long ago) was that we got *married* three years ago, a year after our move to California. We jokingly justified our decision on the basis that our "short" trial period (15 years) was over and that we needed a new set of dishes and a vacuum cleaner. On a more serious note, our main reason for marriage was that we both wanted to start a family. Unfortunately, we encountered and are still undergoing an infertility problem. After many physically and psychologically invasive procedures and a miscarriage, we decided to initiate adoption procedures while we keep trying on our own.

Probably mainly due to the infertility experience as a stimulus for stress, and the move in careers and location, we decided to return to couple therapy about six months ago. This time Larry was equally convinced as Jennifer about the need for the further investigation into our remaining problems with communication and trust. Once again, we both found ways of distancing from one another at times. Larry became more involved in his career and TV, and Jennifer became more engrossed in her medical training and spent more time with girlfriends than before in the evenings. The couple therapist we chose came highly recommended with significant experience in the field (which her fees demonstrate). We've been meeting with her regularly on a weekly basis and believe her expertise (which includes infertility) in analyzing communication and feeling patterns between couples has been quite beneficial so far.

In sum, I believe we as individuals have grown (sometimes asynchronously). Our relationship as a couple has also changed. However, the constant factor has been the caring and love we have for each other. As Larry is fond of saying, "We might not have always liked each other, but we have always loved each other." The key, of course, now is to continue to "like" each other more, through pursuing the work on improving communication and trust. We both feel optimistic about our future together, and feel strengthened by our apparent success at navigating through our past.

THE FOUR INTERVIEWS IN RETROSPECT
(WRITTEN BY JENNIFER)

Peggy Papp: **Rating = 10 (Rating scale 1–10)**

Papp's way of identifying and attempting to solve problems in couples' relationships through fantasy has many merits. First, it allowed us to utilize our creativity in an almost unconscious or preconscious manner (i.e., I was never quite sure why I chose to create the fantasy I created until it had actually begun to unfold). The fantasy allowed for getting closer to the problems and feelings associated with the problems, as well as for possible resolutions, by providing a "safe" forum where we (1) could re-enact an "old script" (i.e., for identifying the problem), and (2) subsequently modify or change the endings (i.e., come up with compromises that would be satisfactory to both of us). This is an important point for couples like us, who feel entrenched in old, destructive patterns and often feel "lost" and *unable to imagine* a positive outcome because we cannot even identify the issues and conflicts in the relationship.

Papp's method of "role reversal" (i.e., having Jennifer play Larry and Larry play Jennifer) was also beneficial in that it allowed for each of us to experience (to the extent that it was feasible, as play-acting) the other's predicament or dilemma. Most importantly, Papp's technique heavily utilized *empathy* and *creativity*. Peggy's *astute and insightful interpretations* helped allay much of my anxiety and feelings of hopelessness regarding the seemingly insurmountable nature of our situation. The task she sent us afterward contained material which was extremely useful (e.g., regarding the competitiveness that existed between Larry and myself and how we could work on the need to "control each other's game").

In retrospect, I feel that Papp would have been *best* suited to help us with our relationship in the long run.[2] I also found her to be warm, genuine, and highly empathic. She seemed to *listen* to us more than the other therapists, who appeared more concerned with adhering to their agendas for illustrating their points.

Jim Framo: **Rating = 7–8**

Jim Framo's approach to couples therapy was to bring in my family of origin. This confrontation (according to Framo) was necessary so that all

---

[2]Jennifer's note: Papp's fantasy technique felt somewhat awkward initially, and, of course, realizing that we were being filmed. However, with time, I believe we could have become more comfortable and spontaneous with this productive technique; it also has the potential for adding a welcomed dimension of levity or fun to the work in therapy—a very useful piece for couples like us who have difficulty in the area of spontaneity and "playfulness."

members would have the opportunity to express feelings (not dealt with to date), face to face, in a "safe" setting with an objective person, to clear up "misconceptions" or "misunderstandings" of the past. (I think here he should have concerned himself more with validating the feelings or perceptions of each family member; perceptions are *not* misconceptions!). This confrontation would then hopefully enable me to feel more liberated as a person with rights, so that I wouldn't have to "apologize for living"—-even to Larry (that statement of Framo's felt almost patronizing).

I remember feeling extremely anxious *before and during* the interview about this potential "emotional Waterloo." There I was, not expecting anything nearly as traumatic as what was about to occur, until I met Framo, feeling powerless, helpless, and unprotected (yes—those horrible, almost unbearable feelings from the past were conjured up) just anticipating the "scapegoating" I was about to re-experience. Throughout this extremely uncomfortable session with my family, I felt vulnerable and at the mercy of this so-called "safe" setting with an objective therapist, whom I barely knew. (We had a very pleasant lunch previous to the family interview, making it even more difficult to oppose the person I had just "broken bread with.") All I could think about was how I could somehow protect myself from the very people who really never listened to me, understood me, or wanted me in the first place (for whatever reasons). I believe the *feelings or perceptions* regarding the past are far *more* important than the *rationale for another's behavior* at the time; feelings need to be worked through first.

Framo clearly made his point—that my parents had difficult childhoods, too, in which emotional deprivation and strict discipline greatly influenced their role as parents. I think it's important to try to understand why one's parents behaved the way they did, and I believe my parents were doing the best they could given their childhoods. However, this realization doesn't take away the rage, hurt, and distrust.

Given the potential intensity of the situation (Framo said he doesn't usually have his clients confront their families of origin until he's worked with them for *several months* beforehand), Framo should have perhaps focused on what he said he was planning to do—to help improve my relationship with my sister. Instead, I felt he used that as the "back door" to launch into an emotional upheaval with all the members. It felt as though once sufficient momentum was generated, one thing led to another (orchestrated by Framo and fueled by my father). I wound up feeling manipulated and violated (all over again). Framo seemed to be violating boundaries and out of control (or am I just projecting, because I felt so out of control?). He appeared to be continually explaining my family's behavior to me (implying justification) without *reciprocally* attempting to explain my behavior (based on what I had told him) to them.

The dynamics of the session, therefore, were skewed. *Thank goodness for Mary Framo's appropriately timed, empathic interjections!* Upon sensing my consternation and terror, Mary's empathy helped me feel "held" and protected by validating the emotional flooding and onslaught of frustration I was experiencing in feeling "attacked" and "misunderstood" as the "patient" or "problem" in the family.

In retrospect, my crying was mixed in nature. Yes, I did experience a certain sense of relief in getting my feelings out in the open. However, I also felt that I *should* feel grateful to Framo for providing this unique opportunity, while at the same time, feeling manipulated and "setup." I was crying because I felt humiliated, ashamed, and extremely vulnerable. I believe that such a direct and terrifying confrontation is warranted only when one has already worked through a lot of the negative feelings towards one's family and the past. Only then can *understanding* and forgiveness truly take place. Because this session was potentially so emotionally laden, volatile, and unpredictable, it would have been nice to have been followed up for a while by the Framos, simply by a few subsequent phone calls. On the other hand, I realize that Framo had a difficult task to accomplish in a short period of time, and I believe his motivation was well intended. On the positive side, I believe that Framo very nicely illustrated how my initial attraction to Larry was in large part because of his large, "warm," zany, and "open" family. More importantly, Framo's session may have influenced the ("intermittent") more open relationship with my mother (see "Jennifer: Personal"). It's difficult to assess whether this change (and, if so, to what degree) resulted from the interview, or whether it occurred because my mother and I felt "safer" sharing our respective hurt and sadness with each other as we grew older. Framo also pointed out how I could continue to improve my relationship with my family, especially with my mother, as formidable and difficult as it seemed.

In sum, I didn't (at the time) nor do I now object to Framo's approach. However, I strongly feel it should have been handled more gently and with greater empathy (especially since he knew that I had never directly expressed my feelings to my family before; there were valid reasons for that). In fact, I think it can be extremely liberating to confront the real targets of one's feelings in the presence of a *highly supportive* and *well-known* (to the patient) therapist, if the client is ready to and can do so without feeling like they will overwhelm him or her.[3]

---

[3]Jennifer's note: The same principle holds in individual therapy in my opinion. A client should not be "hoodwinked," enticed, or coerced into feeling something terribly painful, such as in re-experiencing a trauma he or she is not ready to do. This could create a major setback in therapy, resulting in a serious empathic lapse in the therapeutic alliance, *especially* if the client has issues with trust.

Norman Paul: Rating = 9

Paul very elegantly and successfully demonstrated that we all acquire and/or inherit characteristics of our parents that influence the way we think, feel (especially with respect to sadness and loss), and behave. We unconsciously bring these patterns into relationships with significant others in our lives. Paul's technique of having us watch the interviews with Larry's parents and with the two of us provided a type of "observing ego" or "objective self" for identifying common patterns of interacting, and also for distinguishing between what we think we are (i.e., how we see ourselves) and what we really are (i.e., how others perceive us).

In viewing the tapes of Larry and his parents, I could more readily identify common communication patterns existing in Larry's parents' relationship as well as in ours. I also saw parts of Larry in both of his parents, and noticed how I often reacted either like his mother or father in situations with Larry. For example, when I behaved like Larry's mother in dominating the conversation, Larry, like his father, would retreat or withdraw. (Perhaps if I didn't "push" so hard to "get him" to interact, Larry would feel less threatened and defensive and communicate more spontaneously.)

There were ways, however, in which I felt Paul's technique *could have been more effective for us.* Since communication was mentioned as a major problem in our relationship, he could have focused on ways in which feelings (especially with respect to vulnerability) are experienced in Larry's family. Instead of spending so much time asking seemingly trivial questions (e.g., names, dates, places, etc.), he could have concentrated on some of the "sad" events in Larry's parents' lives to find out how sadness is dealt with. Is it ever talked about, experienced, shared, etc.?

Most of all, I learned how much of Larry's communication style evolved from that of his parents. This *greatly helped me to understand* why Larry communicates with me in the way he does or doesn't. However, too much time was spent on identifying problems that existed in our relationship. There was little attention devoted to possible resolutions (i.e., how to improve or reconcile, via compromise, the "communication conflict" or "barrier"). This can be contrasted with Papp's creative fantasy approach to couples therapy, or with what was oftentimes suggested in Sluzki's language of metaphors.

In all fairness to Paul, he was probably attempting to make us *aware* of the *whys* behind the present behavior, perhaps as the first step for *understanding* change (or simply accepting it).

Finally, I felt that Paul misinterpreted our reason for couples therapy. We were not seeing him to determine our "marriageability," but rather to find out ways to improve communication and overcome the many impasses in our relationship.

Carlos Sluzki: Rating = 8–9

Sluzki was a master at creating a *balance* between the interactions in the "therapeutic triad" (i.e., Larry, Jennifer, and Sluzki). He was able to expertly "manipulate" the situation to elicit a response from Larry or myself to bring each of us "out" equally. He emphasized our complementarity as a positive and unique feature of our and probably many relationships. This implication caused me to view our relationship in a more optimistic light.

At least superficially, Sluzki appeared to be "poking fun" (with a bit of sarcasm) at some of my responses, especially in relation to my pedestrian knowledge of psychotherapy. His subtle teasing or playfulness served to maintain a constant dynamic in the "therapeutic triad." I believe it enabled Larry to be more involved and expressive in what was being discussed.

On a more critical note, I would probably not choose someone like Sluzki as a therapist for us. His approach was too "game-like" in nature (he seemed a bit like a milder version of Fritz Perls in the old Gloria film series). It was difficult to relax at the time, realizing that he was probably several steps ahead of us in his thinking. (Although I wasn't cognizant at the time of how subtly he was "directing" us during the interview, I always had the feeling that he was "up to something.")

In sum, I liked Sluzki's adeptness at instantly "picking up" on our opposite personality traits and integrating them as complementing one another's styles and needs. (Why *do* opposites attract?) Similar to Papp, he also allowed us to experience playing opposite roles, or as Sluzki put it so well, "to speak in each other's language." For example, if Larry were the "amplifier" and Jennifer were the "dampener," what would that be like? How could we come to a closer "meeting point" in our relationship if Larry were not always the "rock" and Jennifer the "balloon"? Sluzki's points were well taken and have *helped me in better appreciating our differences* as a couple.

OUR EXPERIENCE OF THE COUPLES CONFERENCE IN RETROSPECT

Jennifer

I feel that the experience of the couples conference was a positive one in general (much the way I felt at the time). I learned a lot about Larry, myself, our relationship, and how both our families influenced us as individuals and as a couple. It was fascinating to witness first-hand how therapists can use different approaches (given the same information) to illustrate what they deem important in the couple interaction.

With respect to family influences, Paul demonstrated a continuation of patterns in communication (especially in relation to sharing feelings of vulnerability, as a prerequisite to intimacy and "marriageability"). Framo, on the other hand, strongly believed that a direct "feelings" confrontation with one's family of origin facilitates a better understanding of parents' behaviors by "clearing up misconceptions" so that one can be "healthier" in one's present relationship. Because these approaches involving the family of origin differ significantly with respect to theory, orientations, and outcome, I would have liked to have participated in *reciprocal interviews* (i.e., have Larry's family interviewed by Framo and Jennifer's family by Paul). The experiences may have been quite different and interesting. (I believe I would have felt less anxious and upset in a family session with Paul than with Framo, and may have learned as much, perhaps in a different way or from a different perspective.)

Each of the techniques used by the therapists not involving families of origin had its own advantages and disadvantages. Because Papp and Sluzki were also different, it makes it difficult to compare the two approaches. Both were useful in pointing out salient features in our relationship and how to resolve some old established patterns by "being the other" to some extent. In my opinion, a combination of such methods (in an eclectic approach) would probably best benefit Larry and myself. Specifically, I would suggest beginning with Paul's gentle ("seeing it on video is believing it") approach, and following it *perhaps* (at some later point in time) with Framo's more directive, confrontational style. (I believe this could only be successfully accomplished by Framo if I were to have a number of prior sessions in the absence of my family.)

Would I do this again? I honestly don't know, but I'd like to speculate. I would still agree to a biographically fictionalized account and discussion in a book, and hope this benefits other therapists and couples, but I am fairly certain I wouldn't want to have myself on video for thousands of therapists to scrutinize. It's a very personal thing, and my need for privacy has probably grown since the conference.

In ending, I'd like to thank both Dick [Chasin] and Henry [Grunebaum] for their continual support and concern and for giving us this opportunity to learn and help others like ourselves, both therapists and couples alike. I want to especially thank Maggie [Herzig], who I believe understood us best of all.

Larry

As contrasted with Jennifer's fairly in-depth critique of our "couples therapy" experience, I will try to be fairly brief. I believe that it is important to restate the objectives of our experience before we critique it. The main premise was that we would volunteer to be used by each therapist to help demonstrate his or her approaches. There was no promise of therapeutic benefit, but it was understood that there may be some. We also understood that all four would be one-time situations, and thereby quite artificial in setting. It takes many sessions to develop the proper rapport and trust in order to create the necessary foundations for lasting benefit. Even though we knew all of this going in, it did not prevent the experience from affecting us.

Since the experiment was designed as it was (only one session), are we really asking whose technique is more amenable to short-term benefit, rather than which technique is more beneficial and lasting in the long term? Is there any correlation between Jennifer's and my choice of who we felt the most uncomfortable with as a therapist and which one was with our own family of origin? Are we asking the wrong questions with regard to technique? I would propose to answer the question for which I think I *am* an expert. That is, "Who do I believe would help us the most in the long run, and who are we best suited for?" As a corollary question, I would also rather ask "With whom did I feel the best about myself?" rather than "Who did I like the best?"

In answering these last questions, it is important to state that it is six years later, and both Jennifer and I sat through all 12 hours of tape (this, of course, was not so hard for me given my interest in TV and the *interesting* subject matter!). We had not seen them before.* The main question I kept asking myself during the viewing was if I liked that person on the screen that looked like me (only younger). The second question I asked was if any of the myriad of points made about us were accurate with respect to my present perceptions. (In an interesting side note, I thought that Jennifer was quite good and how fortunate I am to be involved with someone as bright as she—something I didn't quite realize during the sessions.)

I seemed to like myself better in the Sluzki and Framo sessions, I felt a little "put on" in the Papp session, and I didn't particularly think I was very good in the Paul session (rating myself a 9, 9, 7, and 5, respectively). Even though I *knew* we were being manipulated by Sluzki (as the

---

*Editor's note: In fact, Larry and Jennifer had viewed tapes in anticipation of their six month followup interview. When this was called to Larry's attention during the editing of this book he said that he had forgotten his earlier viewing of what he guessed must have been the edited tapes.

rest were trying to do but not as expertly), it seemed to be OK because he wasn't trying to hide it. There were no inconsistencies there. With Framo I certainly felt safe because it wasn't my family waiting in the wings, and this provided the setting for (what I believed to be long in coming) communications between Jennifer and her family. I thought (and still do) that if she worked out the many serious problems with her family, especially her mother, our lives would be better for it. I also believe, that if there was a mechanism for follow-up between Jennifer and her family (through Framo or someone else), the benefit here might have been more lasting. Thus another problem with the experiment. In the session with Papp, I felt that it was a bit contrived in that you can make many connections between a "fantasy" and real life (an example being the Freudian-like connection between dreaming of red balloons and wanting sex with your mother). They may not always be valid, and the "horoscope-like" quality was not exactly to my taste. Having said that, however, in reviewing the videotapes of that session, I felt that Peggy had some excellent points with respect to our relationship. Was this due to the use of her "fantasy" technique, or that she is a very bright and empathic therapist?

Finally, I felt awkward with Paul, and I'm not sure why. It could be that I disagreed with the approach (of pigeonholing people in his theory of couples and the family of origin rather than adjusting to the individuals) or the fact that I have my own communication problems with my family (which no doubt I do). The fact that he stated that he "can determine marriageability" of a couple 15 minutes after he meets them (hell, it's taken us upwards of 18 years to figure that out for ourselves) didn't help my perception. It shouldn't be up to the therapist to determine. It should be up to the couple with the aid of the therapist. (We've all seen some pretty weird combinations in our time, but they think they're happy! Who are we to say they are not?)

Last but not least, there were few questions with regard to what we liked about each other. Obviously there are some things; otherwise, why would we be motivated to work things out or stay together as long as we have? And, even more importantly, nobody asked us if we loved each other, or what we mean by that if we do. A strong relationship requires understanding the good things, as well if not better than, understanding the bad. I love Jennifer and she loves me. Finally, someone (I) asked. That is for the record.

REFERENCE

American Psychiatric Association. (1980). *Diagnostic and statistical manual of mental disorders* (3rd ed.). Washington, DC: Author.

APPENDIX
Clinical and Ethical Reflections on Demonstration Interviews and Teaching Tapes

RICHARD CHASIN and HENRY GRUNEBAUM
with MARGARET HERZIG

When we invited four family therapists to demonstrate their approaches with one couple at a Harvard Couple Therapy Conference our purpose was to create a learning experience for others. What we did not realize at the time was that we had embarked upon a significant learning experience for ourselves. Nothing in our training as clinicians and teachers had prepared us to attend to and balance the educational, clinical, and ethical requirements of the elaborate exercise that we designed. Despite the popularity of videotaped demonstration interviews with "real clients," our profession offered little in the way of ethical standards or guidelines for their production and use.

As the process of editing this book was drawing to a close, we realized that we had an opportunity, and perhaps even an obligation, to offer something quite distinct from a set of approaches to couple therapy. We could also contribute the important lessons we learned as creators and conveners of a major teaching conference that utilized videotaped demonstration interviews.

We undertake this appendix to consider four problems:

1. The ethical and therapeutic issues involved in the creation and use of clinical teaching tapes are often inadequately addressed.

2. There are important, inherent tensions between doing good demonstrations and doing good therapy which are likely to affect any therapist who conducts a teaching interview.

3. Demonstration interviews constitute a significant intervention in a client's life and therapy. Those who arrange for these demonstrations may fail to provide adequate preparation and follow-up.

4. How we recruit, interview, tape, and provide follow-up for these clients sets an example for all who attend the conference. The audience, however, is usually told little or nothing about these activities. When these activities are not described, the audience may get the message that the handling of participating clients is unimportant.

In this appendix we will discuss these ethical and clinical issues, describe our experiences as conveners of the Harvard Couple Therapy Conference, and offer a few recommendations. Although our discussions will use a major teaching conference as a case example, we believe that much of what we learned as conveners of that conference is applicable even to the most modest and commonplace of teaching interviews.

THERAPEUTIC AND ETHICAL CONSIDERATIONS IN THE MAKING AND USE OF VIDEOTAPED DEMONSTRATION INTERVIEWS

Therapists generally develop an intuitive grasp of the ethical requirements of their relationships with clients. These requirements are embodied in professional codes and laws governing practice. Underlying these intuitions, codes, and laws are fundamental ethical principles. Beauchamps and Childress (1989) specify four: the principles of autonomy, nonmaleficence, beneficence, and justice. We will refer to these and related principles as we discuss the relationship between therapist and client in clinical demonstrations.

When therapists become teachers of therapy, and particularly when they utilize videotapes of sessions, a new dimension is brought to their relationships with the clients involved. That new dimension arises in part from the business contract that is made for the educational use of the clients' words and images. This dimension is external to the usual therapist-client relationship; it is not a part of the therapy services contracted for by the client. It is our concern that this external dimension can lead even the most compassionate and sensitive of therapists into a void of ethical naivete. Thus, we believe it is important for our profession to consider ways in which its therapeutic and ethical standards can be applied to the making and use of videotapes for teaching.[1]

---

[1] J. Grunebaum's chapter (this volume) discusses the ethics of human relationships and the importance of an ethical approach by the therapist. In particular, she indicates that she

Contracting with Larry and Jennifer

Soon after we conceived the idea for the conference we set out to find the couple. We did this in a fairly traditional manner. We told some of our colleagues and trainees that we were seeking a couple in therapy who would be willing, for compensation, to participate in four demonstration interviews with well-known therapists.[2] In addition, we required that their families of origin be willing to join them for one interview. The therapist who recruited the couple described the interviews to them as demonstrations for a teaching conference—not as therapy sessions *per se*—but also as opportunities for the couple to learn something new about their relationship.

One of the psychiatry residents whom we were supervising referred Larry and Jennifer to us. She said that the couple was intrigued by the proposal, and that Jennifer, in particular, seemed drawn to the drama of the exercise. They both seemed to understand the nature of teaching conferences and the obligations they were assuming. They also indicated that their families were willing to participate.[3] After the couple had had further discussions with the resident, and then with us, we decided that they were well-suited for our exercise. They were unmarried, but had been committed to each other for several years. They insisted, however, on limiting their agreement to a single use of the tapes, and since we had no plans for any other use of the tapes we were satisfied with this arrangement. In fact, we were quite anxious about the single conference and had no thoughts of repeating it, much less of preparing a book about it. We were relieved to have found any couple for the conference, and happy to have found such a bright and pleasant pair of young people.

As mentioned, the distinctive feature of our contract with Larry and Jennifer was that they authorized us to use the tapes only at the particular conference for which they were made; any subsequent use would have to be negotiated later. Thus, after completing the videotaping of the last interview, the couple signed a contract for the showing of the tapes the next day at the Harvard Couple Therapy Conference in

---

would have "thought it urgent to address the ethical aspects of the teaching conference itself early in the session." She states that the " 'business contract' would obscure the clients' vulnerability and, thus, the therapists' responsibility." Utilizing a quite different approach to therapy, Weingarten (this volume) also calls attention to the context of the conference, asking, for example, "Who...has the most on the line at this conference?" and "What discussions have taken place about the handling of the videotaping and the editing of the videotapes?"

[2] We did not suffer from the illusion that we could find an "average" couple. We recognized, for example, that any couple willing to participate would be less shy than most. By itself, this was of little concern to us.

[3] Larry's brother wished to participate, but had unresolvable time conflicts.

Boston. When we sought to conduct another such conference, also in Boston, we contracted with them to release the tapes for that use, and later, for two additional uses at conferences in San Francisco and New York. The couple was paid once for participating in the interviews and four times for the four showings of the tapes.

When it became clear that the couple was unlikely to allow further showings of the tapes, as they became older and more visible in their professions, we focussed our attention on this book. The couple agreed to the use of their case in this book, with fictionalized names and identifying details. In order to be certain that their identities were protected, we asked them to carefully review the final manuscript of each chapter. (We compensated them for their time.) The highly restricted use of the videotapes, and our later decision to retire the videotapes in favor of this book, can be seen as attending to privacy and confidentiality, and as being in accord with the principle of autonomy.

Problems with Typical Contracts for Training Tapes

Our contract with Larry and Jennifer granted them considerable control, much more than clients in training tapes are generally offered or think to request. It is not at all unusual for clients in teaching tapes to be asked to "release any and all interests" in their tapes for an indefinite period of time for a broadly defined and unlimited number of "educational uses." Often the clients are given only a short time during which they are allowed, by contract, to change their minds.

For example, the contract used by the American Association of Marriage and Family Therapy (AAMFT) for its "Masters Consultation" series allows the client only five days after videotaping to change his or her mind, and offers the client no power to limit either the number of uses or the time period during which the tapes can be used. (Of course the tapes in that instance are sold, which gives the makers and the therapists involved little option for recall!) AAMFT's contract represents an improvement over many contracts, however, because it at least specifies what is expected from the users of the tape. It stipulates, for instance, that the presenters of the tape will remind members of the audience that they are "bound to confidentiality as they would be in any other professional interview situation," and that, if they should know the family personally, they should remove themselves from the viewing room.

One of the few widely available (but unfortunately, quite dated) published discussions of client consents for videotape use, a chapter in Milton Berger's 1970 book, *Videotaping Techniques in Psychiatric Training and Treatment*, presents sample consent forms that protect the therapist to a much greater degree than they protect the client. They specify no time limit or escape procedure, and they give broad, imprecise definitions of anticipated uses. In one sample contract the client is asked to allow the therapist to "use the session or any portion thereof in any manner on television or in any other manner or media at any time or times throughout the world and in perpetuity, subject to the restrictions here and above stated." The only important restriction in this contract is that the client's name "shall be retained in confidence" (p. 197). The author of the chapter, Berger's lawyer, however, does recommend that "consents be accompanied by safeguards to protect the patients" (p. 192). Regrettably, these safeguards are not discussed in detail.

Asking clients to sign a one-sided contract seems to us unethical. We recognize that such contracts might not be upheld by the courts if the clients changed their minds. But how many clients, having signed such an agreement, one replete with "legalese," would question whether the terms of the contract would be upheld in court? We would hope that clients who changed their minds would be treated ethically rather than purely legally. Specifically, we think that therapists should not exercise rights granted in a contract if doing so would violate the clients' wishes.

The manner in which clients are approached with contracts may take unjust advantage of the power difference between the therapist and the patient. In the Berger volume (1970), Max Rosenbaum writes about privacy and raises the question of power: "While many therapists feel there is no effect [of recording on the patient], this author questions the assumption. Is there no effect, or no effect that the patient feels free to express? After all, once he has decided to enter treatment he may be considered disruptive if he rejects being observed" (p. 201). In a recent article Sandy Cape (1988) argues that contracts, and/or the ways in which they are presented to clients, often place so much emphasis on the prestige of the therapists involved and the importance of their teaching endeavors that clients may be seduced into feeling that they should be honored to participate on almost any terms.

It is quite possible that we would have been able to gain the consent of the couple for an open-ended contract. Perhaps all we would have had to do would have been to offer them more money. They were students at the time and, like many students, were living in genteel poverty. Demonstration cases are recruited characteristically from groups in the population for whom relatively modest remuneration can be a significant factor in gaining their consent. It is important to consider the ethical problem of using a financial reward as an inducement.

Most private patients and mental health professionals would refuse to participate as clients in a videotaped demonstration interview for use at a conference. This unwillingness should give us pause. Are we taking advantage of others—and perhaps violating the principle of justice—when we use our power to ask them to do what we would refuse to do? Indeed, the families and couples who are videotaped for teaching are frequently viewed by clinicians as "them" as opposed to "us" and are thus dehumanized. The parallel in medical rounds in a teaching hospital is the common practice of referring to a patient as the "heart" in bed 2. We believe that psychotherapists can do better than that for their clients.

Recommendations

Larry's and Jennifer's own foresight made it easy for us to "stay on our toes" as protectors of their privacy. We recommend that other professionals offer the kind of treatment requested by Larry and Jennifer regarding permission to use the tapes and protection of privacy. Specifically, we suggest that contracts be written to cover single or time-limited usage of teaching materials (e.g., one year). We also recommend that participants be told that they can withdraw consent at any time.[4,5]

Preparation of teaching videos takes a lot of time, energy, and money. It is therefore quite tempting for the producer of the videos to try to secure permission for as much use of the tapes as the clients will allow. Contracts with no time limits and with only vague descriptions of intended uses would seem ideal from a practical and economic point of view. From an ethical point of view, however, they should be avoided. Clients change. Their families and friends change. Their locations change. Their professions change. The degree of privacy required for them to maintain their autonomy, therefore, may change over time. The issue of future autonomy is especially important when young people are involved. We should not ask parents to consent to long term use of material showing their children, nor should we ask teens and young adults for long term consent. After all, what would it mean for a young woman of 18 years to give *informed consent* for her case to be shown to professionals for an unlimited time? While she might readily consent at age 18, at age 25 she may be in the conference hall herself as a professional, or be closely associated with members of the audience.[6] Even the conveners and the therapists conducting the demonstration

---

[4]Some conference conveners may feel so vulnerable to the possibility that the clients will withdraw consent at the last minute that they may ask the clients to waive the right to withdraw consent during the two weeks or so before the conference. If consent is withdrawn before that period, the conference conveners and presenters can plan and create an alternative program. For example, they may hire actors to enact the sessions on the tapes, they may use other tapes for which consent has been secured, or they may adapt the material to a lecture format.

[5]When feasible, we recommend that clients be paid separately for the taping session and for each use of the tapes.

[6]This is not to suggest that potential membership in the "professional class" should be a crucial factor in determining how diligently we protect our subject/clients. A teen struggling with severe learning problems may need our protection as much, if not more, than a client who seems more likely to become "one of our own."

may change over the years and become uncomfortable with continued use of tapes that have fallen out of their control.[7]

Larry and Jennifer anticipated that their needs for privacy would change and that their lives might bring them socially and professionally into contact with potential viewers of the tapes at conferences. Not all clients are so astute, and even if they are, not all will be assertive enough to protect themselves in relationships with powerful professionals. The younger and more compliant the clients, the more it is incumbent upon the creators of teaching materials to protect the clients' interests. This protection can and should take many forms.

First, as we have suggested, clients should be asked only for specific, time-limited use of the materials. Second, they should be informed of the specific uses to which the material will be put. What will be the size and nature of the audience? Will audience members be drawn from a particular region other than the clients' own? Will they be students officially enrolled in a course? If the material is to be used at a large conference, will lay people be in attendance, people who may be less accustomed to rules of confidentiality than professionals in the field of mental health? What will the audience be told about the requirements of confidentiality? Will they be asked not to discuss the case outside of the conference room? (Who knows who might be in the lobby of a major hotel!) We recommend that clients be given such information when they are asked to give informed consent for use of the materials.[8]

---

[7]Looking back, we feel a bit uneasy about how we selected interviewers and clients. In the period since 1982, when the demonstration interviews were designed and conducted, gender issues and abuse issues have become salient and richly articulated in the field of family therapy. If we were to conduct a similar conference in 1990 we would have an equal number of male and female therapists serve as presenters (indeed, there are, and have been for some time, roughly even numbers of highly skilled, senior men and women in the field). We would also bring to the task of choosing the couple a heightened sensitivity to issues of abuse and, therefore, we might avoid involving a family like Jennifer's, some of whose clinical needs would not be appropriate to address before a large audience.

It is important to note that if demonstration tapes are widely circulated and used over several years without regard for the changes in the field that have occurred since the making of the tapes, those tapes can have a conservative effect on the training of therapists. It is therefore important that teachers of therapy who use old tapes be well informed about advances in the field. If so, they can utilize the tapes to the students' greatest advantage, for example, by identifying some aspects of the tapes as having enduring value, and other aspects as having primarily comparative or historical value.

[8]Our reflections on informed consent in the preparation of teaching materials have prompted us to consider how little most therapists do in their every day practice to offer clients informed consent about therapy. Increasingly, professional societies are developing guidelines and forms for informed consent for treatment, covering such issues as permission to consult with other professionals; possible risks of therapy (emotional strain/life changes); and limitations on confidentiality imposed by state laws (such as the therapist's legal obligation to report threats of violence). See, for example, AAMFT's Form Book (American Association for Marriage and Family Therapy, 1989). It may be advisable

THE INTERVIEWS: THE DILEMMAS POSED BY
THERAPY "PERFORMANCES"

One of the many lessons we learned from our work with Larry and Jennifer is how difficult it can be for conveners of teaching conferences and for "master therapists"[9] to resist the temptation to make demonstration interviews more complete, compact, or dazzling than the interviews that they typically conduct in the privacy of their own offices. When preparing demonstration videotapes for a teaching conference, especially one that enjoys national prestige and draws a large audience, a therapist who does careful and caring work behind closed doors can easily become a demonstration therapy "performer." Expectations are high in the audience; the therapist's reputation is on the line. Everyone hopes to witness an intervention in which mere mortals manage to "leap tall buildings in a single bound." In such an atmosphere, how likely is it that "good therapy" will be demonstrated?

Ives Hendrick, a founder of the Boston Psychoanalytic Society, often said, "Good medicine is good teaching." If in a demonstration interview you do what the client needs you to do, he said, you will demonstrate good clinical practice. We are convinced of the wisdom of Hendrick's dictum. The educational value of a tape of a "master therapist" working with a couple, for example, on a rainy Thursday morning, in the third of five "stuck" sessions, may be as great if not greater than a demonstration of a perfectly crafted and dazzling intervention, especially if the latter is a bit forced or "performed."

Thus, we recommend taking measures that will limit the impact of the audience on the interviewers and help them, in the spirit of Hendrick's dictum, to place the goal of conducting good therapy well above that of impressing the audience. For example, the interviewers should be urged to have confidence that the interviews will be enlightening or informative in some manner, whether or not what is elicited optimally demonstrates their theory and/or clinical approach. In addition, interviewers should be offered opportunities to describe their theory and practice at the conference, especially when these are not demonstrated well in the taped interview. This would reduce the pressure on the interviewer to

---

not only to provide clients with such information about legal requirements and standard procedures, but also to explain in each phase of treatment how we plan to proceed, and then invite open discussion about the risks and benefits of our plan. By our doing so, clients are likely to experience themselves as protected and respected co-participants in the therapeutic process. This, it seems to us, is not only therapeutic, but ethical. Further remarks on this important topic are outside the purview of this book.

[9]This honorific title bespeaks the belief that family therapy theorists and teachers are "masterful" clinicians. Often what "master therapists" are is well known, i.e., published theorists and teachers.

do whatever he or she is "known for" during the session.[10] Finally, the expectations of the clients and the audience should be tempered with an understanding that they may witness straightforward interviews conducted with quiet simplicity rather than dramatic sessions replete with sophisticated and flashy complexity. They may see the "master" do what many therapists do, or they may see something distinctive. The latter should not be promised, even implicitly. All that should be promised is an attempt to demonstrate "good therapy" within the constraints of the circumstances.

If we were to design another conference during which videotaped demonstration interviews would be used, we would be inclined to give the therapists as many sessions as they felt they needed to demonstrate their approach, commensurate with the needs of the clients and the logistical limitations. At the conference the audience could then view a highly edited tape showing the major points in the work, or the clearest examples of certain techniques.

Why is it so important to aim to conduct good therapy in a demonstration, even when you haven't promised the clients therapy *per se*? One of the reasons is quite simple. The authenticity we ask of the demonstration clients makes them vulnerable and the techniques of therapists, especially very skilled ones, can be quite powerful. Whether the interview is a demonstration or not, the clients will, one hopes, share real pain, conflicts, and hopes. How these feelings are handled by the interviewer will affect the clients, perhaps quite deeply. Consultations by therapists "on stage" sometimes elicit material prematurely, as do ordinary consultations, at times, and leave the clients and their regular therapists to pick up the pieces. Clearly demonstration interviews can violate the principle of nonmaleficence.

The other reason why teaching interviews should be similar to therapy interviews is equally important. Beyond the effects of the demonstration on the clients, there is the effect on the audience. Members of the audience characteristically seek to learn from, to imitate, and to identify with the presenter. What they should identify with is good solid therapy, not theatrics. The presenter has an opportunity to model beneficence, and should not be satisfied simply to avoid maleficence.

While the goal of conducting good therapy should supersede that of "dazzling" teaching, it is important to note that there is a higher principle that should supersede both: that of ethical treatment of the clients. What might be strongly indicated therapeutically for clients in

---

[10]Various scenarios are possible when an invited therapist and a demonstration couple are brought together. If the case is well-suited to the approach of the therapist, then all may go well. But when the case and the approach are a mismatch, and the therapist must choose between teaching the approach and treating the clients, the therapist often teaches the approach. After all, that is what he or she is being paid for (Grunebaum, 1988a).

treatment behind closed doors cannot always be done ethically in a public conference. The dictates of therapy and ethics may conflict, for example, when what is clinically indicated is a painstaking exploration of such sensitive areas as abuse or sexual relations. In such cases the needs of the clients to avoid harmful public exposure should be placed above their therapeutic needs. All participants in demonstration interviews—clients, therapists, and audience members—should understand that some of the therapeutic needs revealed during the course of the demonstration can only be addresssed adequately at a later time in the protected context of private treatment.[11]

Although it might be ethically important for demonstration therapists to avoid certain sensitive areas, this may have unfortunate clinical consequences. When an expert clinician publicly sidesteps an issue like abuse, he or she may serve to reinforce the family's own conscious or unconscious tendency to suppress painful facts. Similarly, a couple's collusion to avoid conflict in their relationship may be unwittingly reinforced through their participation in a demonstration interview in which they succeed in presenting their best face to the world.[12]

PROVIDING ADEQUATE PREPARATION AND FOLLOW-UP

So far we have considered two of the major questions that must be addressed by therapists who design or conduct demonstration interviews: What should the client be asked to agree to contractually, and how can potentially damaging performance pressures be reduced? We now turn to the therapeutic and ethical issues raised by what must come before and after a demonstration interview—preparation and follow-up. Without adequate attention to these phases a demonstration interview might be compared to surgery without pre- and post-operative care.

Preparation

After Larry and Jennifer agreed to participate in the demonstration interviews, Chasin had preparatory phone conversations with Larry's fam-

---

[11]J. Grunebaum's and Weingarten's chapters (this volume) address this issue. Grunebaum writes that she would have sought to "protect the couple from undue exposure and other potential ill effects of their and their families' participation." She expresses a "multipartial" concern for all parties in the exercise, especially the family members who do not have an ongoing relationship with the therapists. Weingarten would have asked before the conference, "What can Jennifer, Larry, and the senior family therapists do during their interviews to protect their own and each other's interests—to safeguard the couple's right to privacy and to 'save face' for the therapists—while promoting everyone's learning?"

[12]We are grateful to Norman Paul and Frances Givelber for raising these issues in discussions we had with them during the drafting of this appendix.

ily members to explain the agreement that Larry and Jennifer had made, and to describe the interview process and the roles that family members would be asked to play in the interviews. Jennifer spoke to her own family and assured us that they were comfortable with our plans. As for Larry and Jennifer, they seemed to share our enthusiasm for our plan and appeared to need little preparation. They, and their couple therapist, felt that the exercise would be interesting and potentially very helpful. We gave only cursory attention to any potential harm to the couple or to their ongoing therapy. We did not discuss with them whether the exercise would benefit or harm them or their families, other than to suggest the possibility that the consultants might have useful input.

If we were to conduct a similar exercise in the future, even with a similarly enthusiastic couple, we would systematically explore with them and their families any misgivings that they might have about participating. We would look for hidden pressures that might induce any of the participants to disclaim their reluctance to cooperate. For example, might Larry's parents have had difficulty refusing to cooperate with their son and potential daughter-in-law, especially given Larry's recent struggle with cancer and given their eagerness for him to marry? Could Jennifer's parents have refused her request for their participation without fearing that their refusal might further impair their relationship with her?

We recommend to others who seek permission from families to make demonstration interviews (or to release videotapes) that they describe the exercise in detail and invite full discussion of all apprehensions and give each participant the right to openly or secretly veto the whole project. Everyone should be told that the project might be cancelled without full explanation, due to the persistent misgivings of any of the participants, including the therapists and conference conveners. This procedure protects all participants (including the therapist) from subtle forces that might abridge their autonomy.[13]

In addition to exercising great care during this preparation stage, it is necessary to delay getting consent for the use of the tapes until the interviews have been conducted. No one can know in advance what they are going to say or what emotions they will express. Moreover, when tapes are edited for teaching purposes, it may be preferable to secure consent after the edited tapes have been made available to the clients for viewing.

We suggest that risks to ongoing therapy be explored even when the

---

[13]Chasin commonly offers secret veto power to families and groups whose sessions have been taped, explaining to them that even an unsigned letter will suffice. The tape will be erased with no explanation offered to the group other than, "someone requested that it be erased."

clients and their regular therapist appear to have no concerns. In fact, Larry and Jennifer stopped their couple therapy soon after the conference. We know little about the reasons for this termination. Unfortunately, we have no systematic research to guide us in informing clients of the potential harm to their ongoing therapy. Our experience suggests, however, that special sessions with "master" therapists can leave the clients' regular therapist feeling inadequate. Regrettably, the clients may share this view.

One way in which risks to ongoing therapy may be minimized is to treat demonstration interviews as consultations (assuming that the regular therapist endorses this idea). The demonstration interviews in our exercise were conducted, for the most part, as though ongoing therapy did not exist; only Sluzki made reference to it. Unfortunately, we have insufficient information to guess what relation, if any, the conference interviews and the conference itself had to the termination of the couple's therapy. All we know is that we scarcely considered the therapy when we designed the conference. This is an omission we would not repeat.

Follow-up

As part of our initial agreement with Larry and Jennifer we offered to be available for consultation to them and their current therapist, to faciliate any follow-up contacts with the interviewers that they might want to make, and, over the longer term, to make any referrals that they might find helpful. We called them immediately after the conference to learn of their reactions to it, and we conducted a pre-arranged, videotaped, follow-up meeting with them six months after the conference. As described in chapter 16, the couple eventually terminated therapy with their original couple therapist and later sought therapy on their own that apparently did not include further work with Jennifer and her family. They indicated in their retrospective reports that they would have liked more follow-up (from some of the interviewers, we believe), yet they never accepted our offer (or Jim Framo's) to arrange for follow-up sessions. We were somewhat perplexed by this.

Upon reflection, we realized that our dual role, of clinician and convener, in relation to the couple was as plagued with inherent tensions as the dual role of clinician and teacher played by the interviewers. Just as the interviewers could aim to provide good therapy, but succeed in doing so only within the constraints of the conference, so too we could aim to provide caring follow-up, but only succeed within the constraints of our non-clinical relationship with the couple. Just as the interviewers could seek to minimize but not eradicate the impact of the audience on their clinical work, so too we could seek to minimize but not eradicate the impact of our educational agenda on our clinical relationship with the couple. When we initiated contacts with the couple they were happy to work with us and Jennifer, in particular, seemed to enjoy the task of providing feedback to us as conference conveners. The couple seemed to have had mixed feelings about using us or the interviewers as clinical consultants. Was this ambivalence due to an incompatability between the role of conference convener/presenter and that of clinician?

If we were to conduct a similar exercise in the future we would communicate to the couple a recognition of the tensions inherent in our unusual relationship with them. We would impress upon them and their families our desire to be helpful after the conference should they want our help. We would also let them know that we would understand if they found that their evolving clinical needs were best kept separate from their relationship with us as conference conveners.

It is impossible to predict what follow-up demonstration clients will desire or require, or what the conveners or interviewers will feel is appropriate to suggest. For example, the clients may desire no services from the therapists associated with the conference. On the other hand, they may seek consultations by those therapists with their regular therapist, or they may request additional sessions with some of the interviewers. The conveners may feel comfortable serving as intermediaries between the clients and the interviewers, or they may judge that some or all of the interviewers should call the clients directly to discuss the impact of his or her interview and to assess any follow-up needs pertaining to it. Plans for follow-up made with clients during the contracting process (and thereafter) must be flexible in order to respond to their emerging needs. These plans should be made with all family members who agree to participate in any interview.

Despite the unpredictability of follow-up needs, we recommend that therapists contracting for demonstration interviews explain to clients the educational and ethical importance of follow-up, and then propose a way for their follow-up needs to be addressed. For example, the convener might indicate an interest in hearing from the clients if they should want to discuss the impact of the interviews, and ask the clients if they would mind being called at certain intervals of time, e.g., one week, six months, and one year after the interviews are conducted. An important ground rule for these therapist-initiated contacts would be that the clients can choose to enter into discussions at the prescribed time or they can decline. The conversations can be simple and brief; the clients can provide updates on the major events in their lives, or if they wish, they can enter into more extensive discussions, e.g., of their retrospective thoughts on the conference experience or of their current clinical needs. If such needs are expressed, the convener should offer to help in whatever manner seems realistic.[14]

Clients who give up their privacy to participate in demonstration interviews make themselves vulnerable for educational purposes. Educators who work with these clients, therefore, owe it to them to avoid harm, and, if possible, to help them. Thoughtful and flexible follow-up procedures can contribute to both of these goals.

MAKING THE RELATIONSHIP WITH THE CLIENTS PART OF WHAT IS TAUGHT

Therapists who convene conferences and conduct demonstration interviews exercise considerable influence, especially on the younger generation of therapists who will one day succeed them. We have become more mindful of this influence through our experiences with Larry and Jennifer. Therapists who hold conferences and conduct demonstrations also model ethical stances toward clients, and it is their responsibility to examine these stances carefully. It is also important for them to report to the audience what was done over the course of the relationship with the clients and to comment on the ethical and clinical issues raised by the interactions. If conference conveners and interviewers fail to describe these relationships adequately, the demonstration interviews become decontextualized and the clients are, in a sense, dehumanized.

Larry and Jennifer asked if they could attend the first conference in Boston. We invited them to do so and they attended on one of the two days. We had alerted the audience that the couple might be among them, and some members of the audience recognized them and went out of their way to thank them. We believe that this knowledge that the couple might be among them had a profound impact on the people in the audience. It heightened the sense of respect, empathy, and concern for privacy with which they discussed the case. We clinicians tend to discuss our work with greater humility and humanity when clients are listening and with greater objectification when they are not. Terms that roll off our tongues when we are with colleagues are suppressed when we are with clients. Our experience with Larry and Jennifer suggests that it is important for teachers and trainees to consider how clients would feel about the ways in which their situation is discussed. Are the clients being treated with respect, dignity, compassion, and with appropriate safeguards to their privacy? Are the standards of good

---

[14]The earliest discussions of follow-up should provide the clients with a general idea of what the conveners would consider to be "realistic" requests. For example, a few additional sessions with a local interviewer or a few phone calls with a distant interviewer might be realistic; free long-term therapy and transcontinental trips might not.

therapy being upheld in the teaching of therapy? If not, the conference conveners and presenters are serving as poor models. At best they are missing an opportunity to help other professionals to become more respectful of clients, and at worst they may be harming the larger community of client–therapist relationships.[15]

ALTERNATIVE METHODS FOR PRODUCING DEMONSTRATION MATERIALS

The recommendations that we have made may seem idealistic, and more of a burden than any conference convener or demonstration interviewer would care to bear. Fortunately, not every situation will require that all of the recommendations be followed. (In any case, we think of our recommendations not as requirements but as guidelines or cautions, particularly at this early stage of professional dialogue on these matters.) The challenge of juggling the needs of the clients and the educational objectives of a conference, while not insurmountable, may be significant. Thus, when asked if we would ever again design and convene a conference like the one we convened in 1983, our answer is this: Only with modifications such as those suggested above, and perhaps with an even more radical difference. If we were to do it again we would seriously consider using actors rather than real clients.[16] Actors could be used in at least two different ways.

We could conduct taped demonstration interviews with clients such as Larry and Jennifer and then have professional actors reenact the sessions as faithfully as possible (with changes of names and identifying details). This would protect the clients' privacy (as has been done in this book) while attaining a level of authenticity similar to, or higher than, that achieved in the exercise we conducted in 1983.

As an alternative, we could provide a case report of a couple (real or fictional) to the therapists and ask them to script a hypothetical session with that couple. The scripted session would then be enacted by professional actors. Such a procedure (which is akin to what several

---

[15]As Lyman Wynne pointed out to us in our discussions of this appendix, asking professionals to discuss cases as if the clients were in the room would not only elevate the group process ethically, but it would also enhance the clinical sophistication of the discussions. It would improve their ability to be fully empathetic with the clients, and to help them to discover clients' competencies and resources. In short, it would serve to inhibit the well-recognized and chronic tendency of clinicians to pathologize all that they see and hear.

[16]In a conversation with Carol Nadelson, past President of The American Psychiatric Association (APA), one of the editors learned that the APA recommends that demonstration videotapes be made with actors whenever feasible.

authors have done in Part III of this book) would place the goal of clear and efficient technique demonstration above the goal of authenticity. In a scripted demonstration several approaches and techniques can be demonstrated in a fairly short period of time. Moreover, "performance pressures" are also reduced. Of course, the tapes would have to be presented to the audience as fictional condensations of work that would be unlikely to occur exactly as portrayed.

Whatever the method chosen to produce the training materials, the people in the audience should understand what they are witnessing. How did the people on the screen get there? What is the clients' understanding of the interview and its use? What were the therapists asked to do? What measures have been taken to uphold the same standards in the exercise that therapists strive to uphold when they conduct therapy? As discussed above, the answers to these questions should be treated as integral parts of the learning experience.

CONCLUSION

When researchers studying therapy outcomes interview clients about their past therapies, what clients recall most often and most clearly are the personal characteristics of the therapist. They describe therapists as caring, warm, or respectful after successful therapies, and as cold, seductive, or rigid after harmful therapies (Grunebaum, 1983; 1986). These descriptions correlate with outcome data from patients who had undergone different kinds of therapy (Grunebaum, 1988b). Clients remember little about the interventions the therapist made. They recall helpful people, not helpful interventions. Similarly, students are likely to look back on the "master therapists" they have watched and remember their attitudes and values as well, if not better than, their techniques and theories. It is wise to assume that trainees will emulate not only what their teachers say and do, but also the attitude and care with which they do it.

Trainees will also learn from conference conveners and interviewers how to treat demonstration clients. It is for this reason that we have called attention to the clinical and ethical dimensions of our work with Larry and Jennifer. We have noted what is lacking in the usual contracts between conference organizers and clients. Indeed, we suggest that the concept of a contract, when construed narrowly as the specifying of an exchange of goods and services, is not adequate. Instead, a broader concept, such as that of a fiduciary relationship, is preferable as it presumes trust, caring, and respect.

Before closing we would like to identify one aspect of the conference exercise that we continue to value highly. Many therapists who attended the conferences said that they found our exercise to be not only intellectually stimulating, but also confidence building. Often, after attending conferences with presentations by "masters," therapists report feeling inadequate by comparison. To see the interviewers at our conference working with a case that was not ideally suited to their methods—one that they would have been unlikely to write about in a journal article or present at a more traditional conference—left many of the therapists in the audience feeling validated in their struggle to find the best way to work with their own cases. They saw the advantages, but also the limitations, of each interviewer's approach. They were able to see how their work was similar in some respects to one interviewer's work and in other respects to the work of another. The gap between "master therapist" and uncelebrated practitioner narrowed somewhat.

We have made a few recommendations, but we have raised many more questions than we have answered. Our hope is that our questions and recommendations will contribute to a growing understanding of the clinical and ethical aspects of demonstration interviews and teaching tapes.

REFERENCES

American Association for Marriage and Family Therapy. (1989). *AMMFT forms book*. Available from AAMFT, 1717 K Street, NW, Suite 407, Washington D.C. 20006.

Berger, M.M. (1970). *Videotape techniques in psychiatric training treatment*. New York: Brunner/Mazel.

Beauchamps, T.L., & Childress, J.F. (1989). *Principles of biomedical ethics*, 3rd ed, Oxford: Oxford University Press.

Cape, S. (1988). The context setting function of the video "consent" form. *Dulwich Centre Newsletter*, Adelaide, South Australia, Autumn, 1988.

Grunebaum, H. (1983). A study of therapists' choice of a therapist. *American Journal of Psychiatry, 140*(10), 1336–1339.

Grunebaum, H. (1986). Harmful psychotherapy experience. *American Journal of Psychotherapy, 40*(2).

Grunebaum, H. (1988a). The relationship of family theory to family therapy. *Journal of Marital and Family Therapy, 14*(1), 1–14.

Grunebaum, H. (1988b). What if family therapy were a kind of psychotherapy? A reading in the Handbook of Psychotherapy and Behavior Change. *Journal of Marital and Family Therapy, 14*(2), 195–199.

Name Index

Acker, J., 196
Ackerman, N., 4n
Ainsworth, M.D.S., 311
Allen, W., 327
American Association of Marriage and
  Family Therapists (AAMFT), 390, 393n
American Psychiatric Association, 401n
Andersen, T., 141
Anderson, H., 141, 149, 150, 165, 196
Argyris, C., 6n
Aring, C., 84
Aristophanes, 332
Auerswald, E.H., 146, 149

Bach, S., 171, 172
Balint, M., 193n, 312
Barbach, L., 241
Barnes, M.L., 310, 315, 322
Barnett, J., 171
Bateson, G., 146–150, 152n, 155, 161,
  161n, 162
Beauchamps, T.L., 386
Baucom, D.H., 229, 231
Becker, E., 89
Bellah, R.N., 197, 323
Berger, M.M., 390–391
Bernal, G., 192
Binstock, W.A., 174
Birdwhistle, P.L., 4n
Blehar, M.C., 311
Boas, G., 274
Bograd, M., 130n, 140, 143
Bohr, N., 307
Boscolo, L., 26, 141, 146, 152n
Boszormenyi-Nagy, I., 173, 174, 176, 182,
  192, 192n, 193, 193n, 194n, 198,
  201–203, 207, 212, 221, 222
Bowen, M., 4n, 25, 182
Bowlby, J., 171, 309, 312
Bradburn, N.M., 179
Bradshaw, D., 310–312
Browning, E.B., 308
Buber, M., 192n, 193n, 194n, 195–200,

208, 211, 212
Buss, D.M., 315, 322

Cambridge Hospital Department of
  Psychiatry, 167
Cancian, F.M., 317
Cape, S., 391
Carter, E., 27, 46
Cecchin, G., 26, 141, 146, 152n
Chasin, R., 4, 4n, 5, 85, 101, 130, 130n,
  131, 140, 216, 225, 230, 237, 297, 334,
  339n, 344n, 349, 350, 384, 397n
Chekhov, A., 85
Childress, J.F., 388
Chodorow, N., 201, 224n, 254, 261
Cohn, C., 195n
Colapinto, J., 293
Collier, J., 197
Collingwood, R.G., 85, 85n
Cotroneo, M., 192
Cowan, P.A., 317
Cuber, J.F., 333

Dacre, H., 322
Dallas, M., 230
Dell, P., 148, 197
deShazer, S., 141n, 155, 294
Dicks, H.W., 25, 50, 171, 173–176, 177,
  180, 188, 312
Dietrich, M., 321
Dinnerstein, D., 224n
Duhl, B., 27, 130n
Duhl, F., 27, 130n
Dunne, H.P., Jr., 209

Eastern Pennsylvania Psychiatric Institute,
  4n
Elwood, R., 230
Epstein, L., 273
Erickson, E., 193n, 205, 224
Erickson, M.H., 138

404

Subject Index

408